LOOK YOUNGER, FEEL HEALTHIER

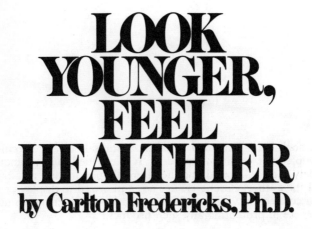

LOOK YOUNGER, FEEL HEALTHIER

by Carlton Fredericks, Ph.D.

Originally published as *Eating Right for You*

Publishers · Grosset & Dunlap · New York

This book is not intended to promote the sale of any specific food, food supplement, or vitamin product. It is intended to be promoted and sold solely as a book containing the personal opinions and recommendations of the author. Purchasers are not authorized to display or sell the book in connection with any food or vitamin product nor to use it for the purpose of promoting any such product.

Copyright © 1972 by Carlton Fredericks
All rights reserved
Published simultaneously in Canada

Library of Congress Catalog Card Number: 74-158745
ISBN: 0-448-11933-1
First paperback edition, 1975
Originally published as Eating Right For You

Printed in the United States of America

To my dear wife Betty without whose encouragement this book would have been long delayed or never written.

CONTENTS

1   For Jack Sprat and His Wife....................... 1
2   For Women Who Are Witches Once a Month....... 23
3   Sometimes It's Not "All in Your Mind"........... 40
4   Diabetes....................................... 54
5   Figures Do Lie................................. 64
6   From Here to Maternity......................... 99
7   Nutrition Versus Mental Disease................. 108
8   Appointment in Damascus....................... 127
9   Shelf Life or Your Life?........................ 145
10 Dietary Supplements............................ 168
11 How to Shop in a Health-Food Store — and Why... 207
12 The Well-Fed Baby.............................. 224
13 Superstition or Fact?........................... 235
14 Nutrition in Prevention and Treatment of Disease..... 250
Appendix
    1 Diet Plan: Hypoglycemics..................... 271
    2 Diet and the Period........................... 278
    3 Cornell Bread Formula........................ 281
    4 Testimony of Dr. Fredericks.................. 283
Index...................................... 301

LOOK YOUNGER, FEEL HEALTHIER

1.

FOR JACK SPRAT
AND HIS WIFE

You eat pie with fourteen teaspoonsful of sugar per portion and add six teaspoonsful more by taking it à la mode. It tastes good — to a degenerated palate. It also rots some of your teeth and loosens the survivors. You devour sweetened Danish pastry, cookies, doughnuts (plain, jelly, or glazed), plastic bread (10 percent sugar), and bubble-gum rolls. You eat foods that are denatured, overprocessed, over-concentrated, oversalted, oversweetened, overcooked, scraped, and devitalized. Meats and milk heated as you heat them and fed to animals will allow but three generations before reproduction stops — but not before the animals have developed allergies, disorders of the nervous system, calcification of the soft tissues, marked irritability, and homo-sexuality plus partial obliteration of the external sexual characteristics that distinguish the male from the female.

Your salad oil, shortening, chewing gum, and cereals are among many foods preserved with an antioxidant known to cause skin cancer in animals, but that is a British research finding, and to our Food and Drug Administration therefore apparently inapplicable to Americans. You enjoy meat dosed with female hormone, chicken fed on antibiotics, fish spiced with toxic mercury, vegetables dusted with pesticides related to nerve gas, and maple syrup containing a *legal* content of formalde-

1

hyde. The foaming agent in your root beer was shown to cause tumors; the dye in your maraschino cherry was demonstrated to cause cancer. You eat frozen packaged dinners with a protein content inadequate to support a senile horsefly, while watching TV advertising of remedies for heartburn, indigestion, hyperacidity, and constipation — yet you are constantly told that Americans are the best-fed people in the world. You engulf pizza, pop, patties, puddings, dumplings, waffles, starches that are first cousins to paperhanger's paste, and nineteen pounds of candy per year, while you sympathize with the malnourished in less advantaged countries. Your chemicalized menus bring you an assortment of over a thousand food additives, with the comfort that nearly a third of them have been tested for safety. The Vitamin E you need to help protect you against the asphyxiating gases you call "air" is removed from virtually all the starches and sugars that comprise half your food intake. You eat at least a thousand meals a year, all selected on a basis of habit, conditioning, family tradition, superstition, myth, folklore, advertising, impulse, seasonal availability, price, convenience, and the death wish — while you view with distaste the antics of the food faddists who try to make their food purchases with some thought to the needs, tolerances, and sanctity of their bodies. Indeed, friend, if you are what you eat, you're a disaster area.

In moments of weakness, you may give lip service to the thought of altering your food habits, but you will cling to them until you reach the genuinely teachable moment, usually when you're horizontal with an illness — at which point, should your doctor suggest that fertile eggs with stale caviar will be therapeutic, you will meekly eat the mess. As a nutritionist who has educated the reluctant American public for thirty years, I can anticipate all the ways in which you will rationalize as you block emotionally when offered the proposition of spicing food selection with biological sanity. Your most telling argument — to you, at least — will be: "I must be eating properly; after all, I'm healthy!" That sounds most reasonable, until you are pressed for a definition of "healthy." Usually, it means to you what it does to so many physicians: the absence of a major disease. This is a lenient standard that allows you to call yourself well if you have nothing more than sinus trouble, postnasal drip, dandruff, indigestion, heartburn, fat intolerance, constipation, allergies, virus attacks, colds, blotchy skin, decayed teeth, gingivitis and recession of the gums, slight decalcification of the jawbone with loosening of the teeth, flat feet, corns, poor posture, weak muscle tone, varicose veins, premenstrual tension and menstrual pain, insomnia, anxiety, irritability, nervousness, a touch of claustrophobia, or constant fatigue. Physicians do not call such ailments *sickness*. Sickness is heart trouble, cancer, high blood pressure, hardening of the arteries, pneumonia, asthma, and multiple sclerosis.

So we know what you mean by being "healthy." It's any state of well-being that allows you to walk upright — provided that the wind is blowing in the right direction. But to a nutritionist, good health is not the absence of major sickness. It's a positive well-being that brings a zest for living and makes of each new day a new adventure. It is enjoyment of good food, with good digestion, proper utilization, and adequate elimination. It is a prolonged prime of life, without the serious degenerative diseases we mistakenly blame on time itself. It is clear skin, fine muscle tone, maximum resistance to stress, infection, and fatigue. It is heightened response to medication when you do become sick, with fewer and less threatening side reactions to drugs. It is living up to your full potential. Now, against *that* standard, are you still healthy? And how many people do you know who really are?

Face the fact: If your canary, pedigreed dog, or thoroughbred horse had but a random sampling of the minor disorders you accept as part of good health, you'd be telephoning the veterinarian. For that matter, if 10 percent of all racehorses were infertile, owners would be urging a federal investigation into the quality of oats and hay. Would the veterinarians urge instead an inquiry into the possibly neurotic relationship between mare and stallion? Note: Ten percent of American marriages are involuntarily barren, yet no one has demanded an organized investigation into American eating habits. I might add that when I spoke before a professional society dedicated to the study of the causes of infertility, I was told I was the *first and only* speaker on the subject of nutrition in the some twenty years of the organization's history.

Your next gambit: "All right, so by that definition I may not be so healthy, but there's nothing seriously wrong — I'm doing all right, so far." That invites a look at the future for those who will survive to stagger through the late sixties — some 60 percent of you. Six in every ten of those who do live that long will have diabetes, heart trouble, high blood pressure, hardening of the arteries, or some other degenerative disease as a companion on their way through the twilight. And when such a disease strikes, you may be sure that at some point in your dismayed conversation with your physician, you will plaintively ask: "What should I eat, doctor?" Ask that question *now*. In most degenerative diseases, a special diet is certain to be part of the prescription. If that diet is in any way helpful, it will be a monument to a lost opportunity for prophylaxis, for what nutrition cures, it prevents; what it mitigates, it may delay or attenuate. That translates into simple, everyday language: You'll reduce your insane intake of sugar when your diagnostician tells you you must. Must you wait?

If you really believe American health to be a testimonial to the excellence of our food choices, you've never taken a searching look at a medicine chest. Why do you superb specimens of glowing health find it difficult to survive without laxatives, decongestants, cold capsules, tranquilizers, psychoenergizers, stimulants, sedatives, painkillers, antihistamines, and remedies for insomnia and headaches?

Next defense of your love affair with gastronomic suicide: If you're right, if our diet is so poor, why are our children so tall and healthy? No single index can be used to appraise a child's nutriture or well-being. Any pediatrician will tell you that height and weight are but two of a dozen standards by which he appraises a child's development and health. Are there not tall children whose sex organs are underdeveloped? Or those whose height and weight appear normal, but whose skeletal maturation is retarded? Our teen-agers *are* taller than the previous generation, but they are anything but healthy. In fact, specializing in teen-age disorders is a new branch of medicine. Physicians aware of the numerous medical problems of the adolescent call this age group the most neglected, healthwise, in the population, just because everyone blithely assumes that the teen years and buoyant health are inextricably linked. Suicide — no testimonial to mental health — is the second leading cause of death among college students. Surveys show that the teen-age girl has the doubtful distinction of being the poorest-fed member of the family, and that an inadequate diet is eaten by four in every ten boys. If she marries one of these, what kind of babies will she bear? *If* she can bear children at all: It is estimated that one pregnancy in every four does not yield a living, healthy baby. In what health category would you place the one teen-ager in every six who is grossly overweight? And where do you place the young draftees who failed their preinduction examinations — 22 percent of them for physical reasons? Height and health don't necessarily walk hand in hand.

Another specious argument against the need for learning how to eat properly brings up the persuasive myth of your "voice of inner wisdom." Translation: What you crave is what you need. Do you really think Nature built into you that yen for Goofies, the cereal that whistles at you from the plate but doesn't feed you? In a world filled with foods Nature neither created nor possibly anticipated, how could such an instinct operate? Animals show it; young babies may; you don't.

If you beam X rays along a channel of a maze, a rat will travel its path but once. Possibly he scents the ozone from ionizing irradiation.

In any case, man in that situation would unknowingly expose himself to a slow death. If you damage the rat's adrenal glands, causing its body to lose salt, it will sip bitter brine and stay alive. Man exercises his craving for salt when it is contributing to his lethal high blood pressure, and conversely, has to be persuaded to swallow salt tablets when intense heat and humidity deplete his supply.

Make a rat deficient in Vitamin B_1, and then offer it access to solutions of various vitamins. It will unerringly choose the one it needs and attack you, tooth and nail, if you try to remove *that* one from the cage. Compare the animal's inner knowledge of its needs with the blindness of a woman, a patient in a sanitarium where I was a staff nutritionist, who could not be persuaded to eat the diet rich in thiamin needed to cure her "nervous breakdown."

Create diabetes in the rat, and it will avoid sugar. Human diabetics offer a striking contrast, for they are notorious for cheating on their diets, and will continue to do so even when they have been warned that the forbidden sweets may be a pathway to cataract, coma, or even death!

There are mice with an hereditary tendency to convulsions, touched off by high-pitched sounds. Given the opportunity, the mice will increase their intake of thiamin by a factor of about nine — and the convulsions fade away. So some animals do have a voice of inner wisdom, but yours is mute, or perished under the impact of your conditioning and your food environment. What, for instance, tells you that your friendly colonic bacteria are dying in response to the antibiotic you are taking? When your tongue turns shiny and magenta? Is it the whisper of your body's wisdom — or a violent diarrhea? And when the physician imprudently overdoses you with cortisone or diuretics, is there any small inner voice to let you know that you are dangerously low in potassium, even to the point where you have lost enough of it in your urine to make you fall flat on your unnutritious face? Do you have a compensatory craving for oranges, bananas, or other rich sources of the potassium you desperately need? If you do have a voice of inner wisdom, it is probably screaming out of pure frustration.

Last refuge of those who continue to dig their graves with knife and fork: If we are badly fed, why are we living longer? We aren't, really — it just seems longer. Life expectancy is an average that is weighted by the newborn babies' chances for survival. Those *have* improved, for infants no longer die by the thousands with croup, diphtheria, polio, and smallpox — for which there is little credit to good nutrition and much to immunization and antibiotics. It's wishful thinking to believe you're going to live longer because little children toss extra years of life expectancy into the pot to be averaged. And it is pertinent here to note that there are twelve countries that better the U.S. record for survival of the newborn in the first thirty days of life — which doesn't speak well for nutrition in (and before) pregnancy, among other factors. At any rate, if you are curious enough to study vital statistics, you'll soon realize that more people are staggering to the sixties, but those achieving the seventies are as yet still a privileged minority, in whose survival a canny choice of ancestors may be a more positive factor than their diets.

On the optimistic assumption that your defenses are now down, and you are emotionally as well as intellectually determined to contaminate your food selection with a dollop of sanity, let us begin our adventure in good nutrition by studying *you*. Because, you see, there's really no answer to the question "Is this a good diet?" unless we know a great deal about the individual who will eat it. For he *is* individual, and so are his needs in nutrients as well as his tolerances for pollution of air and water and his resistance to harmful effects of insecticide residues and food additives. The diet adequate for you may bankrupt me, a statement that jars those who cherish the shibboleth that in all things all men are created equal. Applying this political philosophy to physiological characteristics, biochemistry, and nutritional requirements may well deprive you of the chance for superior health. Uniform menus and tables of "minimum daily vitamin requirements" are as logical as proposals to cut clothing costs by making shoes on one last, and dresses, suits, and bras in one size. It may be disturbing for you to realize at this point that nowhere in this book will you find menus offered as nutritional panaceas applicable to every reader, but this is so.

Let us, therefore, take a close look at some of our individual differences, with emphasis on those that help fix our nutritional requirements. They derive from small distinctions in anatomical structure and great differences in physiological function, enzyme chemistries, and glandular activity. They are shaped by subtle distinctions in the messages conveyed by genes and chromosomes and molded by the physiological insults you have inflicted on yourself in your lifetime.

Consider some facts about smoking and lung cancer. One in every ten smokers develops the disease, which means that nine smokers escape; out of every ten lung-cancer cases, one is a nonsmoker; farmers who smoke are less prone to the disease than urbanites who do. Obviously there are causes of lung cancer other than smoking as well as factors of resistance and susceptibility that remain to be identified. A constitutional tendency is a possibility, which is another way of saying that the soil on which the insult falls is a determinant of the outcome. One of the variables in the equation must be air pollution, which is known to increase your need for Vitamin E. We also know that smoking raises your requirements for both Vitamin C and Vitamin A — indeed, recent evidence shows that in some people an intake of generous amounts of Vitamin A may prevent smoking from causing the initial degenerative changes in the cells that precede lung cancer. On what bases shall we set *your* requirements for these nutrients? On "average need"? Who is average — and does he smoke? What is in the air he breathes?

Millions of women take the birth-control pill, a source of estrogenic (female) hormone, although that has been described by a cancer authority as "playing with fire." In fact, more than twenty years ago a Rockefeller Foundation cancer specialist warned the New York Academy of Medicine that some women *manufacture* so much female hormone (an ingredient of all oral contraceptives) that they may *cause* breast cancer in themselves. Most of the women using the Pill, so far, escape penalty. Thousands develop blood clots, hundreds suffer consequent strokes, and a few die. Medical statistics are people with their tears wiped away. Among the forces that determine the outcome may be the woman's blood type, which is, of course, genetically fixed. Another is certainly her diet, for that plays a dominant role in protecting her against excessive estrogen activity, whether the hormone is self-produced or medically administered. As you will see in Chapter Two, it is the protein and Vitamin-B-Complex content of the diet that keeps the female hormone in check. Requirements for these nutrients are also "averaged" by the Establishment, although estrogen activity in women may vary as much as women themselves differ.

Millions of women eat the average intake of 104 pounds of sugar yearly without apparent harm. Others pay the price in tooth decay and weakening of the supporting structures of the teeth. Millions of women suffer with such agonies in the menstrual cycle that they call it "the Curse"; they never realize that the average sugar intake of one and one third teaspoonsful every half hour is contributing to their troubles.

Psychology will never be accurate in predicting human behavior until more attention is given to the influence of the body on the mind. How can you forecast the reaction of a man to a nude female if you disregard the fact that some men produce *five* times the "average" amount of male hormone? Some psychiatrists place total blame on the slum neighborhood for the juvenile delinquent and the adult criminal, although socially useful citizens also emerge from just such backgrounds.

As high testosterone levels may drive a male to a more intense reaction to a sexual stimulus, so may the pressures of a slum neighborhood become more telling when they fall upon children who are the products of defective germ plasm, inferior diet, or both.

A few doses of a medication may cure another, and half kill you — with the same disease. The reaction to a drug is patently shaped in part by its chemical structures and may rest as heavily on the genetically determined presence or absence of an enzyme process in the body. It may also be influenced by the patient's dietary habits. Dosed with the type of tranquilizer called an MAO inhibitor, the patient may be free of side reactions until he eats sharp cheese or herring. Then the outcome may be a sudden, and possibly lethal, attack of high blood pressure. Others so medicated munch such foods with impunity.

The preceding paragraph mentioned two people with "the same disease." Actually, no sickness is the same in two individuals, because they *are* individuals. Not only will the age, sex, dietary history, and previous sicknesses of a person play a part in shaping the course of a disorder, but so will body structure, as an expression of the genetic inheritance. The outcome of the illness can sometimes be predicted by the characteristics of the body structure of the patient. A disorder tends generally to be more severe in the very tall and the very short — if you are curious, it is best for sick men to be about 5′10″ tall. The more chronic forms of illness tend to befall long, thin women. It is usual for the two sides of the face to be different, as well as the testicles, breasts, and feet, but a child in whom the differences are exaggerated is a more likely candidate for rheumatic fever — and the mere absence of eggs from his diet may be the environmental factor that invites or worsens the disease. Gall-bladder syndrome, predominantly a feminine disorder, tends to occur in the rounded, overstuffed, very feminine woman, and when it occurs in a man, he is likely to have such feminine characteristics in his body structure. Such appraisals of body build versus constitutional susceptibility have been made for stomach ulcer, duodenal ulcer, diabetes, and several other disorders.

In old-age homes, you will find eighty-year-olds enjoying their morning eggs, bacon, toast with butter, and coffee with cream. In medical journals you will encounter articles threatening young men with early heart attacks from exactly such menus. Their theory founders in the face of a multiple reality: Hardening of the arteries and coronary thrombosis are not always the penalties for a way of diet, and when they are, not of a single way. Cholesterol and animal fat may be a threat to some men, but there are obviously those whose organisms do not treat them as such. Which, of course, indicts as sheer numerology the "three-eggs-a-week — no more" advice so many American men receive from their physicians. How beautifully simple all becomes when one ignores the individuality of men and the plurality of disease processes lumped under a single title! Our men of healing often seem to forget the origin of the word "quack," even though they use it frequently. In part, it describes the healer who, like the duck, is guilty of monotonous repetition.

We are not created equal, and our differences are often greater than our similarities. The kidney transplanted from your father to you will almost certainly be rejected as an alien intruder, and your brother's skin tends to shrivel when grafted to yours. Until these differences are fully recognized, untold numbers of us will continue to be unsafe if we accept averages in recommendations of tolerances for medication, radiation, air and water pollution, pesticide residues, food additives — or suboptimal diet.

Nevertheless, many physicians prescribe "average" doses of medications and patients experience reactions ranging from healing to therapeutic failure or death. Dietitians and home economists compile "balanced menus" identical in composition for people who are not, some of whom suffer thereby the effects of dietary deficiencies. Government agencies assure us that the average American diet, whatever *that* may be, is totally adequate (for whom?) and publish tables of "daily vitamin allowances," abdicating their nutritional responsibilities to millions of citizens who are anything but average, and who therefore become dietetic nonpersons, frequently penalized with subnormal health. Food processors manufacture uniform products for a nonuniform public and profess the belief that buoyant well-being is based on consumption of butylhydroxytoluene, butylhydroxyanisole, cornflakes, frozen apple pie, and white bread that is rejected by hungry mice offered the opportunity to eat almost anything else. There are those who eat such foods and additives and go unscarred. They are matched by those who will never enjoy decent health until they learn to avoid such foods and chemicals.

Until *you* accept the concept of your biochemical individuality, you may be condemned to gratuitous risks in your food, water, air, and medication. You and your family may be deprived of the maximum chance for maximum health — mental and physical. Your aged may prematurely be dumped on the scrap heap of senility; your retarded may fall short of even their limited capacities; your sick may grope toward recovery made gratuitously elusive; and you yourself may go through life in a twilight zone, neither truly sick nor truly well, never functioning at your full potential.

Before we continue with an examination of our individual differences, particularly as they are reflected in our dietary requirements, it is surely appropriate now to tell you, unsurprisingly, that this book is biased in favor of the consumer. It profoundly believes what the U.S. Food and Drug Administration once said, that the best protection for the citizen comes not from government agencies, but from his own alertness coupled with understanding. This was an odd admission, considering that it came from an agency that has labeled as "food faddists" those who are wary of overprocessed foods, cryptic chemical additives, and suspect pesticide residues. It was also paradoxical, for the Food and Drug Administration is the agency that has guarded consumers against being well informed, by permitting certain manufacturers to omit from their labeling all indications of ingredients, additives, or nutritional values. Try, for instance, to learn from the labels that mushrooms may legally contain 40 percent more pesticide residue than other foods, or that ice cream contains 16 percent sugar and may contain as many as fifty additives, or that most cereals are so "foodless" as to be a nutritional injustice to the children who largely consume them, or that a cola drink has the acidity of vinegar, masked by five teaspoonsful of sugar and garnished with the caffeine of one-third of a cup of coffee, or that there is in a frozen chicken pie about enough chicken to take care of the protein needs of a (small) kitten! There is full information, of course, on the labels of foods packed for hamsters, cats, turtles, dogs, and guinea pigs.

There are no labels on tap water, which is fortunate for the peace of mind of the inhabitants of some thirty cities where the "drinking" water falls below even the minimum standard of purity. Indeed, repeated distillation of Boston tap water has yielded a residue that was mutagenic to living cells, an action that offers the possibility of cancer-causing potential. What kind of water are you drinking? And why has the Food and Drug Administration used its vast powers to discourage the advertising of bottled (and pure) mineral waters?

Do not think these observations are secrets, ferreted out by this observer alone, and do not believe for a minute that they are thoughtfully received by the authorities and the food industries, or acted upon, however grudgingly. Complaints about American food or water, whether the everyday menus or the medically prescribed diets, invite excommunication of the critic. (Do not be concerned about me. A nutritionist can be excommunicated only so many times.) Why is this so? Physicians may disagree in medical matters and yet part friends. Dentists differ about the treatment of periodontaclasia, without descending to invective. Nuclear physicists clash in the scientific arena, and yet join an hour later to discuss new theoretical approaches to charring the earth to ashes. Only in nutrition seemingly does name calling masquerade as debate. He whose opinions, however justified, are inimical to the sale of processed foods is in danger of being immediately labeled a food faddist. Why is the man attacked rather than the nutritional issue debated? Granted, when one's case is weak, an attack on the man in lieu of a defense of the (often) indefensible can be a useful ploy. But that is not the compelling reason for the hostilities in the field of nutrition. Face the fact that the food market in the United States comprises more than 100 billion dollars a year, a revenue so formidable that those who participate in it must form the most vested of interests. That investment may sweep over professors of nutrition, whose departments are often supported by grants from food processors, exactly as it can envelop those processors who are intolerant of any suggestions that their products might be improved nutritionally. The government agency primarily charged with policing the food industry, the Food and Drug Administration, appears to regard any criticism of the worth of the American food supply as (a) a direct attack on its own competence, (b) a voluntary admission of food faddism, and (c) a gratuitous insult to the giant industry which it seems to feel the need to defend rather than regulate. The better business bureaus find it better business to use their prestige to silence or persecute those they define as food faddists — primarily, it appears, those subversive enough to suggest that American diet is not only less than optimal, but contributes to the disgraceful level of ill health that is average, and thereby misconstrued as normal. The American Medical Association makes periodic forays against nutrition quackery, which it seems to consider the use of health foods and vitamin supplements, though the latter are prominently advertised in its publications, and the former include some praised as excellent nutrition in A.M.A. publications not readily accessible to the public. The nutrition departments of some of our great universities maintain an enthusiasm for poor foods that sometimes appears to be in linear relationship to the size of the grants they receive from the manufacturers. A glaring example appeared in the Senate hearings on breakfast cereals, in which the defense of these triumphs of emasculation of food rested primarily on the eloquence of a Harvard professor of nutrition, whose department, the Senate subcommittee was *not* informed, is housed in a building donated by a giant manufacturer of some of America's most overprocessed foods, including cereals. The university boasted at the time that this was the single largest grant ever made to this educational institution by an industrial organization.

A personal note here may prove illuminating to those readers who cling to the belief that the consumer receives full protection from the government agencies charged with that responsibility. When the Nixon Administration was about to take office, I was queried concerning my possible interest in a "high government position." Investigation revealed that numerous Republicans, disenchanted with the performance of the Food and Drug Administration and aware of my lifetime sympathy for the consumer, were urging my appointment as commissioner of that agency. I refused to apply — not only because I was justifiably certain that the Establishment in medicine, drugs and foods would not tolerate a consumer-biased commissioner, but because — as I informed the Administration — I preferred to retain my independence and integrity. I did make a standing offer, however, to serve in the event that an agency should be created to protect the consumer against the agencies that "protect the consumer." That was not a sarcastic quip, but a sober proposal, based upon thirty years of study of the disservices rendered the American citizen by the Food and Drug Administration and similar agencies, in exercising a distinct bias in favor of the food industry.

Hence this book: It is a manual to help you protect yourself by recognizing your biochemical uniqueness in a world shaped by concepts of the average. In fairness, it should be pointed out that there are risks in acting on such an insight. You may bring down on your head the anxious wrath of the community, in the form of hostility toward behavior that differs from the norms, and it may make you or keep you genuinely healthy. Also, with symptom and sickness no longer ready topics in your conversation, what in the long winter evenings will you do for small talk? If these warnings have not flagged your enthusiasm, let us proceed to examine individual differences that determine nutritional needs. The differences have a common denominator: They are ignored.

Freud once remarked that he found it most difficult to accept the fact that another man might blow his nose in a different way. Social pressures make it difficult, too, to entertain the possibility that you are unique in dietary requirements, out of step with the rest of mankind. In that context, consider the history of a schoolteacher whose great fear was that her unprovoked fits of weeping might cause her dismissal and the loss of her pension. A series of sessions on the psychoanalytic couch made the psychiatrist feel better, but the inexplicable weeping lingered — until the teacher was fortunate enough to fall into the hands of a capable medical nutritionist. A series of injections of the Vitamin B Complex and sustaining doses by mouth and the attacks of crying vanished, and with them a constipation that had forced her to use laxatives almost daily for nearly thirty years. Was her diet poor? Indeed not. She was a victim of a *good* diet, for she had the misfortune of inhabiting a body that needed a *superb* diet — which few achieve. So nutrition adequate for many people was inadequate for her, because she had an elevated need for the B-Complex vitamins. This relative deficiency interfered with the oxidation (burning) of sugar in her nervous system and brain. Unprovoked weeping was the only visible symptom of cerebral starvation. Constipation was the parallel reaction of her gut. Is it not ironic that the Food and Drug Administration has conducted no campaigns against the chronic use of laxatives (or, for that matter, liquor and tobacco) but has spent untold millions to discredit the "food faddists" who take vitamin supplements?

The scientist whose papers taught us much about individual differences in nutritional requirements — Professor Roger Williams, former president of the American Chemical Society — tells of a chemist who suffered from periodic headaches through much of his adult life. By chance, he took a multiple vitamin supplement during one of his attacks, and the headache vanished. Research-minded, he wanted to know which vitamin might have been responsible for the benefit and experimented with each of them in subsequent migraines. Ultimately, he identified Vitamin B_1 as his benefactor and determined that he could remain headache-free if he raised his intake of this food factor to eight or ten times the maximum amount suggested as *the* requirement by the authorities. It would be easy to dismiss this history as a rare one, if analogous experiences had not been reported with other patients, for other disorders, by medical nutritionists of my acquaintance. Just recently one of my students at a community college remarked: "I was rarely free of headaches — I took aspirin almost every day. Since I've been studying nutrition, I raised my intake of Vitamin B Complex, and I don't have headaches anymore. I actually didn't realize it, until it dawned on me that my new aspirin bottle is intact — I haven't taken a dose in the last two months."

Experiments have shown the requirement for calcium in healthy individuals to be as low as 225 mgs. daily, or as high as 1,000 mgs. or more. It sounds like an academic exercise, but it isn't, for a deficit in the mineral is made up by withdrawal from the bone reserves, which means that some people with a high (and unsatisfied) requirement may pay the price with osteoporosis, a crippling and painful bone disease, as the toll for placing their faith in the average diet and the average need.

A variable in calcium requirement is tension: Some people will excrete more of the mineral when they are under emotional pressure, and the calcium need, of course, will rise proportionately. There is the same effect of tension on the requirement for Vitamin C, which is destroyed in the adrenal gland under stress conditions. We have no exact measure of the elevation of the need, knowing only that it must increase — as we know it does in smokers and the allergic. The authorities dismiss all these variables with a simple, sweeping declaration: No one needs more than 100 mgs. of Vitamin C daily, even though there is evidence that for some individuals the requirement may rise as high as 4,000 mgs. daily. (Linus Pauling, Nobel Prize-winning chemist, has suggested that doses of 5000 mgs. of Vitamin C daily will prevent colds and help mental function and resistance to colds, in many adults, as they have for him. E. Cheraskin, M.D., has published evidence that elevated blood levels of Vitamin C are found in those older people whose blood vessels have remained healthy.)

Calcium requirements are also set, in part, by the efficiency of the parathyroid glands, which help to control the metabolism of the mineral. The parathyroids are lobes on the thyroid gland. Some people have only two, some as many as twelve. It is obvious that some of us manage calcium more efficiently than others, and this glandular factor may explain the enormous range in requirements for this nutrient. All very academic, until you're thrown out of your bed in the middle of the night with an agonizing calf-muscle cramp, as a token of spasm induced by low levels of ionized calcium in the blood.

Vitamin D, also needed to help us utilize calcium, is another factor for which the requirement varies — from the first day of life. There are some babies who develop rickets with an intake of the vitamin that completely protects other infants, and these differences must continue as they grow up. In short, no one can tell you with any assurance that *your* calcium need is satisfied by this much milk or that much cheese.

If you think calories and caloric requirements have been studied so long that in this one area of nutrition we must have hard and fast guidelines, consider what happened when NASA assembled a dozen authorities to set up menus for a flight to Mars. To do so, the nutritionists had to estimate the needs of men in space for daily intake of calories, protein, fat, carbohydrate, vitamins, minerals, bulkage, and water. The first item ended the consultation: No agreement could be reached which would fix a spaceman's daily caloric need. If the authorities really don't know how much *food* a person needs under given conditions, what makes them think they can lay down inflexible quotas for the many vitamins, minerals, fatty acids, and other food *components?* This recalls what happened when a pharmaceutical company offered a rich reward to any nutritionist who could determine the exact need of a human being for Vitamin A, or the possible benefits to man of an intake of the vitamin beyond that afforded by a good diet. After many years the prize was withdrawn, no one having claimed it. As it stands now, we suspect that the requirement for Vitamin A varies in man just as it does in rats. Dr. Roger Williams found that one rat may need sixty-four times as much of the vitamin as another.

The need for protein varies greatly, too. Proteins are digested with the help of the enzyme pepsin. Some of us produce 1,000 times as much pepsin as others. The enzyme functions best in the presence of hydrochloric acid. Some of us produce 1,000 times as much of *that* as others; and some produce virtually none. Perhaps these variations explain why there are people whose entire protein need is satisfied by as little as two ounces of meat a day, while others need more than ten ounces. It may be anticipated that similar differences will be found in the human need for amino acids, the building blocks of protein; and this is so. One man may need only 82 mgs. of tryptophane daily; another may need as much as 500 mgs. Requirements for methionine may be as low as 175 mgs. or as high as 1100 mgs. Averaging these needs, or resting adequacy of intake on a "good, mixed diet" is fatuous. But there is one certainty: You will never know optimal health if your need for amino acids is not met in full.

In the pancreas there are little islets of special cells that produce the insulin that helps us burn sugar. Some people have 200,000 such islets; some have 2,500,000. This makes for a profound difference in the ability to "handle" starches and sugars, and the individual whose insulin capacity is low may obviously overtax it by gulping one and one-third teaspoonsful of sugar every thirty-five minutes, twenty-four hours a day. During the years when the pancreas is constantly challenged by the excessive sugar intake, it may be stimulated into overactivity, thereby burning sugar so rapidly that the brain and the nervous system are starved for fuel. This disorder — hypoglycemia, or low blood sugar — can produce many physical symptoms, embellished with neurotic or even psychotic behavior.

If the pancreas ultimately becomes exhausted after years of such punishment, the end of the story might be diabetes, for which hypoglycemia may be a prelude. In such individuals malutilization of sugar may create changes in the blood chemistry that pave the way to atherosclerosis (hardening of the arteries). All this from ingestion of a common food — albeit a poor food — that is well tolerated by others. Individual reactions to sugar sometimes include diarrhea and cramps, which have been traced to an inborn constitutional error — a lack of sucrase, an enzyme needed for digestion of sugar. None of this, however, is reflected in the textbooks, advertisements, and government and industry food charts that assure you that we all need sugar for energy.

Differences in nutritional needs are evident from the first day of life. The experienced pediatrician does not set the same calory intake for a long, thin baby as he does for a wide baby, although their weights may be the same. Some babies are born with an exaggerated need for Vitamin B_6 (a vitamin depleted in the processing of most starches and sugars). If their foods meet the need, all is well; if not, convulsions may develop, culminating in brain damage and mental retardation.

The anatomy our medical students study exists only in textbooks, for variations in the way we are put together are as great as those in our living chemistries. The left coronary artery, site of most thrombosis attacks, is a vivid example of individual differences. Two main coronary branches are common, but they may number three or more, and their size may vary by a factor that could yield the pumping of four times as much blood. The more collateral circulation a man has (to take over the burden when one of the main vessels is blocked by a clot) the better his chance to survive. Sometimes, too, these branches kink; sometimes, they run true; what they do can make a difference in chances to avoid or outlive a heart attack.

Uniform systems of exercise — jogging, bicycling — have been recommended as a virtual panacea for avoiding heart attacks. Yet men differ in their reactions to physical exertion, and a not uncommon result of exercise is an *increased tendency to blood clotting*. What generalizations can we make about exercise, and what predictions about its role in prevention of heart attacks? Vitamin E is the natural anticlotting agent in human blood. What can we say about a uniform need for a uniform quantity of Vitamin E? How shall we reply to the apologists for processed foods who defend the removal of this vitamin from 94 percent of the starches and sugars consumed by Americans?

The giant vessel leaving the heart, the aorta, has three branches normally, but some people have one and some have six. Considering the variations in the sizes and efficiency of the hearts, it is not astonishing that some of us pump three quarts of blood per minute and others pump twelve. Is this difference reflected in certain dietary needs? Answer: No data. And which group will be more susceptible to the numerous disorders in which poor circulation plays a part?

The television advertisements for nasal decongestants give an idealized picture of the sinuses. In some people they are large, well formed, and easily drained. In others they are small and drain with difficulty. The latter are the people who are often more susceptible to sinusitis and postnasal drip — particularly if they are allergic, or if they eat a high carbohydrate (starch and sugar) diet. Have you envied those who do not share your tendency to colds and sinus troubles? You may be able to raise your level of resistance by changing your diet and by raising your intake of Vitamin A.

There is also the matter of infertility, for, despite the population explosion, there are many homes that are involuntarily barren. Reproductive efficiency varies tremendously from woman to woman, man to man. Those at the low end of the reproductive totem pole will need all the exquisite hygienic care and dietary support they can receive; the "fortunate" will reproduce on doughnuts and coffee. Male sex glands may weigh as little as ten grams, as much as forty-five; female ovaries may weigh as little as two grams, as much as ten — and one woman may have thirteen times more ova (egg cells) than the next. Numerous factors in nutrition — many of them arbitrarily removed in food processing — are important to fertility. Experience has taught me that raising the intake of these factors may sometimes counterbalance the inefficiency of the reproductive system in both sexes. Here is an individual difference in dietary needs that may alter a whole family's destiny.

Nothing has yet been said about allergy, though surely this is the height of individuality gone beserk. Little appreciated, save by allergists, is the impact food allergy may have on the efficiency of digestion, necessitating great care in selection of a diet balanced to meet the exaggerated nutritional needs of a digestive tract that utilizes food poorly. Sometimes mistaken for allergy is intolerance, another facet of individual difference. There is the Chinese Restaurant Syndrome — an assortment of gastric complaints and chest pains as a reaction to monosodium glutamate, a flavor enhancer well-tolerated by most people. There is intolerance to milk, predicated on a deficiency in lactase that allows milk sugar to ferment in the digestive tract, creating flatulence, cramps, and diarrhea. The interference with utilization of sugar, created by deficiency in sucrase, has already been mentioned. All these are differences in people, not in properties of foods. They must be recognized and managed if these idiosyncrasies of reaction are not to lead to a restricted and inadequate diet.

We are not all born with the same number of brain cells, and, indeed, their development can be depressed by faulty prenatal diet. Teeth are not the same. There are those hard as marble and resistant to decay; there are those soft as limestone, disintegrating when the diet is high in processed starches and sugars. Lymph systems, important to resistance to infection, are not the same in any two people. The size of the stomach varies tremendously, and therefore, so does the emptying time. How do we keep straight faces as dietitians talk about "three balanced meals a day" when some people need six, and a minority does well on two?

As we age, the time needed to clear fats from the blood lengthens. Blood fat that disappears in a few hours when we are thirty may linger for fifteen hours when we are sixty. No one has ventured to estimate how much fat we need, which is perhaps fortunate, but will not estimates necessarily vary with the age of the individual? Or will we one day be sensible enough to increase in middle age the intake of those nutrients that help the utilization of fats? (Some of them are removed from popular foods.)

The complaint here is not that these questions aren't answered. It is that by and large they are not *asked*. The Establishment is too busy generalizing about the nutritional needs of senior citizens, with statements that the menus that permit you to survive to sixty are obviously a success story and should not be changed.

Some of our differences may be ours alone; others are built into the genes. There are babies born with a sensitivity to an amino acid, leucine, which is essential to growth. Their reaction to milk, in which it is contained, is a lowering of the blood sugar. This in turn may result in convulsions. Adults sometimes show the same aberration of body chemistry, but it manifests itself in constant fatigue and frequent headaches.

Phenylalanine is another essential protein acid; yet its presence in the diet of some children will threaten them with feeblemindedness. Sometimes these inborn errors of metabolism have the opposite effect: Rather than being intolerant of an essential nutrient, one may be born with an inordinate need for it. Earlier in this chapter, examples have been given of moderately elevated nutritional requirements that, unsatisfied, may cause chronic poor health and restricted functioning; but these metabolic errors may be aggravated enough, in rare instances, to cause a disease — sometimes a lethal one. Although the Food and Drug Administration and the American Medical Association agree that intake of vitamins beyond the "minimum daily requirement" is at best, wasted, there are over a dozen serious diseases in children that can be controlled *only* with doses of vitamins from 10 to 100,000 times the "minimum requirement." Most of these result from the genetically determined inability of the body to manufacture vitamin-dependent enzymes needed for the synthesis of vital protein substances. The vitamins involved are B_1, B_2, B_6, B_{12}, and D.

Tested with sugar solutions in varying concentrations, some children will not report the taste as sweet until the concentration of sugar is raised to 20 percent. This reaction, beyond the understanding of those who are sickened by such syrupy sweetness, often identifies children in whose families there is a history of diabetes. Does this individual difference arise because they bear a diabetic tendency, or is the predisposition to the disorder reinforced by the large amount of sugar they must use to satisfy their sweet tooth? And, apropos of a sweet tooth, is there any more sensitive index of individual differences than sensitivity to pain — the dentist's drill, for instance? Some people are stoic; some leap out of the chair. There are areas on your skin where sensitivity to a pinprick is great, and other areas that are insensitive. Charts of these areas, Roger Williams points out, are not the same for any two people.

These constitutional quirks remind us that generalizing about human physiology, biochemistry, or nutritional needs is as risky as assuming universal reactions to individual foods, but this is what we have done. For a century, nutritionists (not I) have grouped all dietary fats and oils. The proposition was logical: Fats are fats, and it could make no difference to your well-being whether you chose olive oil, fried your foods with hydrogenated fats, preferred butter, or elected for peanut oil. It is true that Paccini in the early 1940s insisted that there are profound differences in the body's reactions to certain fats, with particular emphasis on distinctions between animal and vegetable fats. But he made the mistake of pioneering and received no apology from the Establishment when it finally recognized that the differences in the physiological impacts of animal and vegetable fats may be a matter of life and death for *some* people. Of course, once the orthodoxy in medicine had accepted the principle, it promptly swung to the other extreme and announced that animal fats are virtually lethal to *everyone*. As a purely incidental by-product, the subsequent craze for polyunsaturated fats culminated in cases of cancer in some men overdosed with such oils in the hope of preventing heart attacks.

Virtually all nutritionists (not I) have always lumped dietary starches and sugars together. Most still do. Carbohydrate is carbohydrate, and what is the point of making a distinction the body doesn't? After all, starches are turned into sugars in the body. It suddenly became apparent, however, that many of us react differently to starch than to sugar, and the difference could spell immunity or susceptibility to heart and blood-vessel diseases — in *some* people. When the Establishment finally accepts this observation, we can expect that the public will be told that sugar is deadly to *everyone*. While the amount of sugar we eat is biological insanity, this philosophy, unless individual differences in reaction are recognized, could have us dying of malnutrition — with healthy arteries.

The medical profession does not escape criticism when it is guilty of assuming that (a) the same disease has the same impact on all patients, and therefore (b) can be treated with the same diet. Perhaps the most telling warning against such glittering generalities about nutrition came from the organization so frequently guilty of them. An *ad hoc* committee of the American Medical Association Council on Foods surveyed medically restricted diets for digestive disorders and concluded that none of these diets makes scientific sense; all these diets constitute nothing more than ceremonial therapy — the rattling of the witch doctor's bones — and there will be no scientific rationale for such restricted menus until we know something about the actions of individual foods in the digestive tract. In the *individual* digestive tract may be an emphasis supplied by the *ad hoc* committee of tomorrow, let us hope. Meanwhile, hospitals, clinics, and physicians continue to prescribe routine bland diets for highly individual patients with highly individual reactions to their ulcers, colitis, diverticulosis, liver disorders, and pancreatitis. Would it interest you to know that a diet high in meat elicits *less* acid production than the venerable high-milk regime for *some* ulcer patients?

Individual differences in dietary needs and tolerances are academic — until *you* are part of the equation. Take the history, for instance, of a girl who married at sixteen to escape a brutal father. She brought to her wealthy husband — as a price, so the psychiatrists said, for her traumatic childhood — stammering so severe that it was almost impossible for her to communicate. She refused therefore to employ domestic help, would not answer a telephone, and went shopping only if armed with a written list of her wants. If, in one of her rare conversations, a friend tried, however tactfully, to supply the word with which she was struggling, she would retire in tears. Years of psychoanalysis and speech therapy had made her no more fluent. Then came the improbable coincidence. She was listening to one of my radio broadcasts in which I told of the mice with the tendency toward audiogenic seizures; they were relieved only when their extraordinary need for Vitamin B_1 was satisfied. In that program, I asked: "May we go from mouse to man? What would be the equivalent in man of convulsions in mice that are touched off by sound? As epileptic attacks may be touched off by the flicker of a candle or a television set, could stammering be initiated by the overreaction of a human nervous system, hypersensitive to sound for want of a more liberal intake of nutrients important to functioning of the nerves?" I thought this suggestion might offer a challenge to speech therapists, whose concepts of stammering have long been shaped by the mystique of the psychologist.

The stammerer discussed the theory with her physician, whose enthusiasm for nutritional therapy and theory was less than ecstatic. He called me and ended the conversation with the usual damnation with faint praise: "It can't help, but it won't hurt." So the patient began to raise her intake of Vitamin B$_1$ until she reached a dose more than fifty times the "requirement." Her speech gradually became less halting, and the improvement continued until her husband wrote to me in mock anger, "I used to come home to pipe, slippers, and home-cooked meals. Now I'm taking dancing lessons, we're going to Europe, we have four live-in help, I've eaten in restaurants for the last month — and it's all your fault."

Subsequently, I published this history in a nutrition newsletter I edit and received a visit from a young speech therapist who was working toward her Ph.D. She wanted me to know that, her committee willing, she proposed in her doctoral research to explore the possibility that inadequate nutrition, among other nonemotional factors, might be an influence in some speech difficulties.

The history does not imply that all stammering originates with vitamin deficiency — direct or relative to an unusually high requirement that makes a "balanced" diet inadequate. It does remind us again that it's not always "all in your mind," and that there is an "I" in diet and a "me" in menu.

Another example of nutritional needs that were not average occurred in a former Miss America, so dehydrated by persistent vomiting in the first five months of pregnancy that her obstetrician volunteered to call me as a consultant. He was faced with a choice between losing the baby or losing his patient. When this happened, in the 1940s, Vitamin B$_6$ (pyridoxin) was not well known, except to nutritionists; and less understood was the disturbance in its utilization that occurs in pregnant women — in some, raising the need for the vitamin and thereby intensifying and prolonging "morning sickness." I suggested 50 mgs. of pyridoxin daily, a dose then considered heroic. The "baby" is now about thirty.

A dentist developed a crossed eye when he was overtired — the tendency more pronounced in the spring and fall seasons. The symptom terrified him, and with some justice. Who wants his teeth drilled by a cross-eyed dentist? Even though he would have been described by any physician as "well-nourished" — indeed, overfed, if anything — he was able to discard the prisms he had worn, when his intake of vitamins essential to the nervous system was raised. Higher intake of thiamin, pyridoxin, and the Vitamin B Complex rescued him from a dietary deficiency not absolute, but relative to a need greater than the average.

A salesman had a problem shared by millions: too many colds. He had tried immunization unsuccessfully and heavy doses of Vitamin C, again without reward. He fell back on antihistamines, aspirins, and antibiotics. When his intake of Vitamin A was raised to 25,000 units daily, his colds lessened in frequency, severity, and duration. Yet medical pundits vow that vitamins neither prevent nor break colds and prattle about the toxicity of Vitamin A.

Even with nutrients not regarded as essential in the diet of human beings, the factor of individual differences may operate. Take PABA, a B-Complex nutritional factor that increases the fertility of women. Government agencies do not recognize PABA as an essential nutrient, though it is found in many foods as a component of the Vitamin B Complex. Yet hundreds of families, formerly infertile, responded to doses of PABA and improved nutrition with such heightened reproductive efficiency that a bumper crop of healthy babies resulted. In fact, I received a plaintive note from one husband after the third baby was born, asking: "Hey, Doc! How do you turn it off?" So much for the effect on fertility of food factors not always considered vital in human nutrition, in doses beyond quotas — where they exist — set by the authorities.

A pilot's eyesight shows improvement in the fifth decade of his life, when reason and medical experience argue that it should be slowly deteriorating. The government physician who examines him says: "Just what is it you do with your diet?" The pilot tells a story of more judicious selection of foods and the use of nutritional supplements; for once, the medical man does not scoff. (You can be sure that, relative to table of average nutritional requirements, *no* licensed pilot is ever considered malnourished.) This is a real person, living evidence of the individuality of dietary needs. The pilot is my good friend, Bob Cummings, the TV and movie star. Of him I heard a woman say: "Certainly he looks twenty years younger than his age. Why shouldn't he? He's a food faddist!"

You should be ready now to concede that there is a need to strike a compromise between the pleasures of the palate and the needs of the body, which are highly individual. As we journey, you will begin to realize that such a balance does not require a sacrifice of the pleasures of eating; in fact, good food tastes good. So discovered a group of girls, students in my nutrition course at Fairleigh Dickinson University, as we reshaped their menus to spare them the "normal" tortures of the premenstrual week and the painful period. It is a history of the benefits we can achieve by ignoring the dictates of the Nutritional Establishment, by whose standards virtually all Americans — save alcoholics — are well fed. It is also a story of the negative dividends of good nutrition — benefits that accrue in terms of what does *not* happen.

2.

FOR WOMEN WHO ARE WITCHES ONCE A MONTH

To many American women, the "normal" menstrual period brings with it tension, cramps, backache, dizziness, fainting spells, craving for sweets, tenderness of the breasts, water retention and weight gain, nervousness, incoherence, hysteria, weeping spells, and pain. It is equally normal to wait patiently after childbirth for hemorrhaging to subside and the uterus to shrink, unlike the primitive who is able after delivery to return promptly to her work. American women are likewise philosophical about cystic mastitis (cysts of the milk-producing tubules of the breast) and uterine fibroid tumors. All these are the prices a woman must pay for the privilege of being feminine and the biological birthright of having children; and they are all "normal" — because they are average.

Suppose they aren't normal. Suppose they are preventable, or at least can be mitigated. Suppose the prophylactic weapons are on the shelves of your supermarket and health-food store. Suppose you can wipe out premenstrual tension and menstrual pain by selecting your food more intelligently. Will you be willing to brave the wrath of the community by doing what is not average and thereby not "normal?" Are you willing to take the vitamins and eat the foods the Establishment calls "faddist," to achieve such benefits? I have a moral obligation to ask these questions, as a nutritionist who, via the mass media, has helped many women to experience — often for the first time in their lives — menstrual cycles not fraught with pain and tension. I have taught physicians how to block the basic *cause* of cystic mastitis with good nutrition, rather than attack the cyst, which is the symptom, with scalpel and retractor. You'd realize the value of the theory if you were familiar with the lessons taught by the pioneer researchers whose papers, neglected and unread, are gathering dust in the libraries. You'd accept the proposal enthusiastically if you had the opportunity to read the mail I've received from women who read my articles on this subject in such national magazines as *Family Circle*, writing in appreciation to tell me of vanished premenstrual tension and menstrual pain, or to exult in the new infrequency or even disappearance of breast cysts. Nor are those the only dividends, as you will discover if you will ponder on the nutritional chemistry into which this chapter will take you. For here is a means by which better diet may help protect you against cancer of the breast — a statement neither reckless nor undocumented. As you read you will discover that some individual differences in dietetic needs arise from one of the forces that determine how feminine a woman will be.

It is not usual that a study of men should teach us something significant about the chemistry of women; yet what we know about the effects of menus on premenstrual tension and pain comes partially from observations of starved American soldiers, prisoners of the Japanese in World War II. Army doctors, confined with the G.I.'s and sharing their meager food, noticed that the captives were gradually shifting toward the feminine: They were becoming impotent and were losing interest in sex; their beards were growing less rapidly and their breasts were enlarging. Identical symptoms had been recorded in men dosed with female hormone in the treatment of prostate disorders, and this suggested that somehow — by a pathway not then understood — dietary deficiency was provoking a rise in the level of estrogenic (female) hormone activity in the men's bodies. The theory was logical, but there was a disturbing fact: If starvation was actually producing this hormone imbalance, why did the symptoms grow worse when food packages temporarily improved the menus? Captivity itself was not responsible, for the same intensification of the sex shift appeared when the repatriated prisoners were treated with a nourishing diet in Army hospitals — but as the good nutrition was continued, the symptoms gradually subsided, and the men returned to normal.

Unknown to the Army doctors at the time, the chemistry of the sex shift had been explored, during the war years, in the research of a medical nutritionist who had proved — both with animal experiments and in research with women — that sex hormone balances are normally held within narrow boundaries by the liver, which has the ability to break down female hormone into two compounds that are not only less active as female hormones, but largely lose the cancer-producing effects of the original hormone molecule. Required for that function of the liver is a generous supply of protein and Vitamin B Complex — nutrients *not* lavishly supplied by the food choices of millions of women, whose menus are selected with an eye to calories and with little attention to nutritional adequacy.

Oddly, when the diet is not adequate and the breaking down of female hormone falters, the liver still retains its ability to control *male* hormone activity. The result, of course, is a steadily widening gap between the levels of the two hormones, the estrogens rising sharply, the androgens (male hormones) remaining at normal level. In the malnourished man, then, there is enough active female hormone to make him impotent, dilute his sex drive, lighten his beard, and enlarge his breasts. Indeed, from the vantage point of hindsight, it has been suggested that this may explain the lack of sex drive in male alcoholics — as well as the truth of the observation that many male alcoholics, innocent of hygiene and unacquainted with shampoos, still retain more scalp hair than the doctors who examine them. (Retention of hair on the head is more commonly a feminine attribute.) It is also interesting that in cirrhosis of the liver — with or without alcoholism — one of the early symptoms in men is a loss of chest hair — again, a shift toward the feminine — with a demonstrated rise in the levels of female hormone in the body.

The research also answered the remaining question: Why did a short-term supply of good food intensify the prisoner's shift toward the feminine? Because it promptly intensified the production of female hormone. The liver, perhaps the first organ to feel the impact of inadequate diet, is slow to respond when nutrition is improved. In the lag between rise in female hormone level and recovery of the ability of the liver to break down the estrogens, the symptoms of the sex shift were aggravated.

The forces that make a woman very feminine are not purely hormonal, although estrogen levels certainly play a role. Self-image and the culture that shapes it, the genes, and the functioning of the glands also help determine the level of femininity. What happens when a woman eats improperly, so that her estrogen activity increases while her output of male hormone is still under normal regulation by the liver? Here individual differences in response to the insult will again be determined in part by the soil on which it falls. In some women, it might manifest itself as asocial behavior that intensifies as the female hormone level soars from ovulation through the menstrual period — this observation is based upon studies of women in reformatories and prisons, 49 percent of whose crimes, it was shown, were committed in the premenstrual week. Mental acuity may be affected — some girls, taking college examinations just before their periods, earned grades 15 percent below their usual scores. Mental balance may tilt toward psychosis: Forty-six percent of female admissions to mental hospitals come in the week prior to menstruation. The will to live may weaken at that time, when 53 percent of attempts at suicide by women occur. In other women it may manifest itself as cystic mastitis; the number, size, and painfulness of the cysts paralleling the estrogen activity. A common response is intensification of premenstrual tension, with symptoms varying from insomnia to irritability, backache, bloating, nervousness, tenderness and fullness of the breasts, hysteria, blackouts, craving for sweets, weight gain, or the temper tantrums men have come to accept as the price for marrying girls who periodically ride broomsticks. (Apropos of hysteria: The Greeks had a word for it — derived from the Greek term for womb.)

The mischief does not end when the menstrual period starts, nor when the painful first day or two have passed. In the menstruating woman, high estrogen levels may contribute to more severe and more prolonged hemorrhaging. This is the real basis for the television advertisements urging menstruating women to take iron supplements, for the excessive loss of blood may create an iron deficiency as the end of a chain of dietetic errors that started with inadequate intake of protein and Vitamin B Complex. Since a diet low in these factors is automatically low in iron, a vicious circle is apt to develop, which is obviously not broken by the usual medications — diuretics, tranquilizers, sedatives, and pain-killers. Between ovulation and the premenstrual week, cysts of the breast may develop, growing more numerous or larger (or both) until the advent of the period signals a drop in estrogen levels. Then the cysts will disappear, until the next cycle starts. In some women they do not disappear, lingering to cause constant pain, so great in some cases that the sufferer is compelled to sleep with a bra on. Surgery is frequently recommended when these cysts persist, for some gynecologists fear to temporize with a situation they regard as possibly portending breast cancer. The surgery is a philosophical cousin to the tranquilizers and the diuretics, aimed at symptoms that return because the causes are ignored.

These bits and pieces of a technician's thinking in nutrition can now be reduced to simple conclusions, susceptible to practical application. Among the individual differences that determine a woman's needs in her diet is a most neglected factor: how much estrogen she produces. The more she manufactures, the more critical becomes her supply of Vitamin B Complex and protein. If she fails to meet that need, she will also require a greater supply of iron to offset the excessive loss of the mineral during her period, for the hemorrhaging will not only be greater but more prolonged. Indeed, a medical nutritionist who gave this sound nutritional advice to hundreds of women, with the result that the duration of their menstrual periods was reduced by 40 percent, came to the conclusion that the five-day period isn't normal — it is an "average abnormality." He concluded that giving women diets that meet their unique requirements as women would make the three-day menstrual period become the norm. Another medical man found in this application of good nutrition the key to the quick recovery of the primitive woman from the aftermaths of childbirth. Her primitiveness has nothing to do with the rapid return of her uterus to normal and briefness of postchildbirth hemorrhaging. It is simply that inherited wisdom in choice of food gives her a diet that properly supports liver function. There is no inherited wisdom in the American woman's food selections; in fact, if you want a diet that will help liver function, simply follow the average American housewife through the supermarket, buying what she rejects and rejecting what she buys!

If you have now accepted the concept that your menus and your menstrual phenomenon are interlocked, perhaps it has occurred to you that this protection against excessive estrogen activity will extend to the female hormone from any source — medication, the Pill, and the natural estrogens in food. Unfortunately, while the debate rages on about the safety of the birth-control pill, the youngsters who so largely use it patronize the pizza-pop school of nutrition, unaware that there is dietetic protection against mischief caused by estrogens.

Another conclusion is inevitable: When we talk about deficient diets, the Establishment is always quick to point out that beriberi, scurvy, and pellagra are virtually unknown in our cornucopia of plenty. But it is perfectly possible to be malnourished — as millions of American girls and women demonstrate — with nothing more than premenstrual tension and menstrual pain as the visible toll for dietary inadequacy.

This is an important point. It is not necessary to be an alcoholic or to starve yourself into obvious signs of protein and Vitamin-B-Complex deficiency before liver control of estrogen begins to falter. A classic example of that truth occurred in a thirty-two-year-old woman who

was a patient at a medical group practice for which I was a staff
nutritionist, some years ago. By every index — dietary history, physical
appearance, blood chemistry — this young woman was well fed. Her
complaint was cystic mastitis. She had an aggravated case — a total
of seven to eight cysts which would begin to increase in size at ovulation,
until the pain drove her to seek surgical relief. Not being a tactful
nutritionist, I suggested to the surgeon that dietary control of estrogen
activity might be more rewarding than surgery that could bring nothing
more than temporary relief. The result was an intramural battle, which
I would have lost had it not been for a fortunate happenstance: The
director of the practice was a fine medical nutritionist. Administration
of protein supplements between meals, plus substantial doses of liver
concentrate and Vitamin-B-Complex capsules brought complete recovery in a period of four months. At that point the medical director
gave a demonstration that silenced the surgeon, who even then had
remained skeptical. He stopped the nutritional therapy and applied an
estrogen cream to the bust; within three days a new crop of cysts
developed. Renewal of the dietary therapy was followed by their disappearance. This history is one of dozens I could recite.

Some years ago I was teaching nutrition at Fairleigh Dickinson
University, where, taking advantage of the prerogatives of an associate
professor, I organized a study of about 200 female students in my
courses. The group was selected on the basis of its troubles with the
menstrual cycle, although it was not aware that this was the nucleus of
my interest in it. (One must control the factor of the power of suggestion
in all such experiments.) Complaints among the girls included cysts of
the breast, marked premenstrual tension, pain on the first day of the
period, and excessive and prolonged hemorrhaging. Superficially,
most of the students appeared to be well fed, and, in fact, were described
as "well-nourished females" by the physician with whom I collaborated.
Dietary histories were not as prepossessing. Many of the girls ate no
breakfast, in the mistaken belief that this is a means to avoid weight
gain. Others lunched on a sandwich and a bottle of soda. Dinners were
usually selected with an eye on calories rather than on the body's
requirements.

Those girls who had no breakfast were encouraged to take at least
an eggnog, or liquid whole milk reinforced with nonfat milk powder.
Those who skipped lunch, if they could not be persuaded to mend their
ways, were given one of the 225-calorie drinks of the type suggested for
reducers. Some were given brewer's yeast or liver concentrate as supplements to their meals. All were guided in balancing their diets. It
made no difference how the nutrition was bettered; if the result was an

increase in protein and Vitamin B Complex, a majority of the girls, some months later, reported a lessening of menstrual distress. It was easy to evaluate the response when a student remarked: "I used to know my period was arriving because I climbed walls. Now I know it's coming when it arrives. And it's shorter now." Another said: "Ever since I began menstruating, I've had to throw away eight or ten days of each month — I just couldn't function. Now my menstrual has dropped from six days to three, and the cramps and weight gain are gone. I feel like an idiot," she added, "when I realize that simple changes in my food habits could have done this a long time ago." As breast cysts diminished in number and size and in some cases vanished completely, the students expressed their astonishment, startled that this symptom, too, can be an indirect by-product of food choices that do not satisfy the needs of the body.

On the other hand, the technician is not always prepared for the anxiety reflected in one girl's question: "If you wipe out too much of the female hormone, couldn't you make a girl mannish?" This was the point at which she became acquainted with one of the great safeguards inherent in good nutrition: Its direction is always toward the normal. For this same reason, a good diet, high in protein and Vitamin B Complex, will not reduce estrogen activity in the postmenopausal woman, whose supply of the hormone is already diminishing; but it may help her to prolong her prime of life. Likewise, such a diet will not increase the difficulties of the woman who, estrogen-poor, has irregular or missed periods. Conversely, there are factors in nutrition that *increase* the response to female hormone and become useful adjuncts when the physician is treating the girl whose ovaries are lazy.

Often, the woman whose menstrual problems are resolved by improved nutrition will also gain other dividends. Resistance to fatigue increases, and sleep better knits "the raveled sleave of care." Nails improve. Texture, sheen, and manageability of hair are bettered, with the hairdresser often the first to recognize that you're "doing something about your diet." The nervous system may be grateful, with minor irritations becoming more bearable. As one woman, a subject in a study of diet versus the menstrual cycle, put it, "I am still aware of the dripping of the faucet in the next room — but I'm not *compelled* to go and turn it off."

The experience of the captives of the Japanese suggests that these interactions between food and hormone metabolism may affect men in subtle ways that are not usually recognized. In point are observations that go back to 1907, linking actual atrophy of the testicles with nutritional deficiencies in which liver function is disturbed. The late-onset male diabetic is, unhappily, a frequent victim of this interplay between poor nutrition and glandular function. Unfortunately, the tendency of the middle-aged man with diabetes to lose sex drive and to become impotent has been thrown into the medical wastebasket as a "complication of diabetes." It might be more accurately described as the penalty for the failure to meet the diabetic's critical needs in nutrition. It is the price a man's body pays as estrogen levels rise when the liver — the function of which is frequently disturbed in diabetes — is not nourished to meet its qualitative requirements. The process is intensified as the abnormal estrogenic levels feed back to the pituitary gland, causing a drop in male hormone output, so that the process is embellished with a reduction in sperm count and motility. (Do you recall that male minks fed on chicken necks from birds treated with synthetic female hormone became sterile? *This* was promptly investigated and *solved* — mink being the national peasant costume, and minks worth hard cash!) All this has been strikingly demonstrated, to use the researcher's own language, when the diabetic's potency and libido return as his deficiencies in protein and Vitamin B Complex are corrected. The trouble with the remedy is that it's simple, not a wonder drug, involves nutrition, is inexpensive and widely available. In addition, the wife of a diabetic will be more likely to search for an aphrodisiac pill than to believe that her husband's virility will return if she incorporates more protein and Vitamin B Complex in his menus. There is also the risk of his being considered a food faddist, though that's better than having him labeled a cuckold.

Such successes with diabetic men do not draw a road map from the dining room to the bedroom for every diffident lover, for impotence more often springs from the emotions than from the gut or the glands. The specific chemistry of nutrition that we have been discussing is almost certainly the cause of many male diabetics' sexual failures, but it can also be involved in any man who shows recognizable signs of nutritional deficiencies. Unfortunately, such signs may be as subtle as emotional instability, insomnia, and rapid fatigability — easily assigned, like weak libido and impotence, to the emotions rather than to the diet. Others, however, are clearcut warnings of nutritional inadequacy: Bareness and shininess of the tongue, cracks at the corners of the mouth, inflammation of the gums, cobwebbing of the small blood vessels, or painful neuritis. A man with these symptoms who is also lacking sex drive may well have suffered nutritional castration from elevated estrogen levels based on disturbances of liver function — exactly as a woman who is grossly obese may, by a parallel process, become infertile.

Persistent cysts of the breast are regarded as precancerous by some medical men. This is not to say that every woman with this condition will progress to malignancy, but that statistically such women are more prone to than women who are cystfree. If corrected diet in some women can mitigate or cure cystic mastitis, are we not invited — indeed, obligated — to examine the possibility that proper control of female hormone activity may help to protect women against cancers of the two areas of the body that are sensitive to estrogens: the breasts and the uterus?

Such a proposal offered at a medical symposium would invite a bitter storm. There would be those physicians unacquainted with the mechanism of dietary control of estrogen activity. Their numbers would be tripled by those who do not regard the estrogens as cancer-producing hormones. Still others might reject the possibility that, in prescribing birth-control pills, they have been dosing their patients with potentially cancer-causing substances. And among these would be a sizable group unaware that Dr. Roy Hertz, internationally regarded as an authority on the role of endocrine (glandular) substances in cancer, has labeled steady dosage of estrogens as "playing with fire"; and he is not alone in that opinion. It has been said (by me) that the path of safety is the only possible choice for the layman when the scientists disagree. One can, of course, refuse to take the birth-control pill. Or, taking it, at least follow the dietary pattern that helps tame the estrogens. Since Dr. Hertz's warning is both well based and echoed by cancer authorities of comparable scientific standing, such menus may yield the most striking of all bonuses from optimal nutrition: a rise in resistance to precancerous changes. Women are often urged to undergo "preventive" checkups to detect such indications. "Preventive," however, is an ill-chosen adjective, since the mischief has already begun; frequent checkups simply provide early diagnosis. In contrast, the evidence in this chapter offers guidelines to *predictive* medicine coupled with *preventive* nutrition. When the millenium arrives one would hope that all women dosed with estrogens, eating meat from cattle medicated with the hormones, or producing unusually high amounts of these hormones, will receive prescriptions for this nutritional protection. *All* women deserve optimal diet, do they not? If you receive this as a pie-in-the-sky type of thinking, consult the footnote below, citing a paper in the *Journal of the American Medical Association* that flatly declares that normal breakdown of estrogens is the path to heightened resistance to estrogen-dependent cancer. However, the authors reveal no awareness that breaking down of the hormone rests ultimately on the wisdom of the woman's choices in food.*

*H.M. Lemon, et al, "Reduced Estriol Excretion in Patients With Breast Cancer," *Journal of the American Medical Association* (June 27, 1966), p. 13.

Let me quote another of the many references that might be cited to persuade you that this is not academic theory posing as scientific fact. Morton Biskind, M.D., the medical nutritionist who helped establish the role of dietary factors in liver control of estrogens, remarks: "Investigations by many workers have shown that estrogen may be etiologically involved in the production of a variety of neoplasms in tissues responsive to estrogens, notably in the breast and uterus."* Dr. Biskind adds that many workers indict the continuous (rather than the intermittent) bathing of the tissues in estrogen as undesirable. One achieves such a constant estrogen bath by use of the birth-control pill, of course, or by eating an inferior diet that inactivates liver control of the hormone. Ironically, the estrogen bath becomes part of a vicious circle, for the hormone itself can damage liver function. How many women leap into that circle by taking the hormone, overproducing it, and eating improperly?

There is a question that may occur to you while thinking over the relationships among diet, estrogen levels, and susceptibility to cancer in those tissues constantly bathed with female hormone. Should we not view the interplay of these factors from the vantage point of hindsight, by examining women who do have cancer of the uterus or breast? Where are their estrogen levels, and what is their supply of Vitamin B? That thought occurred to two researchers at McGill Medical School twenty-five years ago. Spurred by Biskind's findings, they compared two groups of women matched in age distribution, one group with cancer and the other without. High levels of estrogen and low levels of Vitamin B were characteristics of nearly 95 percent of the cancer group. The same percentage of the healthy women showed lower levels of estrogen and adequate amounts of Vitamin B. It doesn't mar the research that protein intake was not measured, or that other B vitamins were not included in the assays. The evidence is still there, and the conclusions are also applicable to premenstrual tension, to the painful menstrual period, to cystic mastitis, and to the processes leading to estrogen-dependent malignancies of breast and uterus. In America it is estimated that over 200,000 hysterectomies are performed yearly because of uterine fibroid tumors. Here again it appears to be the symptom and not the cause that preoccupies the medical profession. Yet should you explore the thinking of gynecologists, you would find that they often recognize, at least tacitly, that estrogen stimulation is involved in the growth of such tumors. If, for instance, a woman begins to develop fibroids when she is thirty-nine years old, there will be physicians who

---

*M.S. Biskind, "Nutritional Therapy of Endocrine Disturbances," *Vitamins and Hormones,* Vol. 4 (Academic Press, 1946) pp. 147-180.

will suggest that surgery be deferred, if possible, until the menopause arrives. It may bring a drop in estrogen levels that may halt, if not reverse, the progress of the tumors. Similarly, removal of the ovaries to drop estrogen levels in the body and therefore slow the growth of a breast cancer, is an approved surgical procedure. It is regrettable that such surgery constitutes the practice of scientific and ethical medicine, but the proposal to control estrogen activity with good nutrition will, to many physicians, be tainted with "food faddism."

In this book, we examine some of the changes in dietary habits and shopping criteria that will raise your intake of Vitamin B Complex and protein. Accomplishing these goals will require that you lower your quota of overprocessed starches and sugars, thus permitting weight loss when it is needed. Fat women *are* more susceptible to cancer of the breast, for obesity is actually malnourishment conducive to high estrogen activity. That activity explains the infertility of grossly obese women — they manufacture enough female hormone to act as an internal birth control. Incidentally, you will discover that combining optimal nutrition with weight control is not difficult. Why should it be? You had no trouble combining poor nutrition with weight gain, did you?

FULFILLING A WOMAN'S UNIQUE NEEDS IN NUTRITION

All competent nutritionists know that whole-wheat bread is a better food than white bread. Realistic nutritionists are also aware that we've been able to persuade only 6 percent of the public to eat whole-wheat bread. It is obviously an academic exercise for us to eulogize the superior nutritional values of foods you refuse to consume, but if I can't persuade you to bake with whole-wheat flour or to buy whole-wheat bread, I'll settle by teaching you how to raise the Vitamin-B-Complex and Vitamin-E values of such processed carbohydrates as white flour. Brown rice is better food than converted rice, which is better food than white rice, but I'll set my sights on the converted rice when I know that you may balk at the more distinct flavor, longer cooking time, and adhesiveness of whole-grain rice. It would be nice to think that the evidence in this chapter will motivate you into eating topnotch nutritious food at every meal, but as a pragmatist, I know you'll sin — and realizing that temptation is sometimes the only thing you can't resist, I'll supplement your diet with concentrates of Vitamin B Complex,

Vitamin E, and protein. This simple philosophy outrages the orthodox diet experts, who are committed to the proposal that we all share the same nutritional needs, and that ideal nutrition can be achieved by a "good, mixed diet." Since my compromises grudgingly sanction continued consumption of some of the mischief-making carbohydrates, there are nutritionists who are alienated by my "leniency," despite my use of supplements to compensate for the inadequacies of these over-milled starches and sugars. Scientifically, they have a case; realistically, they must learn to bend a little before the winds of stubborn dietary and food preferences. So long as the compromises lead you to the nutritional goal, I have no apologies to make to either group and assume that you now need no further justification for the recommendations that follow.

Selecting Foods Rich In Vitamin B Complex

An authority on the metabolism of starches and sugars has remarked that man opened a Pandora's box of troubles when he learned how to break the relationship between the Vitamin B Complex and the starches and sugars with which it is normally associated. He was referring to the overprocessing that removes this group of vitamins from the wheat, corn, rye, barley, rice, sugar and other carbohydrates that contribute 50 percent of the calories to most modern diets. Industry shrugs off such criticism by pointing out that it supplies what the consumer wants, which calls for hosannas because the consumer has not yet insisted on breakfast rolls spiced with heroin. If the responsibility *is* the consumer's, another indictment of your shopping habits should be added: In the butcher shop, you do your best to avoid the meats that are rich in the Vitamin B Complex by directing your buying to the muscle meats (steaks, chops, roasts) and by neglecting the organs (liver, kidney, brains) that are infinitely richer in B-vitamin values. Accept a dogmatic statement here: The word "healthy" means "whole." A whole food is healthful. A fractionated food isn't — and it can contribute to fractionated health. If you respect the sanctity of the body, eat *whole* grains, like whole wheat; and eat the *whole* animal, muscles *and* organs.

Selecting Supplements Rich In Vitamin B Complex

This group of vitamins is called a "complex" because it consists of many factors that are usually found together in the same foods. These include thiamin, riboflavin, niacin, pyridoxin, PABA, pantothenic acid, folic acid, inositol, choline, B_{12}, pangamic acid, and a large group of unknowns — their presence assured, their identity not established. Among these is an antifatigue factor, found in liver, and an antiestrogen factor. (Obviously, the liver must create a specific agent to break down estrogens.) The Vitamin B Complex is concentrated in the germ of the grain, which is the site of the new life when the seed sprouts. Industry removes this germ to "improve shelf life." Whatever it does for shelf life, it does not do for human life. Enrichment consists of the restoration of *three* of these vitamins to flour. The term "enrichment" is obviously flattering.

The best sources of the entire Vitamin B Complex in supplements are brewer's yeast and liver, but buying these requires an understanding of differences among the many commercial versions of these B-Complex concentrates. There are two main types of brewer's yeast — primary and secondary. *Primary* refers to a yeast that is grown specifically for use as a supplement to the diet. *Secondary* refers to yeast that is grown initially for use in brewing — the spent yeast debittered and freed of the taste of hops and salt and sold as a supplement. Since the brewer cares not at all about nutritional values, the yeast he uses is selected solely for its efficiency in the fermenting of alcoholic beverages. Secondary yeasts are therefore good sources of protein and Vitamin B Complex, but the primary yeasts, grown specifically for these values, supply more of both. In addition, tailoring a yeast for use as a supplement by human beings allows the producer to choose varieties not only higher in nutritional values, but distinctly better in taste.

All this information reduces to a simple suggestion. Use brewer's yeast that is labeled *primary*, in preference to the secondary type or torula. Use tablets or powder, and select your brand for protein and vitamin values and for taste. Some varieties run as high as 62 percent protein, others run lower in protein, but are still a good source. They offer especially high values of certain B Vitamins, or of the sulphur-containing amino acids (protein building blocks) that are not usually well supplied by yeast. Still others are fortified with Vitamin B_{12}, which is usually only supplied by animal proteins. All are excellent foods and valuable supplements. The powder form can be mixed with tomato juice or incorporated into baked recipes. Begin with a modest amount — say, one percent of the weight of the flour.

I hear a faint sputtering. Are you asking how much you should use? You swallowed degerminated cornflakes and 104 pounds of sugar per year, yet you never made anxious inquiries about overdoses. But when I come to you with something especially nutritious, your anxieties bristle! Some people run into flatulence or laxative action if they overdo brewer's yeast; others are grateful for the laxative effect. Some can take unlimited quantities. Dr. Tom Spies, in his pioneering research on pellagra, fed his patients one quarter pound of brewer's yeast daily, plus one quarter pound of liver concentrate! You'll do fine with less, but you might learn something from this fine medical nutritionist, for he discovered early in his treatment of the malnourished that the synthetic vitamins alone are simply not enough. The "unknowns," the cofactors of yeast and liver hold healing in their chemistry. So in addition to organ meats, try a dozen tablets of yeast or a few teaspoonsful of the powder daily. Baker's yeast is taboo: Living yeast *needs* vitamins and borrows from you.

Liver concentrates are also not alike. They are available in two main types: solvent extracted and desiccated. There are those who prefer the solvent-extract variety because they do not wish to consume the fat and the cholesterol which, in this process, are completely removed. Other nutritionists lean toward liver desiccated (dried) under vacuum, for they prefer to retain the nutrients contained in the liver fat. Vacuum drying permits "heating" at about room temperature. Oven-dried liver concentrates are not desirable, for the high temperature will denature the protein, changing its characteristics. A handful of such liver tablets or two tablespoonsful of the powder constitute a fine supplement of the entire Vitamin B Complex in natural form. The powder may be blended with any liquid or food in which you find it palatable; don't cook it. Should you use both liver and brewer's yeast? If you will, it's better for you; if you're going to use only one, make it liver.

A third source of the Vitamin B Complex is the germ of the grain, for this gives you Vitamin E, inadequately supplied by the other two. Wheat germ is the most popular form. Eat the raw germ if you enjoy it; buy the toasted if you prefer its flavor. It loses a little in the toasting, but it's still a magnificent food, supplying, in addition to the vitamins already named, a high concentration of protein and excellent amounts of minerals and polyunsaturated fats — including a group that may be the body's starting point for synthesis of the newly discovered prostaglandins. These are factors vital to muscle function — including the heart. Always buy wheat germ vacuum-packed, for like all fine foods, it is perishable. (Buy foods that spoil and eat them before they do. If a food keeps, throw it out.) Wheat germ may be eaten as a cereal, or a spoonful may be added to each portion of cereal. It may be mixed with bread crumbs as breading, or added to each cup of flour used for waffles, pancakes, and baking — one teaspoonful per cup. Don't go overboard — this will give you cookies, cakes, or bread with more than a family resemblance to a lump of lead. If you are nutritionally unwise enough to buy cake mixes, make up for some of their deficits by adding about a teaspoonful of wheat germ for each cup of mix. Actually, the sugar and bleached-flour content of these products and the additives that make their labels look like prescriptions, should dampen the buying enthusiasm of anyone but a malnourished masochist.

Meals and Snacks

If there is any meal more important than the others, it is breakfast. Good diet wobbles when supported on only two legs. In fact, six small meals daily are often better for you than three large ones. Weight control is easier for most people on a six-meal pattern, for cheating becomes unnecessary when you're never more than a few hours from a snack or a meal.

Your snacks and meals will be aimed at a low starch, low sugar, high protein diet, with about 20 percent of the fat in the polyunsaturated (vegetable) form. Each day have two glasses of nonfat milk, three slices of whole-wheat bread (or the equivalent in whole-wheat, whole-rye, or brown-rice crackers), and any combination of margarine and vegetable oil adding up to five teaspoonsful daily. The oil should not be used in cooking, but as salad dressing. Serve organ meats frequently.

In each snack include a protein of animal origin — eggs, milk, cheese, meat, fish, fowl, or yogurt. Not the yogurts messed up with fruits or jam — their calory value in sugar far outruns the calories from yogurt. Use your imagination. Sample of imagination: Soften cottage cheese with a little yogurt or milk. Sprinkle with anise, caraway, or chopped chives. Wrap in thin slice of ham, tongue, or leftover meat. Drink tomato or mixed vegetable juice. (The fruit juices tend toward high sugar content.) Don't forget the milk quota.

For breakfast: If weight is not a problem, use four ounces of citrus juice or the equivalent in whole fruit. Weight unwatchers may choose a whole-grain cereal — such as whole-wheat or oatmeal — with a teaspoonful of wheat germ, plus a bit of honey for sweetening, if desired. It's still sugar, but sweeter than the other types, and you'll learn to use less. It also contains fruit sugar, which burdens your pancreas less, and it has some vitamin value. In the health-food store, you'll find a variety of honey produced by bees fed a high-vitamin diet; they obligingly transmit the extra values to the honey. For protein, two small eggs, or at least four ounces (uncooked weight) of any animal protein — sausage, fish, hamburger, or breakfast steak. One slice of whole-wheat bread or the equivalent in whole-grain crackers — whole-rye, whole-wheat, or brown-rice, with one teaspoonful of margarine. If you choose pancakes or waffles, weight gain obviously doesn't worry you; but fortify your recipe with a teaspoonful of wheat germ per cup. If you must use a mix, use one with unbleached flour and soy. At least one such brand already contains added wheat germ. *Read labels:* The goal set in this chapter makes it worthwhile. It takes less effort than enduring cramps or surgery. Beverage at breakfast: Nonfat milk, if you choose this time for it. Decaffeinated coffee — caffeine does more mischief than you know.

For lunch: Repeat the breakfast pattern with four ounces of animal protein (uncooked weight), with a slice of whole-grain bread with one teaspoonful of margarine. Low-starch vegetables, if you choose. Salad with any dressing containing vegetable oil. Dessert such as whole gelatin (not the flavored varieties, which are 85 percent sugar) with fruit, or fruit and cheese, or Bavarian whip made with whole gelatin, or high-protein cookies (available at any health-food store). Beverage of your choice.

Dinner may offer melon, or shrimp or crabmeat cocktail, or fresh fruit cocktail (unsweetened); two vegetables, one leafy; and four ounces of any animal protein (uncooked weight). Dessert should, as always, be low in sugar and starch, and if that generalization throws you for a loss, consult Chapter 5 for suggestions. Remember your need each day for vegetable oil and margarine in any combination adding up to five teaspoonsful. Mayonnaise may occasionally be substituted for part of the vegetable-oil requirement. Keep in mind, too, your need for three slices daily of whole-wheat bread or the equivalent in whole-grain crackers. If you can't conquer your white-bread habit, check out the improved white breads in the health-food stores — and don't hesitate: Their patronage today is no longer confined to little old ladies in tennis shoes. In whole-grain crackers, brown-rice make a good choice — about ten of them are equivalent to one slice of bread. Crisped in the oven a bit, they are quite palatable. They're available in most supermarkets and health-food stores.

While these menus are framed for the needs of women, the men will benefit by the improved nutrition, too, requiring only a uniform increase in the sizes of portions in proportion to their caloric needs. Women who have the common twin problems — excess weight and fat in the wrong places — should reduce the bread to two slices daily. A low-carbohydrate diet of this type, with the indicated amount of vegetable fat, is not only conducive to weight loss, but has a striking effect in causing loss of inches out of proportion to the loss in pounds — and in the stubborn areas, at that. If you don't wish to lose, or the weight loss is greater or more rapid than you desire, the starch content of the diet is the variable that lets you control the process — upping the starches (not the sugar) if you wish to stabilize your poundage.

You'll miss the commercial cakes, cookies, pies, sodas, and puddings at first, but your appetite for starches and sugars will decline, week by week. You'll find whole-grain breads and cereals perhaps a little strange, because they all have a flavor. This is an innovation! American white bread is deliberately made flavorless, since it's used as a vehicle for other things — butter, jam, or whatever — and bakers apparently fear that two tastes simultaneously might upset one-track minds. Some bakers now offer bread sliced in half the usual thickness, which, incidentally, is the only way to bring down the caloric value of bread. There is no such thing as a low-calory bread, no matter what the advertising says.

Don't Forget Your Supplements: The Estrogens Don't Forget*

It's obvious that I dislike the term "average," but if there *is* a characteristic of the American woman that is average, it is impatience in matters dietetic. She spends ten years piling on excess fat and wants a blitz diet to remove it in three weeks, or preferably less. She has eaten like a biological idiot for decades, but wants to know after two weeks of corrected diet why she is not rejuvenated. Be a little patient. The body neither collapses quickly with inferior diet — or you wouldn't have the strength to be impatient — nor responds magically when nutrition is corrected. The dividends *will* come.

*For women with menstrual and related problems, see Appendix 2.

3.
SOMETIMES IT'S NOT "ALL IN YOUR MIND"

There are those with deep, inexplicable anxieties and fears who are *not* emotionally disturbed, although that is the usual diagnosis — and it brings them to unneeded and ineffective psychiatric treatment. There are sufferers with claustrophobia who are *not* mentally disturbed, even though this symptom, too, is usually interpreted as a sign of neurosis or worse. There are those who are melancholy, who endure fears that make no sense even to them and whose troubles are *not* purely mental. These unfortunates are victims of an individual difference in reaction to the common pattern of American diet. Their troubles spring ultimately from stress upon liver, pancreas, and nervous-system function, initiated or aggravated by an excessive intake of sugar and caffeine and triggered by stresses that leave others unwounded. They should be upright at a lunch counter, rather than horizontal on a psychiatric couch. This is the actual story of such an anxiety-ridden woman as she pleaded for help from a physician, the fifth she had consulted. Behind her was a trail of prescriptions for tranquilizers and referrals to psychiatrists.

"I'm worn out when I open my eyes in the morning. I'm more tired than I was when I went to bed," she said. "And it isn't from the insomnia — I'm exhausted even when I have a good night's sleep, which is rare."

The doctor asked: "What do you mean by insomnia?"

"It's a peculiar kind," she responded. "I have no trouble going to sleep at all — most people with insomnia do, don't they? But I wake up at about two in the morning, and that's it. I toss until dawn, or read, and never really get back to sleep again. Sometimes, while I'm lying there I find myself crying, and I really don't have anything to cry about. I have a constant feeling of something dreadful about to happen, and there's no reason to feel that way. When the phone rings, I'm two feet off the floor, and I'm always positive it's a call to tell me something awful has happened to my husband or the children, and I don't know why I expect that — I have no reason. . . ." Her voice trailed off in a sob.

As she talked, the doctor was scribbling brief notes labeling her as a typical neurotic, a hypochondriac, with free-floating anxiety without cause, drifting like a balloon until it snagged on something. Too, there was the classic list of indefinite complaints, with the usual background of constant fatigue. What would he prescribe? MAO inhibitor — psychoenergizer — stimulant — sleeping drug — or would it be better to refer her to a psychiatrist? He disliked the last choice. Why was it, he wondered, that the patient most in need of psychological support flees from it as from the devil?

The patient was thinking: "If he tells me it's the 'tired housewife blues' I'm going to scream!" Aloud, she said: "My temper is unbelievable, and it's not like me, but I'm always so tired that I'm always irritable. I've even slapped my children on the face, and that's something I never do. And then there's the feeling that the walls of the house are closing in on me. It's worse when I go shopping. If the store or the bus is crowded, the feeling gets unbearable and I have to leave."

The doctor's note read: "Claustrophobia." He reflected that his waiting room was filled with people who were really ill, and fate would have it that the "well patient who feels sick" would pop up on a busy day.

Her recital of complaints was not ended. "I sigh all the time," she said, "and for no reason. I feel faint — like greying out, not a blackout. My vision gets dim. Then my heart starts to beat so fast it frightens me, and then it feels as if it's skipping beats. Are you sure, doctor, I don't have heart disease?" she asked pleadingly, as though, he thought, she would welcome such a diagnosis.

He shook his head. "Your electrocardiogram is normal."

She stemmed her tears with a handkerchief and heard herself voicing her secret fear. "You're not going to tell me I'm a neurotic, like the other doctors, are you? I must get help, I can't stand feeling nervous and worn out all the time. Do you know what it's like, feeling as if there are two of you in one body, one watching the other?" she asked.

The doctor put down his pen; his decision was being made for him. She was describing depersonalization, a red flag warning of the possible onset of serious mental disease. This case, he reflected, now fell outside his province as an internist. Before he could decide how to break the news to her gently, yet firmly enough to discourage her from trying to escape psychiatric treatment by visiting more medical men, she made the critical remark that changed her destiny. "It's unbelievable," she added, "that my tiredness never goes away. I can't finish my housework without lying down. I drink coffee by the gallon and keep nibbling on candy to keep up my strength, but nothing helps."

"You didn't tell me about that," the doctor chided her. "How long have you had a sweet tooth?"

"It's more than a sweet tooth," she protested. "I really *need* the sweets. I do crave them. It started after my last pregnancy, I remember. Does it mean something? I thought maybe I began to nibble because I was nervous."

The doctor thought, "It might be she's making herself nervous by nibbling." He knew there is a condition called "hypoglycemia" (which means "low blood sugar") that causes a craving for sweets plus numerous other symptoms that seem purely neurotic — perpetual fatigue, irritability, insomnia, anxiety, weeping, forgetfulness, claustrophobia, depression, depersonalization, and physical disturbances simulating heart disease, allergies, eczema, stomach ulcer, migraine headaches, and arthritis. As the sweet tooth it causes (in most patients) is indulged, the symptoms worsen. The trouble partially results from an overactive pancreas, which responds to a rise in blood sugar by producing excessive amounts of insulin, the hormone that "burns" sugar. The result is that a hypoglycemic who eats foods rich in sugar ultimately suffers a drop rather than a rise in his blood-sugar level. Since sugar is the one fuel the brain and nervous system require, the condition is easily capable of simulating neurosis or psychosis. The onset is often triggered by a strong stress, such as pregnancy, surgery, a protracted illness, or a prolonged period of great tension and anxiety; and it is fanned and perpetuated by improper eating habits — skipped meals, low intake of protein, excessive amounts of sugar and caffeine. This patient had many of the symptoms. Moreover, the tests he had given her had not included one for hypoglycemia: That takes six hours, involves six or seven samplings of blood, and, after all that, may still turn out negative.

The physician disliked subjecting her to the expense and inconvenience, but, he reflected, unneeded psychiatric treatment is costly and protracted, too. He scheduled the test. If it came out positive, he thought, he'd tackle the job of explaining why eating sugar makes low blood sugar *lower* — a paradox physicians themselves were slow to comprehend.

Functional low blood sugar was first recognized by Dr. Seale Harris in 1923. Like most physicians of his day, he was dismayed by the unpredictable reactions of diabetics to injections of the new drug that lowered blood-sugar levels — insulin. It was already apparent that insulin treatment sometimes dropped blood sugar too much and too fast, with the patient going into "insulin shock." But Dr. Harris suddenly realized that he was seeing insulin shock in patients who were not diabetic and not taking insulin injections. Obviously, such people had a condition opposite to that of the diabetics — they were overproducing, rather than underproducing insulin. What, pondered Dr. Harris, would make the pancreas go wild, responding to a rise in blood sugar with such excessive output of insulin that the patient — his brain and nervous system frantic for lack of fuel — would become weak, faint, pale, nervous, and sweaty? The answers ultimately were found in two dietary stimulants to pancreatic function that Americans take in excess. Dr. Harris blamed sugar. Later research also indicted caffeine and similar stimulants.

Further studies showed that emotional tension could also initiate low blood sugar by continually stimulating the pancreas through the nervous system and the adrenal glands. Then, through the research of such pioneers as Dr. Stephen Gyland and Dr. Harry Salzer, a neuropsychiatrist, it became apparent that this could become a vicious circle — anxiety, tension, and fatigue causing low blood sugar, which in turn causes fatigue, tension, and anxiety. These symptoms are logically the result of hypoglycemia, for the brain and nervous system depend for *existence* as well as function on a mere two teaspoonsful of sugar in the entire blood circulation. It requires only a slight drop in blood sugar to imperil them, and only a little, constant overactivity of the pancreas to make the threat a hazard. In over 80 percent of these sufferers, the drop in blood sugar is followed by a craving for sweets; yielding to it stimulates the pancreas into producing more insulin. The result is obvious: The more sugar such people eat, the more they crave; the faster they burn it, the less they have. That is why the treatment is based on a diet as free of sugar and caffeine as possible, low in starch, high in protein and fat, and served in six small meals daily. The objective is to keep the sugar levels as even as possible, for it is enduring rather than quick energy that is sought. Have you reflected that Americans are stuffed with "quick energy" foods yet fatigue is perhaps our most common problem?

The "well patient who felt sick," now her old vivacious self, asked, "Now that I'm well again, how long must I stay on the diet?"

"Maybe forever," the doctor answered soberly. "At least until you are far enough along to try a little experimenting. Some people are cured, but more are merely arrested, and if they overdo sugar and caffeine, or skip meals, their troubles come back. Some people do well so long as emotional pressures and physical stresses aren't too great. And there are people who can never cheat at all — for them, a little sugar is like a little poison."

"I always thought," his patient commented, "that we all need sugar for energy."

"We do," the doctor agreed, "but not necessarily *as* sugar. Man had energy before the sugar bowl was invented. He manufactured sugar in his body, from other foods. That's what you're doing now, and it gives your pancreas a rest, because it doesn't have to rise to the challenge of producing insulin to take care of a teaspoonful and a third of sugar every thirty minutes — which is what you were eating."

"Where did I get that much sugar, doctor? I did eat candy and sweeten my coffee, but that's a lot of sugar!"

The doctor said, "I go through this with every hypoglycemic patient. How about eighteen teaspoonsful of sugar in one portion of apple pie à la mode? That was in one of your menus. The cherry pie — fourteen teaspoonsful of sugar. How about the chewing gum — a half teaspoonful per slice? The glazed doughnuts? The salad dressings and ketchup, full of sugar? Shall I go on?"

"I'll stick to the diet if it kills me," his patient said grimly. "Will I gain weight?"

"Not likely," the doctor assured her. "You didn't gain on the sugar because you were burning it too fast to store it. As your liver function returns to normal, you'll begin to control your estrogens properly. That will let your thyroid function as it should. With good nutrition you'll find that the direction will be toward the normal; the overweight tend to lose, and the underweight gain."

As stress, tension, and anxiety can pave the path to low blood sugar, so can apathy cause a parallel breakdown in the body's management of starch and sugar. The trigger here is frustration, monotony, a feeling of aimlessness, and lack of goal and achievement. This list reads like a lengthy description of the housewife's frame of mind; it is a mental set that may also push a woman toward psychiatric treatment as a victim of the "tired-housewife syndrome," a phrase that concentrates on the emotional but ignores the physical aspects of the disorder. The woman who suffers from constant fatigue, morning headaches, weakness, internal trembling, and sudden attacks of anxiety will be assured that these are purely the products of emotional letdown, the results of duties less challenging than those of an elevator operator. But Franz Alexander, a psychiatrist, identified a type of low blood sugar that is caused by apathy, rather than anxiety and tension, and in turn contributes to emotional letdown. He pointed out that routine activity without emotional participation is much more fatiguing than strenuous activity based on strong emotional drive. If you think about that, you'll realize that dancing tires you less than doing laundry, shopping for a new dress less than mending. So it is that routine and unenjoyed tasks lead to emotional letdown, which in turn causes an interference with the mechanism that controls the concentration of sugar in the blood. Your fatigue from emotional bankruptcy combines with your weariness from low blood sugar and then your housework becomes that much harder. Since you'd love to leave it behind anyway, you're well on the road toward a charter membership in the society of apathetic, tired housewives.

The type of low blood sugar that this emotional letdown causes does not reflect sudden, excessive outpouring of insulin from the pancreas, but rather a state of steady, slight overproduction. This flattens the rise in blood sugar that should follow eating. Thus the blood-sugar levels never drop far enough to make you act neurotic, nor rise high enough to give you relief from mental and physical fatigue. Now you exist, rather than live, in the greyness of a twilight zone, neither truly sick nor truly well, but genuinely unhappy and always weary.

Abstention from sugar and caffeine is a must in this type of low blood sugar, too; your meals must be frequent, and high in protein and in fat. But your recovery — which may be amazingly quick — will not be permanent unless you change your mental perspective and find a challenge in your responsibilities. Otherwise apathy will continue to derange the chemistry of sugar in the body, and the resulting disturbance will feed back to the brain and nervous system as silent fuel for the fire of your discontent. So it is that the physician who treats your "flat sugar-tolerance curve" may suggest that you also seek help from a psychiatrist, a community guidance service, or your pastor. Only thus, he knows, will you find your way back to zestful living as did a housewife, nearing forty, who came to her physician to complain that she was so weak that she couldn't move. "Life has lost all significance for me," she admitted. "I simply don't know what to do with myself!"

Her physician administered the six-hour sugar-tolerance test, found a "flat curve," and prescribed a low-sugar, high-protein, high-fat diet to avoid burdening the already disturbed mechanism of sugar management in her body. With medication to slow down the absorption of sugar, and thereby to avoid stimulating the oversensitive pancreas, this plan brought relief from all symptoms in just *one week*. But her doctor knew that he had quieted only half, the physical half, of the storm that started with the emotions and referred her to a psychiatrist. Under his guidance she came to realize that her troubles began after her son died, and her husband unexpectedly refused to adopt another child. It was then that her life and her contributions to her marriage became meaningless, creating the apathy that caused malfunction of her body's regulation of blood sugar. With the clarity of hindsight, she was able to describe the process in apt terms: "I had a terrible let-down feeling in my mind," she confessed, "and it caused a sit-down strike in my body, and each made the other worse." When she seasoned her new diet with a recaptured zest in living, her cure became permanent.

Although the histories in this chapter have concerned women who were victims of hypoglycemia, the disorder doesn't spare men. The wage earner may not complain of a "let-down" feeling, having arrived at a quiet desperation in his life on the male treadmill; but the rebellion may disturb his body's management of sugar, too, and the resulting deficit in fuel for brain and nervous system will make his daily tasks that much more difficult to fulfill. Men who are genuinely neurotic, men who pursue callings marked by tension, deadlines, and irregular meals — these are some of the candidates for low blood sugar. When it strikes, unfortunately it is likely to be tagged for anything but what it is. Hypoglycemia may choose to appear only in the form of constant fatigue, or headaches; it may masquerade as neurosis or aggravate it; it may initiate or worsen asthma and allergies. Low blood sugar can touch off deep (and even suicidal) melancholia unwarranted by the life situation. It can mimic epilepsy or trigger the attacks of the real disease. The disorder is present in many schizophrenics, making them less responsive to therapy; it contributes to the troubles of many autistic children. One type of alcoholism may directly be caused by hypoglycemia, and I believe that it is sometimes the pathway to drug addiction. Pediatricians blame hypoglycemia for the learning difficulties and behavioral disturbances of some children. Yet the condition often goes undiagnosed. Why?

There are many reasons for the failure of the physician to recognize low blood sugar — other than the obvious one: You don't find what you're not seeking. The symptoms irresistibly suggest neurosis or even psychosis, and prescribing tranquilizers or psychoenergizers is the path of least resistance. Physicians and patients alike are not enthusiastic about the long, involved test for low blood sugar; yet the shorter tests may completely mask the condition, for the trouble may not become apparent until the fifth or the sixth hour of the test. But three hours is the usual period — and that is more often ordered in a search for diabetes, rather than the opposite condition. When diabetes does not appear — which usually can be determined by the second hour — the medical man sighs in relief and terminates the examination.

Should the patient escape these diagnostic errors, he is still not in the clear. It is tempting to use simple logic and prescribe sugar for low blood sugar. When this worsens the condition, both patient and physician lose their enthusiasm, and the door slams on possible help. And that help is critically needed, as you may judge from the following list, a description of the symptoms of hypoglycemia as reported by 600 patients suffering with the condition:

SYMPTOMS

Percentages of patients complaining of these particular symptoms

Nervousness	94%
Irritability	89%
Exhaustion	87%
Faintness, dizziness, tremor, cold sweats, weak spells	86%
Depression	77%
Vertigo, dizziness	73%
Drowsiness	72%
Headaches	71%
Digestive disturbances	69%
Forgetfulness	67%
Insomnia (awakening and inability to return to sleep)	62%
Constant worrying, unprovoked anxieties	62%
Mental confusion	57%
Internal trembling	57%
Palpitation of heart, rapid pulse	54%
Muscle pains	53%
Numbness	51%
Unsocial, asocial, antisocial behavior	47%
Indecisiveness	50%
Crying spells	46%

Lack of sex drive (females)	44%
Allergies	43%
Incoordination	43%
Leg cramps	43%
Lack of concentration	42%
Blurred vision	40%
Twitching and jerking of muscles	40%
Itching and crawling sensations on skin	39%
Gasping for breath	37%
Smothering spells	34%
Staggering	34%
Sighing and yawning	30%
Impotence (males)	29%
Unconsciousness	27%
Night terrors, nightmares	27%
Rheumatoid arthritis	24%
Phobias, fears	23%
Neurodermatitis	21%
Suicidal intent	20%
Nervous breakdown	17%
Convulsions	2%

The patients also commented on changes in personality in the form of unaccustomed lapses in moral conduct, carelessness in dress, and tendencies to drug and alcohol addiction.

On learning that excessive use of sugar and constant intake of caffeine can contribute to symptoms like these, my reader will, predictably, plead guilty to the caffeine and deny any exorbitant intake of sweets. To scotch that defense, consider this chart of the refined sugar content of many popular foods.

Approximate Refined Carbohydrate Content of Popular Foods
Expressed in Amounts Equivalent to Teaspoonsful of Sugar
100 grams = 20 teaspoonsful = 3½ ounces = 400 calories

Food	Amount	Serving	Sugar Equiv- alent
CANDY			
Hershey Bar	60 gm.	(10¢ size)	7 tsp.
Chocolate cream	13 gm.	(35 to lb.)	2 tsp.
Chocolate fudge	30 gm.	1½ inches sq. (15 to 1 lb.)	4 tsp.
Chewing gum		1¢ stick	1/3 tsp.
Lifesaver		1 usual size	1/3 tsp.

Food	Amount	Serving	Sugar Equivalent
CAKE			
Chocolate cake	100 gm.	2 layer icing (1/12 cake)	15 tsp.
Angel cake	45 gm.	1 pc. (1/12 large cake)	6 tsp.
Sponge cake	50 gm.	1/10 of average cake	6 tsp.
Cream puff (iced)	80 gm.	1 average custard filled	5 tsp.
Doughnut plain	40 gm.	3 inches in diameter	4 tsp.
COOKIES			
Macaroons	25 gm.	1 large or 2 small	3 tsp.
Gingersnaps	6 gm.	1 medium	1 tsp.
Brownies	20 gm.	2x2x¾ inches	3 tsp.
CUSTARDS			
Custard, baked		½ cup	4 tsp.
Gelatin		½ cup	4 tsp.
Junket		⅛ quart	3 tsp.
ICE CREAM			
Ice cream		⅛ quart	5 to 6 tsp.
Water ice		⅛ quart	6 to 8 tsp.
PIE			
Apple pie		1/6 of med. pie	12 tsp.
Cherry pie		1/6 of med. pie	14 tsp.
Custard, coconut pie		1/6 of med. pie	10 tsp.
Pumpkin pie		1/6 of med. pie	10 tsp.
SAUCE			
Chocolate sauce	30 gm.	1 tsp. thick heaping	4½ tsp.
Marshmallow	7.6 gm.	1 aver. (60 to 1 lb.)	1½ tsp.
SPREADS			
Jam	20 gm.	1 tablespoon level or 1 heaping tsp.	3 tsp.
Jelly	20 gm.	1 tbsp. level or 1 heaping tsp.	2½ tsp.
Marmalade	20 gm.	1 tbsp. level or 1 heaping tsp.	3 tsp.
Honey	20 gm.	1 tbsp. level or 1 heaping tsp.	3 tsp.
MILK DRINKS			
Chocolate (all milk)		1 cup, 5 oz. milk	6 tsp.
Cocoa (all milk)		1 cup, 5 oz. milk	4 tsp.
Cocomalt (all milk)		1 glass, 8 oz. milk	4 tsp.
SOFT DRINKS			
Coca Cola	180 gm.	1 bottle, 6 oz.	4-1/3 tsp.
Ginger ale	180 gm.	6 oz. glass	4-1/3 tsp.
COOKED FRUITS			
Peaches, canned in syrup	10 gm.	2 halves, 1 tbsp. juice	3½ tsp.
Rhubarb, stewed	100 gm.	½ cup sweetened	8 tsp.
Apple sauce (no added sugar)	100 gm.	½ cup scant	2 tsp.
Prunes, stewed, sweetened	100 gm.	4 to 5 med., 2 tbsp. juice	8 tsp.

Food	Amount	Serving	Sugar Equiv-alent
DRIED FRUITS			
Apricots, dried	30 gm.	4 to 6 halves	4 tsp.
Prunes, dried	30 gm.	3 to 4 medium	4 tsp.
Dates, dried	30 gm.	3 to 4 stoned	4½ tsp.
Figs, dried	30 gm.	1½ to 2 small	4 tsp.
Raisins	30 gm.	¼ cup	4 tsp.
FRUITS AND FRUIT JUICES			
Fruit cocktail	120 gm.	½ cup, scant	5 tsp.
Orange juice	100 gm.	½ cup, scant	2 tsp.
Grapefruit juice, unsweetened	100 gm.	½ cup, scant	2-1/5 tsp.
Grapejuice, commercial	100 gm.	½ cup, scant	3-2/3 tsp.
Pineapple juice, unsweetened	100 gm.	½ cup, scant	2-3/5 tsp.

Our caffeine intake is the largest in the world. Caffeine and related stimulants are found not only in our bottomless cup of coffee, but also in tea, in coffee liqueurs and candies, in chocolate, in cocoa, in cola beverages (with the caffeine of one-third of a cup of coffee per small bottle), and in the stimulant tablets advertised for sale without prescription. Our sugar intake has been stated as an average of 104 pounds per person per year, but that is deceptive, for little babies, diabetics, hypoglycemics who know what is wrong with them, reducers, the dietetically sane, and (hopefully) sufferers with arteriosclerosis eat much less. So we find many Americans eating more than their share — as many as forty teaspoonsful of sugar daily, so that this one empty food supplies nearly one-third of their total caloric intake. Sugar is not only a source of nothing but calories, but is also a food the nervous system and brain cannot "burn" without three vitamins, and these are not supplied by sugar. Thus this strange condiment has not only displaced more valuable foods in the diet, it has increased vitamin requirement — and lowered the supply. Attempting to oxidize sugar in the body without the vitamins leads to the formation of "clinkers" in the body furnace, toxic intermediate products of interrupted combustion of carbohydrate, and these can cause symptoms identical with those of low blood sugar. It matters not whether the problem is too little fuel for the brain (hypoglycemia) or fuel it cannot properly utilize because of vitamin deficiency, the end of the story will be a complex of symptoms indistinguishable from those once called "nervous breakdown." Such symptoms often are misinterpreted, as are those of hypoglycemia. The physician tends to think of vitamin deficiency in terms of beriberi, pellagra, or scurvy, the "classical" deficiency diseases that are rarely seen. These are actually the terminating (and premortal) stages of dietary inadequacy. More common are the "twilight zone" deficiencies, not severe enough to cause the textbook *physical* symptoms, but very effective in interfering with function of the nervous system and the brain. This impact of vitamin deficiency on the personality was long ago recognized by Wilder, of the Mayo Clinic, and Spies, of the Hillman Clinic in Alabama, but their truths have been obscured by a barrage of propaganda that paints America as superbly well fed. Wilder tells us of a group of patients who volunteered to eat a diet low in thiamin (Vitamin B_1) to allow physicians to determine the nervous and mental disturbances that originate with a degree of deficiency not severe enough to cause beriberi. The diet used in that experiment consisted of lean meat, cheese, skim milk, fruits, and vegetables. It was supplemented with brewer's yeast, from which the Vitamin B_1 had been removed, plus Vitamins A, C, and D. The food plan is deceptive. It is, in fact, close to the reducing diet voluntarily eaten by millions of women who take no supplements with it and blame their irritability and nervousness on the frustrations of weight-loss menus. Here is a condensation of the history of one of the volunteers in the experiment, whose reactions are typical of the group.

Prior to the experiment, the patient had no symptoms. She was appraised by the consulting psychiatrists as well adjusted, congenial, industrious, efficient, and vigorous. After two months on the deficient diet, she worked slowly and negligently, followed instructions inaccurately and became forgetful, irritable, and quarrelsome. Her appetite flickered. Three months more and the doctor noted: "She wept and laughed alternately. She was critical of herself. She displayed apathy, confusion, and fatigue. She complained of indigestion and of numbness of the hands and feet." Two months later, she was unable to work because of dizziness and weakness. She described herself as feeling "helpless." She was confused and bewildered, and said decisions were difficult to make. Here the experimental diet was ended, and the missing vitamin intake supplied. "The improvement," the doctor's diary noted, "was gradual. The patient still tired easily and was alternately cheerful and apathetic, sleeping poorly." At the end of four months of corrected diet with two months of supplementing Vitamin B_1, the patient "became congenial, cooperative, and industrious. She no longer complained."

In more severe deficiencies of this vitamin which is needed to burn carbohydrate in the brain and nervous system, behavioral changes are even more dramatic. Here is the actual history of such a breakdown in personality, based on inadequate diet. A forty-nine-year-old woman is brought to a hospital in a state of mental confusion. She does not know where she is, what day or what year it is. She is restless and frightened. She thinks people are trying to poison her. She sees imaginary insects and snakes. Her history is one of gradually developing and progressively increasing nervousness, marked by insomnia, by-products of a long list of food aversions that led to a sharply restricted and inadequate diet. For three months there had been a marked loss of appetite, and for two weeks she had refused virtually all food. In the hospital this woman's treatment consisted of food and vitamins, particularly the Vitamin B Complex, with emphasis on thiamin (B_1) and niacin. On the third day she was mentally clear, entirely rational, no longer had delusions or hallucinations, and was normally cheerful. The important point, other than the impact of dietary deficiency on cerebral and nervous-system functions, lies in her freedom from *physical* signs of deficiency. She had the *mental* symptoms of pellagra, without the diarrhea, the painful tongue, the cracked corners of the mouth, and the butterfly rash that spell pellagra as the medical textbooks describe it. The report of the physician who cured her is illuminating: "It has long been recognized by most physicians who have studied pellagra that many patients had minor, vague, and indefinite complaints that usually existed for years before the classical symptoms of pellagra appeared. *Mild mental disturbances are almost always the first evidence of chronic partial deficiency of niacin.*" (Emphasis supplied.)

Unfortunately, medical men are the victims of inadequate training in nutrition; they also suffer from indoctrination that leads them to believe that there is virtually immediate transition from normal health to full-blown deficiency states, with no intermediate stages. Yet Dr. Tom Spies long ago recognized the subtle alterations in personality that precede by years the blatant physical symptoms caused by inadequate diet. He described patients in this twilight zone of dietary deficiency as easily startled, excited, or irritated. They become hypersensitive to noise and are upset by the shrill voices of children, or the monotone of the radio. They are easily offended or hurt, and they grow angry or cry with little provocation. They are easily frightened and worry a great deal, without justification.

Anxiety is as striking a symptom of this deficiency as it is of low blood sugar. It is as though the emotional brain grows hysterical when its fuel supply is inadequate or cannot, for lack of vitamins, be properly utilized. The condition ranges from vague feelings of uneasiness and apprehension to severe and clear-cut attacks of unjustified anxiety, with marked heart and breathing symptoms that lead, understandably, to fear of impending death. These victims of borderline dietary deficiency sleep poorly and suffer with nightmares from which they awaken dripping with perspiration, with a sense of constriction across their chests, as though an iron band were binding them and interfering with breathing. They imagine things — someone coming up the walk, someone calling them, some intruder in the room. They are melancholy without knowing why and cry without cause. They prefer, like hypoglycemics, to avoid crowds, noise, and company. The hallmark of the deficiency is the feeling, as numerous victims have put it, of "swimmy-headedness." Fatigue is always present, too, as it is in hypoglycemia, and the degree of the weariness is likely to parallel the degree of the other symptoms, among which is one so subtle that it mocks the competence of the medical man who thinks of dietary inadequacy in terms of swelling of the ankles, butterfly rashes, hemorrhaging, diarrhea, or delirium — for the very early sign of deficiency in niacin may be nothing more than loss of a sense of humor!

You now know how hypoglycemia can ravage personality and wreck the function of brain and nervous system. You see the parallel symptoms that torture the victim of mild, chronic deficiencies in the vitamins needed to metabolize sugar (and starch). Picture what may happen when the two disorders are combined! And they *do* combine, for the excessive intake of sugar and the skipped meals that are prelude to hypoglycemia are virtually a guarantee of vitamin deficiency. It takes about 100 mgs. of thiamin to "burn" the amount of sugar an American eats, each year — 100 mgs. of Vitamin B₁ that sugar does *not* supply. Where is it to come from? The thiamin contained in other foods is needed to help metabolize those foods; there is no surplus to compensate for the vitamin vacuum of sugar.

4.
DIABETES

If hypoglycemia is one side of the coin in individual differences in reaction to food, diabetes is the other, and of this disease a specialist recently remarked: "The man who is prediabetic and whose physician does not discover it is lucky!" Yet when insulin was introduced in the treatment of this ancient disorder, it was hailed as the gallant knight on the classic white horse, charging to the rescue of the diabetic. The oral drugs that lower blood sugar were likewise saluted. What touched off the specialist's cynical remark?

The story is painfully familiar and familiarly painful, for you have lived through it again and again with many "wonder drugs" with side effects unforeseen upon their introduction. In the case of diabetes, the happy promises for the "magic" of insulin and the oral drugs had to be invalid. Control of blood sugar is not control of diabetes, although this is the usual medical yardstick. Recycling of sugar reserves is not control of diabetes. Rendering the cell wall more permeable to the passage of sugar is not control of diabetes. Yet these are the actions of medications prescribed for this disease. The truth is that diabetes is a classic example of a complex disorder that has long been treated as if it were solely a problem of malutilization of sugar caused by a deficiency in internal production of insulin. In actuality, diabetes is a disorder involving sugar, protein, fat, vitamin, mineral, and (in one type) water metabolism. Simple underactivity of the pancreas cells that produce insulin doesn't explain the disease; in fact, many diabetics have a normal pancreatic output of the hormone and some actually overproduce it. The major error in the management of diabetes is committed when the pancreas alone is made the prime culprit. The liver inevitably is involved and quite probably is more important in controlling blood sugar than is the pancreas; yet this organ is not a direct target of treatment.

None of this justifies the physician's concept that he is "controlling" diabetes by monitoring blood and urine levels of sugar, which would be academic if by this concept and treatment of the disease he somehow blundered through to a solution of the diabetic's problems; but he does not. Blind reliance on drug therapy has created blind diabetics. "Controlled" diabetes can progress — and sometimes does — into uncontrolled circulatory disorders, including hardening of the arteries and hypertension, kidney disease, hemorrhages of the eyes (now the most frequent cause of blindness in the United States), heart attacks, and cancer — which are dismissed as "complications of the disease." In the opinion of some medical authorities, they are complications of the *treatment* rather than the disease, the inevitable results of therapy that is misconceived, misdirected, and inadequate.

Although insulin therapy has been indicted as a prime contributor to the numerous "complications" of diabetes, it may be, when compared with the oral drugs, the lesser evil. Insulin has several physiological effects; the oral drugs are aimed at nothing more than reduction of the level of blood sugar. As early as 1962, the oral drugs were known to cause such side reactions as muscular weakness, allergic responses, sudden hypoglycemia, granulomas, and cirrhosis of the liver. It was recently discovered that diabetics "controlled" with these tablets developed more heart attacks than those treated with insulin plus diet, or diet alone. Physicians reacted to this authoritative report by continuing to prescribe the oral drugs, or professed themselves to be irked because this frightening information had been released to the public. One is compelled to speculate on the basic anxieties that motivate the practitioner who wants to keep secret the fact that his prescriptions for diabetics represent a "calculated risk" — the calculations, after all, are his; the risks are the diabetics'. No wonder the pharmaceutical suppliers have been described by one diabetic authority as being engaged in a "horsepower" race, striving to dominate the market by discovering more and more potent unphysiological blood-sugar-lowering agents! Lest all this be attributed to the clarity of hindsight, let me note that I published a warning on the side reactions of the oral drugs in 1963, pointing out that they cannot be used for juvenile diabetics, who are too unstable; and they are usually unnecessary for the mature diabetic. The report on their contribution to heart attacks came eight years later. The information on which I drew was not privileged. It came to me from members of the medical profession itself, specialists who were sorely troubled by the increasing use of these agents.

That control of blood sugar is not control of diabetes is evidenced by the observation, well-established, that mothers of heavy babies (over twelve pounds at birth) are frequently candidates for diabetes in later years. The obesity of these infants is a testimonial to a grave disturbance in the mothers' metabolism of carbohydrates; yet diabetes itself is not present, by any clinical standard.

Since diabetes itself is not fully understood, it is apparent that no one knows why oral drugs that lower blood sugar should contribute to the incidence of heart disease. (At least one of these oral medications also appears to encourage premature aging, but I seem to be alone in observing *that*.) Explanations of the side effects of insulin therapy, however, are available. Somogyi, a scientist respected for research in diabetes that dates back five decades to the introduction of insulin, has pointed out that insulin dosage can never be exact and must often drop the blood sugar below the level normal for the individual. This does not refer to doses that cause shock by inducing drastic and sudden decline in blood sugar — with these every diabetic is familiar — but to comparatively minor overdosage that produces no recognizable symptoms. After all, no one knows how much the blood sugar will be lowered by a given dose of insulin, for estimates of the amount of sugar "burned" by a unit of insulin range from one gram to twenty grams. Since dosage must obviously be only approximate, it is understandable that the diabetic must occasionally suffer shock when the blood sugar drops too far and too fast, but he will also suffer *delayed* penalties when it falls just a little too much. How much is "a little too much"? Somogyi labels it as 2 milligrams percent below the level desirable for the patient — which represents a deficit of only 1/15,000 of an ounce of sugar in three ounces of blood! Minute as this drop is, it triggers a compensatory effort by the adrenal glands, touched off by a warning from the pituitary, to offset the excessive insulin effect by production of the several adrenal hormones that raise blood sugar. This makes the body a battleground in a clash between the sugar-lowering hormone (insulin) and the sugar-raising hormones (epinephrine, cortisone) produced by the adrenals. If the adrenal glands succeed in meeting the insulin challenge, the patient will be considered insulin-resistant, for doses of the hormone will no longer satisfactorily lower the blood sugar. The frequent "solution" for this problem is an increase in the insulin dose, posing a higher-level challenge for the overworked adrenals. If again these glands are able to step up the output of hormones that raise blood sugar, the surgeon may now enter the scene with a new "solution": removing the pituitary gland. This leaves the adrenals "blind" to the level of the blood sugar. Let it be noted that this surgery — the long-term results of which are totally unknown — has been hailed as another of medicine's advances.

Should the adrenals become exhausted in meeting the challenge of the excessive insulin doses, the price for their surrender may include high blood pressure, retinal hemorrhage, heart attack, hardening of the arteries, infection, kidney disease, or cancer. Not by chance, these are the diseases Dr. Hans Selye attributes to the "stress adaptation syndrome" — his term for the disorders that develop when the adrenals are unable to cope with continuous and overwhelming insults. In the diabetic, though, these disorders are fatalistically shrugged away as "complications of the disease."

In the light of the preceding explanation, how shall we judge the medical philosophy of the physician who tells the diabetic, "I'm putting you on more generous amounts of insulin to let you have more carbohydrate in your diet"?

Somogyi noted that the adrenals are often grossly enlarged — a sign of excessive stress — in diabetics with the "complications of the disease," and he remarked that these are some of the consequences one might anticipate when you give a solo position to a single instrument in the glandular orchestra. He specifically indicts insulin therapy as responsible for the collateral troubles of diabetics.

As for his concept of the toll for allowing insulin a dominating position in a glandular orchestra, just consider the interplay of the forces that control sugar metabolism: The pituitary growth hormone, glucagon (a pancreatic hormone antagonistic to the insulin effect) epinephrine (adrenalin), insulin, cyclic adenosine monophosphate, the B vitamins, zinc, chromium — and who knows what unidentified hormones, nutrients, and metabolites? When a shot of insulin or a dose of a sulfa derivative is called "diabetic therapy," what are we doing? More important: What are we not doing?

Without extrapolation — merely on the basis of what is already known — we can conclude that the overemphasis on drug therapy tends totally to obscure the importance of zinc, chromium, and B vitamins to diabetics. Insulin is obviously but one link in a very long chain. Mature-onset diabetics may well survive without doses of insulin or oral drugs, and in the old days many perforce did; but without adequate intake of the Vitamin B Complex and trace minerals, they cannot live. Yet, in every sense, each dose of insulin is a raid on the reserves of the B vitamins in the cells, for they are used for the manufacture of enzymes indispensable in "burning" sugar. Supply of these enzymes in diabetics is often low because the diabetic diet is frequently a poor source of the vitamins from which the enzymes are made. After all, it is *not* insulin that "burns" sugar. Sugar yields energy only after it is chemically treated in a long series of reactions within the body; and in these equations, B vitamins and minerals are essential components.

Why is the dominant emphasis in diabetic therapy placed on the drugs? Why are diabetic diets analyzed only for percentages of carbohydrates, protein, and fat? When diabetics are given lists of foods that may be "exchanged" for other foods, why are the equivalents evaluated only in terms of protein, fat, sugar, and starch values? Why do diabetic diets from world-famous clinics and specialists make no meaningful distinctions between white and whole-wheat breads, when the whole-grain is a much better source of the Vitamin B Complex and Vitamin E, and yet supplies no more starch or sugar than the overprocessed varieties? In short, why are these diets not routinely supplemented with foods and concentrates rich in the factors that can lower the insulin need? If sugar deserves and demands attention because added carbohydrate will increase the insulin requirement, should not equal attention be given to vitamins that may decrease it? Has no one reflected over Samuel Soskin's statement that the separation of carbohydrates from the Vitamin B Complex (as is practiced in processing 50 percent of the foods a diabetic eats) has been a fruitful source of troubles for man? He urges that everyone, therefore, use Vitamin-B-Complex supplements. If it is important for the healthy, is it not trebly important for the diabetic? Soskin has also demonstrated in animals that the liver more than the pancreas dominates in control of blood sugar; yet diabetic therapy is preoccupied with function of the pancreas. This, even though autopsies have shown that the liver is structurally abnormal in a large percentage of diabetics!

All this sounds like academic hairsplitting, but its truths are confirmed by experience with hundreds of diabetics in research in which I participated for more than twenty years, conducted by competent internists. Let me tell the story of a single patient. She was fifty-nine years old, diabetic for fourteen years. She was regarded by her physician as a "controlled" diabetic, for her blood sugar was not alarmingly high, and she infrequently "spilled" sugar in her urine. She developed a typical diabetic neuropathy — a disturbance of her nervous system, with pain. This was followed by a reduction of circulation in her legs, more marked in the left leg. A small infection on her heel unleashed its fangs, and when Dr. Wolfgang Seligmann and I saw her, the heel was gangrenous and amputation was under discussion. The area was so painful that she could not stand the pressure of a wet dressing, and the physician spent the better part of a night spraying the lesion with a germicidal agent (developed in our joint research) that was a local anesthetic and also had the property of dissolving dead tissue. Simultaneously, she was given large doses of Vitamin E, with smaller amounts of niacin, calcium, and glycine — a nutritional therapy aimed at improving circulation. Vitamin B Complex by mouth and by injection, together with the insulin she had been taking, completed the treatment. She escaped the amputation. The neuropathy was brought under control. Her blood sugar was lowered though her insulin dose was also lowered. I can say positively that without the intervention of the medical nutritionist that woman would have finished her days as a cripple.

So it is that diabetic treatment is partial and lopsided. All diabetics should receive supplements of the Vitamin B Complex, supplying more than the usual token amounts of pantothenic acid, choline, inositol, and pyridoxin (Vitamin B_6). To augment the beneficial effect of these B vitamins on liver function, raw liver tablets — solvent extracted or vacuum-dried — are needed. Dried pancreatic tissue, prepared from the residue after insulin is extracted, should be among the supplements, for there is hope that as a consequence, the antineuritic factor will be supplied, which may possibly spare the diabetic the "complication" of painful nervous system disorders. For the failure to round out the therapy in this way, the diabetic may pay a price in progressive debility and disease, premature aging, and death via complications.

As I write these lines, I am reminded that with the enthusiasm of youth, I suggested that — without credit to the participating physicians and me — a world-famous clinic devoted to diabetics take over our research, pursue it exhaustively, and publish their findings. The reply I received to my overture was: "We are sorry that we have no facilities for such research." I have the impression that their facilities are monopolized by dispensers of insulin injections and by dietitians, busy counting carbohydrates and calories in diabetic diets.

Yet, given the benefit of more comprehensive nutritional therapies such as I have described, the diabetic will often respond with increased carbohydrate tolerance, permitting a reduction of insulin or oral medication — surely, in the light of the evidence, a consummation devoutly to be pursued. The impotence of the middle-aged diabetic, by way of demonstrating that this, too, is *not* a complication of diabetes, often responds to nutritional therapy, indicating that the liver when it is properly nourished resumes its normal role of holding down excessive activity of the female hormone.

The proposal is neither a panacea nor is it new. Liver was prescribed medicinally for diabetics more than fifty years ago — specifically, to help lower blood sugar. In fact, physicians attempted then to establish the amount of liver equivalent to a given dosage of insulin. Brewer's yeast was used as a helpful supplement for the diabetic diet more than a century ago. The following letter was written to me by an internist, more than a quarter of a century ago:

This patient is sixty years old. She gives a history of suffering from diabetes mellitus for the past fifteen years and has been taking thirty units of globin insulin for control of the diabetes. Her last record of a blood sugar that she can remember is 183 mg. percent. Examination reveals an adult white female who does not appear acutely or chronically ill. The examination was essentially within normal limits, except for the blood sugar which, when taken two months after her remembered record, was 142 mg. percent. She has been taking thirty units of insulin since this examination. I placed her on the following regimen:

1. A high choline-inositol Vitamin-B-Complex syrup.
2. Mixed tocopherols.
3. Multiple vitamin-mineral supplements supplying zinc.
4. Vitamin C, 250 mgs. daily.
5. A diabetic diet of 2,000 calories together with B-Complex injections once weekly.

She continued to show sugar in the urine but to a lesser concentration for the next three weeks. In the fourth week, the urine was entirely negative for four daily samples. The insulin was dropped to ten units daily. However, the following week showed $3/4$ of 1 percent sugar in the urine, and the insulin was raised to fifteen units daily. After one week on fifteen units, she was placed on ten units and the urine remained free from sugar.* For the next three weeks, the insulin was reduced to five units per day, and the patient at the present writing is not receiving any insulin and the urine remains negative. A blood sugar taken three months after the first examination was 148 mg. percent and no urinary sugar.

In summation, this is a sixty-year-old female with a history of known diabetes for fifteen years who is placed on vitamin supplements

*In the early stages of such vitamin treatment of the diabetic, spilling of sugar in the urine may be induced by the treatment itself. It does not ordinarily reflect elevation of the blood sugar.

as recommended by Carlton Fredericks, and who is able to maintain herself on a 2,000-calorie diet without the use of insulin after having required as much as thirty units of globin insulin daily. This is an example of control* of a metabolic disease with the use of vitamin supplements.

Name withheld, M.D.

After I read that letter in a network broadcast, a physician wrote: "Now for the first time I understand why an accustomed dose of insulin sends patients into shock after I've put them on brewer's yeast for a while."

The reduction of insulin requirements is obviously a goal to be cherished, but the use of Vitamin-B-Complex supplements for diabetics is not aimed alone at this or the increase in carbohydrate tolerance that it implies. Several of the B vitamins have important effects on the metabolism of both protein and fat. Several are indispensable to the nervous system, disease of which is again one of the "complications" of diabetes, for long before painful neuritis tortures the diabetic, he will betray the early impact on nervous system function by becoming insensitive to vibration in parts of the body. Yet it is only when the neuritis finally appears that the Vitamin B_{12} and B Complex may be administered. Why must we wait for pathology to flower when what nutrition helps or cures, it mitigates or prevents?

There are millions of diabetics who have the disease and do not yet know it. There are millions of hypoglycemics, some of whom will become diabetics. Millions of diabetics who are aware of their disease are matched by more millions who are prediabetic — a tendency that grows with the years, appearing in perhaps one in every four reaching the mid- or late fifties. The cause of the disease is partially genetic. But some cases are associated with obesity in a way that suggests that the sugar-metabolizing machinery of the body can be abused into misfunction. Other cases may be the price for the dietary experiment in which we have been engaged for some 25,000 years. We have been eating large amounts of starches and sugars, in a concentrated form unknown in Nature, for only 250 centuries — not a very long period for a long-lived species. At the time of the caveman, there was no sugar bowl nor any bread, cake, cookies, cereal, candy, spaghetti, macaroni, pretzels, nor "gelatin" desserts that are 85 percent sugar. The prehistoric man needed sugar to feed his nervous system and brain as we do, and survival of the fittest selected an organism that could

---

*"Control" is not the term the author would choose.

maintain its blood sugar at a functioning level in an environment that offered no predictable meals and no concentrated sugar or starch. Such an organism today would be called at least prediabetic! Move it — with the caveman's genes — into the twentieth century and dump into it a teaspoonful and a third of sugar every thirty minutes, garnished with two hundred pounds yearly of bread, cereals, and other starches, all this going into a body gaited for highly efficient utilization of *very little* starch and sugar, and what might be the predictable results? A deleterious effect on liver function for want of the B-Complex vitamins removed from these processed carbohydrates. (Not by chance, function of the liver is disturbed in at least 50 percent of diabetic patients, and in perhaps an equal percentage of hypoglycemics.) The flood of starch and sugar may easily contribute to obesity — not only because of the burden of excess caloric intake, but because carbohydrates for "cavemen" induce retention of salt and thereby retention of water. Obesity is meaningfully associated with diabetes and with hardening of the arteries, high blood pressure, and cancer. It has been said, apropos of these associations, that the physician who carefully examines diabetics will find undiagnosed heart disease; and, examining victims of coronary thrombosis, will similarly find unrecognized diabetes, so meaningful are these relationships. The tide of sugar and starch may drive the pancreas into overactivity, yielding low blood sugar, and this in turn may lead to diabetes, with some people managing to suffer from both conditions simultaneously. The burden upon the adrenals, arising from pancreatic hyperfunction, could conceivably be a pathway to the allergies that — increasingly — plague us.

Along with our ruinous and experimental modern diet, we have introduced another innovation: the three-meal pattern of eating. Man was originally a nibbling animal. Three meals a day are a concession to the exigencies of business and school. How much nibbling is more physiologically sound may be judged by one statement: Many diabetics whose blood sugar is abnormally high on three meals a day, show a drop — sometimes to normal — when they are fed the same amount of food in six meals daily.

We have also garnished the problem with persistent use of caffeine, of which we Americans have the highest intake in the world. This stimulant prods the adrenals into raiding the liver for stored sugar (glycogen). When that sugar reaches the blood, it is as much a challenge for pancreas and liver as sweets from any external source.

The genetically transmitted type of diabetes may be inevitable when our choice in mates is dictated by biological urge with a thin veneer of sentimentality. The mature-onset type, however, is another matter. We certainly can reduce its incidence and its severity, and may even prevent some of it. But that will call for changes in meal frequency, food processing, the percentage of carbohydrates in our menus, and for the injection of sanity in the criteria of food selection. It will also demand restoration of our vitamin intake to the levels enjoyed by primitive man, who ate the whole — and not the fractionated — food.

5.

FIGURES DO LIE

Weight loss is as much a matter of individual difference as weight gain. There are those who will lose perhaps two pounds a week by dropping their calories to 1,200 daily. There are those who violate all the laws of the arithmetic of calories: They *don't* lose on 1,200 calories a day. And there are those whose weight is normal, but it's in the wrong places, and the lumps, bumps, and bicycle tires at the midriff refuse to depart even with significant weight loss.

Just as there is no pat formula and no single diet for universal well-being, there is no one reducing diet that is a panacea — nor any drugs that are a magic pathway to ideal weight. So it is that this chapter presents four different ways to reshape your architecture to your heart's desire. The first is for those who can resist everything except temptation. It is the diet for those who lose slowly or not at all on the ordinary reducing diet. It is ideal for the chronic nibbler and raider of the refrigerator in the small of the night. The second is for those who are happy losing weight on three fairly generous, well-balanced meals daily. The third procedure must be medically supervised: It is for the grossly obese who have never been successful in reducing, and for those whose problem also includes maldistribution of fat on the body. The fourth is for a small group who are normal in weight, but have some of it in the wrong places. Astonishingly, we do sometimes succeed in meeting that difficult requirement.

A sizable group are those who insist that they don't cheat yet don't lose on a 1,200 calorie diet. Within the group is another who drive nutritionists frantic, because they manage to *gain* on a diet which should burn fat at the rate of several pounds weekly. That ordinarily leads to investigation of their thyroids — what else? The gland, actually, is rarely implicated. In fact, the situation drove me to doggerel:

> I don't understand women —
> They puzzle most of the males.
> They purchase a diet,
> Refuse to live by it,
> And holler "My glands!" when it fails!

But that isn't the explanation. They usually aren't cheating, don't have a glandular problem, and *can* be helped. Their problem is biochemical: They are the modern version of the caveman and the cavewoman who aren't gaited metabolically for turning starches and sugars into energy, as most of us do. Instead, with great efficiency they convert these carbohydrates into fat and store it in unbecoming places. A reducing diet that contains 50 percent carbohydrate, as most conventional diets do, obviously does nothing for such people.

In addition, as an exhibition of another biochemical difference, the cave people have a tendency to store salt when they eat sugars and starches. This in turn induces retention of fluid, which is unfortunate because the objective in all reducing is to convert body fat into water — and get rid of it. If you insist on retaining the water because you are retaining salt because you are eating starches and sugars, the long and short of it is that you will remain fat. And however unaware you are of the biochemistry, you will unerringly point to your peculiarity by remarking, "She can eat pie, and nothing happens. I *smell* it and put on a pound or two!"

Some ten years ago I began to experiment with high-fat, high-protein reducing diets, very low in starches and sugars. Navy nutritionists had proved that eating fat makes you burn fat, whereas fasting, interestingly, makes you burn *tissues*. The water that is formed by oxidizing body fat, I realized, will not be retained when salt is not. Getting rid of much of the carbohydrate in the reducing diet was the key to avoiding salt retention — this device has been used in the treatment of diseases where, ordinarily, the patient is placed on a low-salt diet. Gradually, I realized that Dr. Herman Taller was perfectly right when he said that calories don't count. They don't — for many reducers — when the calories come from protein and fat. Experience taught me that the diet low in starches and sugars is more effective when about 20 percent of the fat is in the polyunsaturated (vegetable) form. And all this information explains, in part, the effectiveness of the diet that follows.

Another consideration is the timing of the meals. The menu plan in this chapter is for six meals daily. It is an aid to willpower, for you're never far from a feeding. It also helps weight loss directly, for the body is less efficient in utilizing small meals, which means losing faster on six meals a day than you would by taking the identical amount of food in three larger meals. The lowered efficiency of utilization of food couples with the amount of polyunsaturated fat in the diet to yield another dividend: better regulation of blood cholesterol. Finally, a most interesting by-product of a diet of this type is a loss in inches that is often out of proportion to the loss in weight.

At first glance, the menus will seem too generous to permit weight loss, but for most people (and *all* cave people) they do. There are, however, some guidelines to be followed.

The menus specify five ounces (uncooked weight — cooked weight, four ounces) of most of the protein foods, such as meat, fish, or fowl. Some reducers can increase these to their regular portions and still lose weight, but it is best to start with the specified amounts and experiment later. You'll not be hungry with these portions, anyhow.

The whole family can use the one menu; limitations on portions and on carbohydrate intake apply to the reducer only. Nonreducers will have their usual desserts, protein portions, and high-carbohydrate foods that are banned for the weight loser.

The French, Italian, and other fancy recipes in these menus are not mandatory Any protein main dish can be substituted for any other, meaning that meat, fish, fowl, cheese, and egg *main* dishes are interchangeable, and steak can, of course, be substituted for Shrimp Delectable, or hamburger for a doughless pizza. Do not tamper with the vegetable oil, margarine, and salad dressings. They supply the polyunsaturated fat without which this diet is much less effective. Any protein can be substituted for any other in the snack meals, but if you reduce the cheese or the skim-milk intake significantly, it would be wise to use a calcium supplement supplying one-half gram of calcium daily.

There have been versions of this diet in which the public has been told that twelve eggs at breakfast are not too much; that a pound of steak is a permissible portion at a main meal; that unlimited intake of hard liquor is allowable. Nonsense is not the stuff of which safe reduction is made.

The skim milk frequently specified in these menus is most economical in the form of nonfat milk powder. Choose brands specifically labeled as "low-heat processed." If you can find any that aren't "instant dissolving," use them. The quick dissolving requires double processing and double heating by the manufacturer, and protein doesn't profit by all this. If price doesn't matter, buy the liquid skim milk. Don't worry about the vitamins removed in the cream, for vitamin supplements are mandatory with any of the author's reducing diets. Better safe than sorry, no matter how well diets are balanced.

The brown-rice crackers mentioned in the menus are available in both grocery and health-food stores. They are recommended because ten of them supply the carbohydrate found in just one slice of bread and are more satisfying to a stubborn sweet-and-starch tooth. They are more palatable when crisped in the oven. When you use other crackers, choose whole-grain (whole-wheat or whole-rye) and eat portions that are equivalent. A slice of bread weighs about one ounce.

Stay away from the scales. A diet like this sometimes is marked by plateaus — periods when weight loss temporarily slows. Frequent weighing can be discouraging, which is unnecessary, for the trend over the weeks will be downward. Weigh yourself when you start and every ten days thereafter, always in the morning. Losses on the diet vary, depending on how active the reducer is, but I have seen losses of nine to ten pounds in ten to fourteen days and watched one man reduce more than 100 pounds with this diet — without bagging, sagging, or pouching.

Built into this diet is protection against becoming a "yo-yo" reducer. We've all seen the people who lose — and regain — forty pounds a year. That is the hazard in blitz diets. Because of their very nature, you cannot continue to use them when you've reached your desirable weight; inevitably you return to the old dietetic pattern that gave you haunch, paunch, midriff bulge, and jowl. I contributed chapters to a book written by a man who had spent his life on such "wonder" diets, titled *I Lost a Thousand Pounds!* You'll not, on the caveman's diet, be .he subject for such a text for once you've reached your ideal weight, ʲou cautiously increase your starches and sugars and remain on the diet as a lifetime support for normal figure and well-being.

Don't go overboard and restrict portions below the levels specified and above all, don't try to lose faster by cutting more starches and sugars than the diet does. I know you've read about diets with no carbohydrates. Some people can tolerate this, but let me assure you that unless you are certain your health is normal, such diets may not be safe and, of course, cannot be maintained indefinitely, which means they fall into the classification of — and have the disadvantages of — the blitz diets. The author of one such distorted menu also endorses the "ice cream" and "banana-milk" regimes, which is as good a measure as any of his willingness to cater to fads. There are people who can do with fewer — or more — carbohydrates than the caveman diet offers; but it is a good and sane compromise.

Apropos of sanity: The menus that follow are adequate in protein, vitamins, and minerals — particularly in protein, even if the requirement is high. Vitamin-mineral intake should be insured with supplements. A multiple-vitamin, multiple-mineral, and a B-Complex supplement from a natural source, such as vacuum-dried or solvent-extracted liver, are excellent protection against the risks of deficiency. A different pattern of supplementing is described later in this chapter for use when the problem is one of fat redistribution. Both procedures protect even those with an unusually high need for these factors.

Most people find these tested menus more than adequate to bolster their willpower. If in the first two weeks you find that old yen for sweets haunting you, or the siren voice of the refrigerator calling in the small hours of the night, reach for an extra bit of cheese or a small piece of meat as an addition to the programmed meals and snacks. As the high intake of protein is continued, the desire for sweets will decline proportionately. For those who need an additional backstop, try taking three ounces of unsweetened wine just before dinner. For no discernible good reason, this weakens the late-night appetite.

Some people with hypoglycemia are overweight. Most are not — they burn sugar too fast to convert it into fat. The overweight person with low blood sugar can use these menus almost intact, but must delete all sources of caffeine or alcohol.

As questions have been raised concerning the safety of the cyclamates and saccharin, these subjects are discussed elsewhere in this book. Suffice it to say, the use of artificial sweeteners in small quantities is not, in the author's opinion, necessarily hazardous, but their use is certainly not mandatory.

Substitutions other than those listed for items in the menus are taboo. Your scale ultimately should tell you that these prohibitions are valid. And now, to the menus:

TEN DAYS OF THE CAVEMAN REDUCING MENUS
An asterisk (*) indicates that the recipe is supplied

FIRST DAY

BREAKFAST
V-8 or Vegemato juice, 4 oz.
Hamburger, broiled, 4 oz., cooked weight
½ slice whole-wheat bread, 1 tsp. soft margarine
Coffee or substitute, or tea, with optional half-and-half, light cream,
  milk, or lemon — no sugar

SNACK
8 oz. skim milk
¼ cup cottage cheese with chopped chives, onion, dill, caraway, poppy
  seeds, or garden vegetables

LUNCH
Tomato juice, minimum 4 oz., dash of lemon, lime, Tabasco, celery
  salt, and onion salt, or Worcestershire sauce
Sautéed beef liver strips with browned onions, 4 oz., cooked weight*
Brown-rice crackers (5) with 1 tsp. soft margarine
Beverage of choice as at breakfast

SNACK
4 oz. skim milk, with ham horn*

DINNER
Crabmeat cocktail
Meat loaf, 4 oz., cooked weight*
Leaf spinach in butter sauce, tarragon
Romaine lettuce, plum tomatoes, scallions, French dressing (made
  with vegetable oil)
Coupe au Black Cherry*
Beverage as at breakfast

SNACK
4 oz. skim milk
½ cucumber, hollowed out and stuffed with cream cheese and chives

RECIPES FIRST DAY

SAUTÉED LIVER STRIPS: With very sharp knife, cut beef liver (best buy!)
into noodle-thick strips. Melt soft margarine (*not* butter!) at low
temperature, add seasoning and chopped onions. When onions begin

browning, add liver strips. (Watch carefully — they cook quickly!) Before serving, sprinkle with a little wheat germ and garnish with parsley.

HAM HORN: Press pot cheese through strainer, adding unflavored yogurt or buttermilk in sufficient quantities to work it to a soft paste. Add chopped dill pickle. Roll ¾ oz. cheese in very thin slice ham and secure with toothpick.

MEAT LOAF: Your recipe — but remember not to stretch it with bread crumbs. If you must stretch it, use wheat germ.

COUPE AU BLACK CHERRY: Sprinkle 1 envelope whole (unflavored) gelatin into ½ cup cold water in top of double boiler. Stir over hot water until gelatin dissolves, remove from heat, and blend in 1½ cups sugar-free black cherry soda. Divide 1 cup black cherries, fresh or canned (sugar-free), among 4 sherbet glasses, and pour gelatin mixture over fruit. Chill until firm. Serve with whipped cream (optional).

SECOND DAY

BREAKFAST
½ sliced orange
1 poached egg with 3 slices crisp bacon
½ slice whole-wheat bread with 1 tsp. soft margarine
Beverages as in first-day breakfast

SNACK
4 oz. skim milk*
Leftover meat loaf or boned chicken on slice of Swiss cheese (thin), 1 oz. total

LUNCH
Sugar-free cranberry juice, 4 oz.
Shrimp Delectable, 4 oz., cooked weight*
Pineapple chunks, canned, self-juice, no sugar, ⅓ cup
5 brown-rice or thin, small whole-wheat crackers, 1 tsp. soft margarine
Green salad, oil and vinegar dressing
Coffee, tea, or bouillon

SNACK
½ small apple or pear with one wedge Gruyère cheese

DINNER
Artichoke hearts, lemon or vinegar
Ham and mushrooms, 4 oz., cooked weight*
Waldorf salad
Sugar-free prepared gelatin dessert
Coffee or tea

SNACK
Any ham left? 1 oz. on 2 brown-rice, ½ whole-wheat, or ½ whole-rye
crackers (small) with a little soft margarine

RECIPES SECOND DAY

SKIM MILK: Vary this by adding vanilla or almond extract to taste.

SHRIMP DELECTABLE: Sauté 1½ lbs. fresh or frozen cleaned shrimp in
vegetable oil until shrimp begin to whiten. Add salt, garlic, and
chopped parsley to taste. Stir all together over high heat for 2 minutes
and add lemon juice before serving. Serves 4.

HAM AND MUSHROOMS: Make small cubes of 1 pound of precooked
smoked ham. Render in skillet, discarding rendered fat. Add 1 lb.
sliced mushrooms, stirring continuously over low fire. When mushrooms begin to color, add 2 tbs. sherry and ⅛ tsp. nutmeg. Serves 4.

THIRD DAY

BREAKFAST
Apple juice, 4 oz.
Fillet of sole, broiled, 4 oz., with margarine and paprika
½ slice whole-wheat bread with 1 tsp. soft margarine
Usual beverage

SNACK
Celery stalk stuffed with 1 oz. Brie cheese
4 oz. skim milk

LUNCH
Tomato juice
Eggs in nests — 2 for you*
½ slice whole-wheat bread with 1 tsp. soft margarine
Usual beverage

SNACK
Cucumber slices, topped with 1 oz. Neufchâtel cheese
Vegetable juice cocktail

DINNER
Melon (⅛ slice)
Pot roast, 4 oz.
Grilled tomatoes, sesame
Verithin carrots*
Strawberry "soda"*
Usual beverage

SNACK
1 oz. pot roast on 4 brown-rice crackers or 1 whole-rye cracker,
1 tsp. soft margarine
4 oz. skim milk or low-fat buttermilk

RECIPES THIRD DAY

EGGS IN NESTS: 4 eggs, 2 tbs. nonfat dry milk, ¼ tsp. tarragon, seasoning to taste. Separate whites and whole yolks. Beat whites to stiffness, add powdered milk, seasoning, and beat again until peaks form. Pile whites into oven cups. Make depressions in middle, place yolks there, top with dash tarragon, and bake until yolks set and whites turn golden brown — about 20 minutes at 375° — 2 eggs for you.

TOMATOES, SESAME: Thick-slice firm tomatoes and arrange on *lightly* oiled baking sheet. Dust with pepper, salt, thyme, or oregano, basil, or mustard. Broil, don't overcook, under medium flame until hot. Add ⅛ tsp. sesame seed per slice.

VERITHIN CARROTS: With very sharp knife, slice carrots razor thin. Melt butter or soft margarine, add carrots, and cook until yellow color runs into fat. Season to taste.

STRAWBERRY "SODA": Use blender. Blend 8 large (unsugared) fresh or frozen strawberries with enough skim milk to fill an 8-oz. glass.

FOURTH DAY

BREAKFAST
½ small grapefruit
2 sausages with 1 oz. Canadian bacon, well-cooked

½ slice whole-wheat bread with 1 tsp. soft margarine
Usual beverage

SNACK

Plain yogurt, 4 oz., with vanilla or almond extract or cinnamon added
to taste
2 brown-rice or whole-wheat crackers (small) with 1 tsp. soft margarine

LUNCH

Carrot sticks*
Doughless pizza, 4 oz., cooked weight*
Green salad, oil dressing
Apricots (3), canned, sugar-free, or artificially sweetened
Whole-rye cracker (1) with soft margarine
Usual beverage

SNACK

1 oz. Velveeta cheese on 4 brown-rice crackers with soft margarine
4 oz. low-fat buttermilk or skim milk

DINNER

Dietetic fruit cup (2 oz.)
Chicken, broiled in orange juice, 4 oz., cooked weight*
Shoestring eggplant (2 tablespoonsful)*
Pineapple-lime salad*
Baked custard*
Usual beverage

SNACK

Fill depression in ½ small pear with soft Camembert cheese
4 oz. skim milk

RECIPES FOURTH DAY

CARROT STICKS: 1 large carrot, ½ cup lemon juice, salt to taste, 1 tsp.
chopped parsley. Scrub carrot, halve, slice into sticks, dip in juice, salt
lightly, roll in parsley.

DOUGHLESS PIZZA: ½ lb. lean beef, ground; ¼ small can tomato paste;
2 fresh tomatoes; 1 medium onion; 1 pinch pepper; ⅛ tsp. each of
sweet basil, oregano, and paprika. Pepper and lightly knead meat,
then line oven dish with it. Chop tomatoes with onions, mix with
tomato paste and spices, and fill meat shell with mixture. Add touch
of oregano on top, plus dash (optional) olive oil. Bake to preferred
doneness at 350°. Serves 2.

CHICKEN, BROILED IN ORANGE JUICE: 1 3-lb. broiling chicken, cut into equal halves; 2 cups orange juice; 1 clove garlic, halved; ½ tsp. tarragon; ½ cup chopped scallions; salt and pepper to taste. Rub each half of chicken with cut half of garlic clove, tarragon, salt, and pepper. Place chicken, skin side up, in shallow oven dish. Pour 1 cup orange juice over chicken and sprinkle on scallions. Broil brown on each side, adding more juice if needed.

EGGPLANT, SHOESTRING: 1 small eggplant, 1 beaten egg, 1 tbs. water, 1 cup bread crumbs and wheat germ (half and half). Salt to taste. Pare eggplant, cut into slices ½ inch thick. Soak in cold salted water for 30 minutes and dry, then dip into egg that has been diluted with 1 tbs. water. Roll in wheat-germ-bread-crumb mixture and fry in about ½ inch hot cottonseed oil, until golden brown. Drain on paper, sprinkle with salt.

PINEAPPLE-LIME SALAD: 1 cup canned, sugar-free, cubed pineapple; 1 tsp. each diced celery and chopped pimiento; salt to taste; 1 tbs. vinegar; 1 envelope lime gelatin, sugar-free; and ½ cup hot water. Measure other ingredients. In vinegar and salt, marinate celery, pimientos, and fruit. Dissolve gelatin in hot water. When it begins to set, add marinated fruit and vegetables, put into individual molds, and let stand until set. Serve on crisp green lettuce leaf. Serves 3 to 4.

BAKED CUSTARD: ½ cup whole milk, 1 egg, ⅛ tsp. almond or vanilla extract, nutmeg to taste. Scald milk. Beat egg slightly, add milk, and mix well. Stir in extract. Pour into custard cup that has been rinsed out with cold water and bake in moderately slow oven (325°) for about 45 minutes, or until pointed silver knife inserted into custard comes out clean. Improved texture and flavor result if custard cups are set in water while baking. Recipe for 1 portion.

FIFTH DAY

BREAKFAST
Cantaloupe (⅛ slice)
Egg, fried in soft margarine, with 1 thin slice fried ham
½ slice whole-wheat bread, with 1 tsp. soft margarine
Usual beverage

SNACK
Macaroons (4)*
8 oz. skim milk

LUNCH
Vegetable juice
Chicken livers and mushrooms, sauté, 4 oz., cooked weight*
Whole-wheat crackers (thin, small, 2) with 1 tsp. soft margarine
Usual beverage

SNACK
Stuffed celery stick with 1 oz. pot cheese*

DINNER
Bouillon
Sukiyaki, 6 oz., cooked weight*
Brown-rice crackers (2) with soft margarine
Snow pudding*
Chinese tea

SNACK
1 oz. smoked oyster on ½ whole-rye cracker with soft margarine
1 glass any diet soda

RECIPES FIFTH DAY

MACAROONS: 1 egg white, 6 small walnuts, liquid artificial sweetener to taste. Add liquid sweetener to egg white and beat stiff. Chop nuts quite fine and fold them into egg white. Drop mixture by spoonful onto wax paper on cookie sheet, dividing it into four equal parts. Brown in moderate oven.

CHICKEN LIVER AND MUSHROOMS, SAUTÉ: 1¼ lbs. chicken livers; ¼ lb. mushrooms, sliced; 2 tbs. soft margarine; 1 medium onion, grated; 1 tbs. flour; ½ cup chicken bouillon (cube may be used, dissolved in water); ½ cup dry white wine; 1 bay leaf; pinch thyme; salt; pepper; nutmeg to taste; 1 tbs. chopped parsley. Sauté livers and mushrooms in margarine over low flame. Add onion, cook with stirring for 3 or 4 minutes. Sprinkle with flour, and stirring constantly, add bouillon and wine. Add bay leaf, thyme, salt, and pepper. Cover, simmer for 10 minutes, occasionally stirring. Pour into serving dish, sprinkle with a little nutmeg, and decorate with parsley.

STUFFED CELERY STICK: Note that this nibble can be made varied and palatable by combining with the pot cheese: Worcestershire sauce, Tabasco, mint, oregano, mustard, garlic salt, chili, curry, dill pickle, watercress, capers, green pepper, or pimiento.

SUKIYAKI: The bamboo shoots and water chestnuts specified in this recipe are not essential, but do add palatability and good nutrition, and can be bought canned or frozen. Chinese cabbage, using the long, green outer leaves, is specified, but tender spinach can be substituted. Remember that the vegetables aren't cooked in the conventional sense, but should taste like a hot salad.

Cook for 5 minutes, in a large, heavy skillet, at boiling temperature: ½ cup chicken bouillon; ¼ cup soy sauce; 1 clove (halved) garlic; 2 small onions cut in thin wedges; ½ cup sliced mushrooms; 2 leeks cut in 1-inch lengths; 2 stalks celery, in 1-inch lengths; ½ cup each of water chestnuts and bamboo shoots.

When onions are half done, add Chinese cabbage or tender spinach. When greens look transparent, make room in skillet for 1 lb. tender beef, such as steak, sliced *very* thin, in pieces about 1 by 2 inches. When beef is lightly browned and hot, mix with vegetables and serve promptly.

SNOW PUDDING: 1 package lemon-flavored, sugar-free gelatin dessert, and 2 egg whites. Prepare gelatin as usual. Chill until slightly thickened, then add two egg whites. Set bowl in pan cooled with cold water and ice cubes. Whip with rotary eggbeater until consistency of whipped cream.

SIXTH DAY

BREAKFAST
Cranberry juice, sugar-free, 4 oz.
Ham slice with orange*
½ slice whole-wheat toast with 1 tsp. soft margarine
Usual beverage

SNACK
Thin-sliced smoked salmon with whipped cream cheese, total 1 oz., on 2 brown-rice crackers
4 oz. skim milk

LUNCH
Cottage cheese omelet*
½ Rye Krisp with 1 tsp. soft margarine
Green salad, plum tomatoes, Russian dressing
Usual beverage

SNACK
Bleu cheese (1 oz.) on two small, thin whole-wheat crackers
4 oz. skim milk

DINNER
Clam-tomato soup*
Kidneys with wine, 4 oz., cooked weight*
Zucchini, Neapolitan*
Raw mushroom salad*
Frozen coffee whip*
Usual beverage

SNACK
½ small apple
1 oz. Velveeta cheese
4 oz. skim milk

RECIPES SIXTH DAY

HAM SLICE WITH ORANGE: The evening before, trim fat from 1 lb.
cooked ham, 1 inch thick. Cover with slices unpeeled orange, spiced
with a few cloves and a dusting of cinnamon. For breakfast, place in
oven dish, cover with ½ cup water, and bake at 350°. When orange
rind is tender, ham should be done. Remove ham, remove fat from
remaining liquid, add pinch allspice and liquid artificial sweetener
equivalent to 1 tsp. sugar, and pour over meat. Gravy can be stretched
with a little orange juice. ¼ slice for you.

COTTAGE CHEESE OMELET: 1 egg, 3 tbs. cottage cheese, 1 tsp. soft margarine, and 2 tsp. water, per person. Separate yolk and white. Add
water to yolk and beat until thick and lemon-colored. Add cottage
cheese, with salt and pepper to taste. Beat white of egg stiff and fold
mixture of cottage cheese and egg yolk carefully into white. Melt
margarine in small frying pan and pour in mixture. Brown lightly till
omelet is set, then place under broiler flame to brown top. Fold and
serve promptly.

CLAM-TOMATO SOUP: 1 cup canned clam juice, 1 #2-can tomato juice
(2½ cups), 1 tsp. Worcestershire sauce, 2 tbs. margarine, and parsley
sprigs (optional). In saucepan, combine juices, Worcestershire, and
margarine. Heat to boiling. To serve, sprinkle with parsley sprigs.
Makes 4 servings.

KIDNEYS WITH WINE: 6 lamb kidneys, 1 tbs. soft margarine, 1 tbs. unbleached flour, ½ tsp. salt, ¾ cup hot water, and 2 tbs. dry sherry. Skin kidneys, remove membranes, and cut in pieces 1 inch by ½ inch. Sauté five minutes in sizzling margarine over hot flame, turning at least twice. Stir in salt and flour. Brown 1 minute. Slowly stir in hot water, simmer 2 minutes more. Add sherry, serve immediately on toast, which you omit. Recipe is ordinarily for 2, but you take 4 oz.

ZUCCHINI, NEAPOLITAN: Wash green squash, do not peel, cut into rounds about ⅓ inch thick. Place in heavy pan with pinch oregano, 1 split clove garlic, dash pepper and salt. At lowest flame, cook under tight cover for 15 minutes until squash is tender but does not disintegrate. Remove garlic and serve. Serves 4.

RAW MUSHROOM SALAD: 1 lb. mushrooms; ¼ cup white wine vinegar; ½ cup olive oil; dash cayenne pepper; salt and pepper to taste; lettuce leaves; 1 tbs. minced pimiento; 1 tbs. pickles or capers, washed and drained; 2 hard-boiled eggs. Peel mushroom caps, slice thin, and in covered vessel marinate them in vinegar, oil, and seasonings for 1 hour in refrigerator. Chill lettuce leaves at the same time. Arrange lettuce in bowl and mound mushrooms in center. Pour over marinade, decorate with pimiento and capers, and ring mushrooms with eggs quartered lengthwise. Serve cold. Serves 4.

FROZEN COFFEE WHIP: 1 cup ice water, 2 tsp. liquid artificial sweetener, 2 tsp. instant coffee powder, ½ cup nonfat dry milk powder, 1 (unbeaten) egg white. In blender, slowly beat ice water and nonfat milk powder. Add liquid sweetener and powdered instant coffee, and blend at high speed for about 5 minutes until light and fluffy. Add egg white, continue beating one minute more. Place in six half-cup molds, freeze until firm — at least four hours. Loosen cream with knife edge and tap lightly to unmold. Serves 6. Half of one of these molds can be added to 1 snack a day, if you're craving something sweet.

SEVENTH DAY

BREAKFAST
¼ cup pineapple chunks (self-juice, sugar-free)
Eggs (2), poached in tomato juice*
½ slice whole-wheat toast with 1 tsp. soft margarine
Usual beverage

SNACK
Anchovies (1 oz.) on thin, small whole-wheat crackers (2) with 1 tsp.
  soft margarine
4 oz. skim milk

LUNCH
Cheese-hearted hamburgers, 4 oz., cooked weight*
Spinach, Chinese*
Brown-rice crackers (2) with soft margarine and (optional) dietetic
  jam or jelly
Usual beverage

SNACK
½ all-beef frankfurter with mustard (optional) (These can be obtained
  without the usual sodium nitrate, nitrite, and cheap sugars in most
  health-food stores.)
1 glass dietetic soda

DINNER
Lamb Dolmas, 1 for you*
Heart pot roast, 4 oz., cooked weight*
Asparagus vinaigrette*
Lettuce salad (1 head), oil and vinegar dressing
Pears with ginger jelly, ½*
Café au lait*

SNACK
Herring fillet in wine sauce, 1 oz., on whole-rye or whole-wheat crackers
  (2, thin, small) with 1 tsp. soft margarine
8 oz. skim milk

RECIPES SEVENTH DAY

EGGS POACHED IN TOMATO JUICE: 4 eggs, 1¾ cups tomato juice, 4
sprigs parsley, salt and pepper to taste. Fill poacher or small pot with
tomato juice and bring to boil. Break eggs singly, then drop in one at a
time. Cook to taste. Season and serve with garnish of parsley. Two eggs
for you.

CHEESE-HEARTED HAMBURGERS: ½ lb. lean ground beef, 1 small diced
onion, ¼ lb. pot cheese, 1 level tbs. chopped tarragon or chives, salt
and pepper to taste. Knead meat gently with diced onion, salt,
and pepper. Form into two large, flat patties. Mash pot cheese with

chives or tarragon and divide between patties, pressing cheese into the center of each. Pull sides up to semi-enclose cheese. Broil. Serves 2.

SPINACH, CHINESE: Heat cottonseed oil with seasoning to taste, just below smoking point. Turn over spinach in hot oil until leaves wilt, then *stop*. Serve.

LAMB DOLMAS: Use grape leaves, lettuce, or tender cabbage leaves. Drop leaves in boiling water and cook until just limp enough to fold without cracking. Drain and stuff each leaf with two tbs. of the following mixture: ½ lb. ground lean lamb; ½ cup minced onions; 1 cup carrots, ground; 1 tbs. parsley, minced; 3 tbs. tomato paste; 1 tbs. lemon juice; dash of oregano; pepper and salt to taste. Place dolmas side by side in lightly oiled pan with end of fold down. Bake 45 minutes in 350° oven and serve with topping of yogurt, stirred for smoothness. Serves 4.

HEART POT ROAST: Remove blood vessels of 3 lbs. beef heart, place in porcelain or enamel pot, and marinate overnight with: 1 cup dry red wine, 1 cup hot water in which you have dissolved 2 bouillon cubes, 1 clove minced garlic, 1 bay leaf, 3 cloves, pinch thyme, 6 cracked peppercorns, ½ tsp. celery salt. Then bring to boil and simmer covered for about 3 hours, or until meat is almost tender. In last 30 minutes, for each person to be served, add 3 whole small onions, 3 carrots in small pieces, 3 small turnips, and 3 mushroom caps. Add Worcestershire (optional). Slice and serve heart surrounded with vegetables.

ASPARAGUS VINAIGRETTE: Make marinade of ½ cup herb vinegar, ½ cup water, ¼ tsp. paprika, pinch of powdered garlic, pepper to taste. Soak canned asparagus overnight in marinade and sprinkle with chopped, hard-boiled egg white before serving.

PEARS WITH GINGER JELLY: 1 envelope unflavored gelatin, ¼ cup cold water, ¼ cup ginger brandy, 1½ cups noncaloric ginger ale, 6 fresh or canned (sugar-free) pears. Let gelatin stand for 5 minutes in cold water. Then stir over hot water until thoroughly dissolved. Remove from heat, add ginger brandy, ginger ale, and blend. Peel and slice ripe pears, one for each person (one-half for you), or drain and slice canned pears. Sprinkle with a little ginger brandy, cover, and chill. Arrange pears at serving time in glass or china bowl, break jelly into bits, and top pears.

café au lait: Dilute nonfat milk powder with half amount of water ordinarily used. Heat ⅓ cup of this double strength skim milk to just short of boiling and add coffee to taste.

EIGHTH DAY

BREAKFAST
Grapefruit juice, unsweetened, 4 oz.
1 scrambled egg, 3 strips smoked beef fry, well done
½ slice whole-wheat bread, 1 tsp. soft margarine
Usual beverage

SNACK
½ small pear
1 oz. Gouda cheese

LUNCH
Hot spiced apple juice, 4 oz.*
Stuffed tomato with crabmeat*
Brown-rice crackers (2) with soft margarine
Beverage

SNACK
Neufchâtel cheese in ham horn, 1 oz. total
8 oz. skim milk

DINNER
Cream of spinach soup*
London Broil, 4 oz., cooked weight*
Carrots anise*
Romaine and escarole salad, scallions, tomatoes, any oil dressing
Junket with berries*
Beverage

SNACK
1 oz. London Broil on 4 brown-rice crackers with 1 tsp. soft margarine
4 oz. skim milk

RECIPES EIGHTH DAY

HOT SPICED APPLE JUICE: 2 cups unsweetened apple juice, 1 stick cinnamon bark, dash of ground nutmeg. Boil juice with cinnamon. Strain. Serve hot or chilled, with nutmeg over each drink just before serving.

STUFFED TOMATO WITH CRABMEAT: 1 medium tomato; ½ cup crab-meat — canned or frozen; salt to taste; lemon juice; 1 tsp. mayonnaise; and 1 leaf lettuce. Mix crabmeat, mayonnaise, salt, and lemon juice. Cut top off tomato, scoop out center, fill with crabmeat mixture, and chill thoroughly. Serve garnished with parsley on lettuce leaf.

CREAM OF SPINACH SOUP: Dissolve ½ cup nonfat milk powder in 2 cups lukewarm water, whipping with beater. When dissolved, beat in 1 egg yolk, pinch of onion powder, dash of white or red pepper. Stir in ¼ cup pureed spinach (baby-food type is fine). Simmer with *constant* stirring, but don't boil.

LONDON BROIL: This chuck cut should be pierced with fork, sprinkled with tenderizer, and covered with mixture of a little Kitchen Bouquet, garlic, paprika, marjoram, and any of the commercial French salad dressings, or golden mushroom soup. Broil at medium heat until tender, but not well done.

CARROTS ANISE: Cook whole carrots in smallest possible amount boiling water. Drain. Sprinkle on a few anise seeds for interesting lico-rice taste.

JUNKET: This is basic recipe for 2 servings for those who want to reduce their intake of cream and sugar. Use 1 cup double-strength skim milk. (See café au lait recipe under Seventh Day.) Also, 4 ¼-grain saccharin tablets and ½ tsp. vanilla. Warm slowly, stir constantly, and when just at baby-feeding temperature, remove from heat and add 1 Junket tablet (not powder, which contains sugar) that has been dissolved in ½ tbs. cold water. Stir quickly for a few seconds, pour immediately into dessert dishes, wait ten minutes, then put into refrigerator to chill. Top with strawberries (6 for you).

NINTH DAY

BREAKFAST
Orange juice, unsweetened, 4 oz.
Cube steak, broiled with 1 strip bacon
½ slice whole-wheat toast with 1 tsp. soft margarine and optional dietetic jelly
Beverage

SNACK
Cornucopia of thin-sliced meat or chicken, 1 oz., filled with cole slaw
8 oz. skim milk

LUNCH
Tomato juice, 4 oz.
Swiss cheese eggs*
Brown-rice crackers (4) with 1 tsp. soft margarine
Beverage

SNACK
Yogurt fizz: ½ cup (4 oz.) plain yogurt, fizzed with club soda
Tomato, cucumber, or celery nibble

DINNER
Dietetic fruit cocktail (3 oz.)
Chinese pork with vegetables, 4 oz., cooked weight*
Chicory, escarole, lettuce salad with any oil and vinegar dressing
Apple fritter*
Beverage

SNACK
Deviled ham on Swiss cheese, total 1 oz.
4 oz. skim milk

RECIPES NINTH DAY

SWISS CHEESE EGGS: 2 eggs, ⅛ lb. Swiss cheese, ¼ tsp. pepper, ¼ tsp.
dry mustard, 1 tsp. salt, dash paprika, garlic salt, cayenne pepper.
Grate cheese and separate eggs. Add most of cheese and remaining
ingredients to egg yolks. Beat in whites. Top with remaining grated
cheese in oven dish and bake slowly until brown on top. Serves 2.

CHINESE PORK WITH VEGETABLES: 1 lb. lean pork, cut into pieces 1
inch wide, 2 inches long, ¼ inch thick. Simmer meat in: ½ cup soy
sauce, 2 ¼-grain saccharin tablets, 1 tsp. vinegar, 1 cup canned bouillon, 1 teaspoon monosodium glutamate, and 2 gloves garlic. After 20
minutes remove meat and add to broth: 1 cup canned bouillon; 2 cups
celery in 1-inch pieces; 4 large onions, cut in eighths; 1 cup tender
spinach or Chinese cabbage, cut in ½-inch widths. Boil, covered, for
5 minutes or less — vegetables should be crisp, like a hot salad. Add 1
green pepper, seeds removed, cut in bite-size pieces. Now boil for 1

minute and return cooked pork to the vegetable-sauce mixture before serving.

APPLE FRITTER: ½ cup dry nonfat milk powder, 2 eggs, 2 tbs. skim milk (liquid), ¼ tsp. vanilla extract, 20 grains saccharin crystals, 1 pinch salt, 1 apple, powdered artificial sweetener to taste. Put powdered milk in bowl. Separate eggs, beat whites stiff and yolks until thick, and add to powdered milk, with vanilla, liquid milk, saccharin crystals, and salt. Mix to smoothness with wooden spoon. Pare, core, and slice apple crosswise. Heat griddle until water dropped on it forms immediately into bubbles. Continue heating over medium flame. Dip apple slices into batter and brown on either side on griddle. Sprinkle powdered sugarless sweetener on each fritter before serving (optional).

TENTH DAY

BREAKFAST
Melon (⅛ slice)
Jelly omelet (dietetic jelly) — 1 egg
½ slice whole-wheat toast, 1 tsp. soft margarine
Beverage

SNACK
Shrimp cocktail, 1 oz., with 2 thin, small whole-wheat crackers and soft margarine
Tomato juice, 4 oz.

LUNCH
Broiled halibut, 4 oz., cooked weight, with lemon-butter
Romaine, fenuche, tomato salad with Thousand Island Dressing
2 brown-rice crackers, 1 tsp. soft margarine
Dietetic apricots (3)
Beverage

SNACK
Grilled cheese (1 oz.) on ½ slice whole-wheat, 1 tsp. soft margarine
Tomato (optional)
8 oz. skim milk

DINNER
V-8 juice (4 oz.)
Broiled steak, fried onions (soft margarine), 4 oz.
Roasted sweet peppers*

Mixed green salad, Roquefort or Bleu cheese dressing
Cranberry sherbet*
Beverage

SNACK
Cold steak, 1 oz., on ½ Rye Krisp, with soft margarine
4 oz. skim milk

RECIPES TENTH DAY

ROASTED SWEET PEPPERS: 4 big red or green peppers, split lengthwise. Remove seeds and fleshy white ribs. Place in very lightly oiled baking dish. Add white pepper and 1 split clove of garlic. Cover tightly, put in hot oven, turn down to 275°, and bake for half hour or until peppers are tender but not completely limp.

CRANBERRY SHERBET: 4 cups cranberries fresh or frozen, 1 tsp. cinnamon, 2¾ cups water, 2 tbs. artificial sweetener (or equivalent of 1 cup sugar), 1 envelope whole gelatin, ⅓ cup cold water, ¼ cup lemon juice, 6 tsp. chopped walnuts for garnish. Cook 4 cups cranberries with 1 tsp. cinnamon in 2¾ cups water until all berries pop. Puree in blender or food mill. Add liquid sweetener and 1 envelope gelatin which has been softened in ⅓ cup cold water; heat until gelatin is thoroughly dissolved. Stir in ¼ cup lemon juice. Pour into ice-cube tray and freeze until mushy. Beat well with fork, return to refrigerator ice-cube compartment, and freeze until firm. Garnish with chopped walnuts at serving time.

For those who merely need the discipline of an ordinary reducing diet while eating three well-balanced meals, select from the following menu outlines the diet that will help you reach the desired weight, at a calorie value that will not test your willpower too severely.

The percentages appended to the vegetable and fruits listed in the following diets refer to the carbohydrate content of these foods. A chart of these values follows the diets.

CONSTRUCTIVE REDUCING DIET FOR
EXPECTED WEIGHT OF 120 POUNDS*

800 Calories

BREAKFAST:

Fruit, 10%**...1 serving
Bacon..2 slices, crisp
Egg..1
Cream, 20%....................................2 tablespoons
Beverage — Coffee or Tea

LUNCH:

Meat..1 serving
Vegetables, 3%...............................2 small servings
Margarine...½ square
Fruit, 5%..1 serving
Milk (skim)...¾ glass

DINNER:

Meat..1 serving
Vegetables, 3%..................................1 small serving
Salad: Vegetable, 3%...........................1 small serving
Margarine...½ square
Fruit, 5%..1 serving
Milk (skim)...¾ glass

1,000 Calories

BREAKFAST:

Fruit, 10%...1 serving
Bacon..2 slices, crisp
Egg..1
Margarine...½ square
Cream, 20%....................................2 tablespoons
Beverages — Coffee or Tea

*All reducing diets — any restricted diet should be supplemented with multiple vitamins and minerals, and a Vitamin-B-Complex concentrate.

**See *Carbohydrate Content of Fruits and Vegetables.*

LUNCH:

Meat..1 serving
Vegetables, 3%.............................2 small servings
Margarine..1 square
Fruit, 5%..1 serving
Milk..¾ glass

DINNER:

Meat..1 serving
Vegetables, 3%..............................1 small serving
Salad: Vegetable, 3%........................1 small serving
Margarine..1 square
Fruit, 5%..1 serving
Milk..¾ glass

1,200 Calories

BREAKFAST:

Fruit, 10%...1 serving
Bacon......................................2 slices, crisp
Egg...1
Margarine...½ square
Cream, 20%.................................2 tablespoons
Beverage — Coffee or Tea

LUNCH:

Meat..1 serving
Vegetables, 3%.............................2 small servings
Margarine.......................................1½ squares
Fruit, 5%..1 serving
Milk..¾ glass

DINNER:

Meat..1 serving
Vegetables, 3%..............................1 small serving
Salad:
    Fresh Vegetables, 3%....................1 small serving
    Salad dressing with oil.........................1 tablespoon

Margarine..1½ squares
Fruit, 5%...1 serving
Milk..¾ glass

REDUCING DIET FOR EXPECTED WEIGHT
OF 160 POUNDS

800 Calories

BREAKFAST:

Fruit, 10%..1 serving
Egg..1
Egg whites...2
Bread..½ thin slice
Margarine..¼ square
Beverage — Coffee or Tea

LUNCH:

Meat (low in fat).......................................1 large serving
Vegetables, 6%...1 small serving
Fruit, 5%...1 serving
Milk (skim)..1 glass

DINNER:

Meat (lean)..1 large serving
Vegetables, 6%...1 small serving
Salad: Vegetable, 3%...................................1 small serving
Fruit, 10%..1 serving
Milk (skim)..1 glass

1,000 Calories

BREAKFAST:

Fruit, 10%..1 serving
Bacon..1 slice, crisp
Egg..1
Bread..½ thin slice
Margarine..½ square
Beverage — Coffee or Tea

LUNCH:

Meat...1 large serving
Vegetables, 3%.............................2 small servings
Margarine....................................½ square
Fruit, 10%...................................1 serving
Milk (skim)..................................1 glass

DINNER:

Meat...1 large serving
Vegetables, 6%.............................1 small serving
Salad: Vegetables, 3%.....................1 small serving
Margarine....................................½ square
Fruit, 5%.....................................1 serving
Milk (skim)..................................1 glass

1,200 Calories

BREAKFAST:

Fruit, 10%...................................1 serving
Bacon...1 slice, crisp
Egg..1
Bread...½ thin slice
Margarine....................................1 square
Cream, 20%..................................1 tablespoon
Beverage — Coffee or Tea

LUNCH:

Meat...1 large serving
Vegetables, 3%.............................2 small servings
Margarine....................................1½ squares
Fruit, 10%...................................1 serving
Milk (skim)..................................1 glass

DINNER:

Meat...1 large serving
Vegetables, 6%.............................1 small serving
Salad: Vegetables, 3%.....................1 small serving
Margarine....................................1½ squares

Fruit, 5%...1 serving
Milk (skim)...1 glass

REDUCING DIET FOR EXPECTED WEIGHT
OF 200 POUNDS

1,000 Calories

BREAKFAST:

Fruit, 10%..1 serving
Bacon...1 slice, crisp
Eggs...2
Bread..½ thin slice
Beverage — Coffee or Tea

LUNCH:

Meat (lean).....................................1 large serving
Vegetables, 3%...................................2 servings
Bread..½ thin slice
Fruit, 5%..1 serving
Milk (skim)...1 glass

DINNER:

Meat (low in fat)...............................1 large serving
Vegetables, 6%....................................1 serving
Salad: Vegetables, 3%.............................1 serving
Bread..½ thin slice
Fruit, 10%...1 serving
Milk (skim)...1 glass

1,200 Calories

BREAKFAST:

Fruit, 10%...1 serving
Bacon..2 slices, crisp
Egg..1
Bread..½ thin slice

Margarine...½ square
Cream, 20%......................................1 tablespoon
Beverage — Coffee or Tea

LUNCH:

Meat (lean)...............................1 very large serving
Vegetables, 3%...................................2 servings
Bread...½ thin slice
Fruit, 5%...1 serving
Milk (skim)..1 glass

DINNER:

Meat (lean)...............................1 very large serving
Vegetables, 6%....................................1 serving
Salad: Vegetables, 3%.............................1 serving
Bread...½ thin slice
Fruit, 10%..1 serving
Milk (skim)..1 glass

1,400 Calories

BREAKFAST:

Fruit, 10%.............................. ....1 serving
Bacon..2 slices, crisp
Egg...1
Bread...½ thin slice
Margarine...1 square
Cream, 20%......................................1 tablespoon
Beverage — Coffee or Tea

LUNCH:

Meat (lean)...............................1 very large serving
Vegetables, 3%...................................2 servings
Bread...½ thin slice
Margarine...1 square
Fruit, 5%...1 serving
Milk (skim)..1 glass

DINNER:

Meat (lean)	1 very large serving
Vegetables, 6%	1 serving
Salad: Vegetables, 3%	1 serving
Bread	½ thin slice
Margarine	1 square
Fruit, 10%	1 serving
Milk (skim)	1 glass

CARBOHYDRATE CONTENT OF FRUITS AND VEGETABLES

Vegetables:

3%
Asparagus
Beet Greens
Broccoli
Brussels Sprouts
Cabbage
Chinese Cabbage
Cauliflower
Celery
Cucumber
Eggplant
Endive
Lettuce
Mustard Greens
Green Pepper
Okra
Radish
Sauerkraut
Sorrel
Spinach
String Bean (tiny)
Summer Squash
Tomato

Watercress
Zucchini
6%
Artichokes — French
Beet
Carrot
Celeriac
Dandelion Greens
Kale
Kohl Rabi
Leeks
Onions
Parsley
Pea (tiny)
Pumpkin
Rutabaga
String Bean (mature)
Squash
Turnip
15%
Parsnip
Salsify
Pea

20%   Horseradish Root
Corn   Potato
Garlic   Shelled Bean

Fruits

5%	15%
Muskmelon	Apple
Honeydew	Apricot
Watermelon	Blueberry
Rhubarb	Cherry
Avocado	Currant
10%	Grape
Blackberry	Guava
Cranberry	Huckleberry
Gooseberry	Nectarine
Grapefruit	Papaw
Lemon	Pear
Lime	Plum
Orange	Quince
Papaya	Raspberry
Peach	**20%**
Pineapple	Banana
Strawberry	Fig (fresh)
Tangerine	Grape Juice
	Fresh Prune

The following is a low carbohydrate diet that is severely restricted in starches and sugars. It is a livable diet when used for a short period of time by those who merely wish to lose a few pounds. However, for those who are grossly overweight, and who will necessarily diet for extended periods, this procedure should be medically supervised.

When the problem includes maldistribution of fat, or when there is a tendency to retain fat in the wrong places even after losing weight, or in those instances when weight is normal but maldistributed, the following supplements will help in two possible ways:

(a) by distributing weight loss more evenly, or

(b) by redistributing body fat even in the absence of weight loss.

The supplements include a multiple vitamin and multiple mineral concentrate, together with a Vitamin B Complex high in inositol and choline. In addition to generous amounts of the other B vitamins, the latter supplements should supply at least a gram of choline and a half gram of inositol in the recommended daily dose of the concentrate.

A tablespoonful of lecithin and 100 mgs. of Vitamin E should also be taken daily.

Green salads may be freely consumed.

MENU FRAMEWORK

BREAKFAST

Fruit or juice

1 egg

1 ounce meat

½ slice whole-wheat bread with 1 teaspoonful margarine (part used with egg — not for frying it)

MORNING SNACK

1 cup skim milk. (Add a little vanilla, if desired.)

1 ounce meat

LUNCH

3 ounces meat

Vegetable serving

2 teaspoonsful cottonseed oil. (Take it right from the spoon, or use it on the vegetable.)

AFTERNOON SNACK

2 ounces meat or meat substitute

½ cup skim milk

DINNER

3 ounces meat

Vegetable

2 teaspoonsful oil

1 serving fruit

EVENING SNACK

½ cup skim milk

1 ounce meat

FIRST DAY

BREAKFAST

½ grapefruit
1 poached egg
1 ounce chicken
½ slice toast
1 tsp. margarine

LUNCH

Chicken salad with 3 oz. chicken
   (¾ cup)
2 tsp. mayonnaise
Chopped celery
Green beans with 1 tsp. margarine
Sliced tomatoes

SUPPER

3 oz. steak

Cauliflower — 1 tsp. margarine
Tossed salad with 4 tsp. paprika
   dressing, plus
2 halves canned peaches
   (waterpacked)

MORNING SNACK

1 cup skim milk
¼ cup creamed cottage cheese

AFTERNOON SNACK

½ cup skim milk
1 oz. American cheese

EVENING SNACK

½ cup skim milk
1 oz. chicken or meat

SECOND DAY

BREAKFAST

½ cup orange juice
1 soft-boiled egg
1 oz. pork pattie
½ slice toast
1 tsp. margarine

LUNCH

Tomato juice
3 oz. beef pattie
Lettuce with 2 tsp. oil
Vinegar

SUPPER

3 oz. pork chop
Spinach — 1 tsp. margarine
Sliced tomatoes with

1 tsp. mayonnaise
½ cup unsweetened applesauce

MORNING SNACK

1 cup skim milk
1 oz. chicken

AFTERNOON SNACK

½ cup skim milk
Egg salad with 1 egg
1 tsp. mayonnaise and
   chopped celery

EVENING SNACK

½ cup skim milk
1 oz. chicken
Lettuce — lemon and oil

THIRD DAY

BREAKFAST

1 cup fresh strawberries
1 poached egg
1 oz. pork pattie
½ slice toast
1 tsp. margarine

LUNCH

3 oz. lamb chops
Asparagus
Tossed salad with
4 tsp. paprika dressing

SUPPER

Tomato juice
3 oz. baked chicken
Broccoli — 2 tsp. margarine
Molded D-Zerta with

10 unsweetened Royal
Anne cherries

MORNING SNACK

1 cup skim milk
½ oz. American cheese

AFTERNOON SNACK

½ cup skim milk
Chicken salad with
2 oz. chicken (½ cup)
2 tsp. mayonnaise
Chopped celery

EVENING SNACK

½ cup skim milk
1 oz. tuna (¼ cup)
Lettuce with lemon and
1 tsp. oil

FOURTH DAY

BREAKFAST

½ grapefruit
1 soft-boiled egg
1 oz. chicken
½ slice toast
1 tsp. margarine

LUNCH

3 oz. broiled liver
Stewed tomatoes
Lettuce with
4 tsp. paprika dressing

SUPPER

3 oz. roast turkey
Wax beans — 1 tsp. margarine
Sliced cucumbers with
2 tsp. paprika dressing

⅛ honeydew melon

MORNING SNACK

1 cup skim milk
Celery sticks
1 tbs. peanut butter

AFTERNOON SNACK

½ cup skim milk
Salmon salad with
2 oz. salmon (½ cup)
4 tsp. mayonnaise
Chopped celery

EVENING SNACK

½ cup skim milk
1 oz. turkey

FIFTH DAY

BREAKFAST

½ cup orange juice
1 poached egg
1 oz. turkey
½ slice toast
1 tsp. margarine

LUNCH

3 oz. beef steak
Tossed salad with
4 tsp. paprika dressing

SUPPER

3 oz. roast pork
Cauliflower — 1 tsp. margarine
Coleslaw with
2 tsp. oil and vinegar
½ cup pineapple (unsweetened)

MORNING SNACK

1 cup skim milk
¼ cup creamed cottage cheese

AFTERNOON SNACK

½ cup skim milk
1 hard-cooked egg

EVENING SNACK

½ cup skim milk
Turkey salad with
1 oz. turkey (¼ cup)
2 tsp. mayonnaise
Chopped celery

SIXTH DAY

BREAKFAST

½ cup grapefruit juice
1 soft-boiled egg
1 oz. roast pork

LUNCH

3 oz. beef pattie
½ cup carrots — 2 tsp. margarine
Lettuce with
4 tsp. paprika dressing

SUPPER

3 oz. baked fish
Green beans — 2 tsp. margarine
Sliced tomatoes

1 small fresh apple

MORNING SNACK

1 cup skim milk
1 oz. pork pattie

AFTERNOON SNACK

½ cup skim milk
Chicken salad with
2 oz. chicken (½ cup)
2 tsp. mayonnaise
Chopped celery

EVENING SNACK

½ cup skim milk
1 oz. chicken or meat

SEVENTH DAY

BREAKFAST

¼ cantaloupe
1 poached egg
1 oz. pork pattie
½ slice toast
1 tsp. margarine

LUNCH

Fat-free broth
3 oz. veal steak
Tossed salad with
2 tsp. oil and vinegar

SUPPER

3 oz. pork chops
Broccoli — 2 tsp. margarine

Molded D-Zerta — 2 halves
   unsweetened pear on lettuce
2 tsp. mayonnaise

MORNING SNACK

1 cup skim milk
1 oz. chicken

AFTERNOON SNACK

½ cup skim milk
1 oz. Swiss cheese

EVENING SNACK

½ cup skim milk
1 tbs. peanut butter
Celery sticks

The fat-redistributing supplements sound too good to be true — particularly when we use them to reshape the figure *without weight loss*. However, this claim is not based on theory. Dr. Harry Swartz and I recognized this action many years ago and tested it on large numbers of volunteers in a carefully controlled experiment. We showed that the action is demonstrated on approximately one-third of the subjects — meaning normalization of fat distribution without change in body weight. The others benefited, too, in improved hair, skin, nails, and general well-being.

This chapter has now pointed out all the sane ways in which to lose weight. It has also supplied "won't" power in the form of menus that recognize the frailties of the flesh. The rest is up to you.

6.
FROM HERE
TO MATERNITY

Whenever I have written or given broadcasts concerning pregnancy, I have always discussed the penalties for mother and baby if nutritional preparation for reproduction is inadequate. In response, I have always received letters reminding me that pregnant women should be spared unpleasant thoughts. This begs the question, for the diet properly must begin before pregnancy begins. Ideally, it starts when a girl is born. Since we rarely are given *that* opportunity, we try for a compromise: Let us feed the would-be mother *and* father for a year before conception is attempted.

While our resources in and knowledge of nutrition for efficient reproduction are considerable, they are not great enough to cope with the situation in which a teen-ager prepares for marriage on a diet of pot, pizza, and pop, becomes pregnant a few months later and then asks the obstetrician for a diet that will simultaneously make up for her past mistakes, supply her current elevated needs, and protect the baby. All this assumes that she does in fact visit an obstetrician early in pregnancy. She may wait until she "feels life," on the grounds that she has been told that in the first few months, the baby is so small that its nutritional needs are microscopic and automatically fulfilled by any diet that will allow the mother to remain upright.

It is unfortunate that this is untrue — unfortunate for both mother and child. The more serious mistake is the belief that nutrition becomes critical only after conception has taken place. If you examine this belief, you find that it means the germ plasm is somehow locked away in the body and immune to all malign influences until sperm meets ovum. This notion is, to put it mildly, ridiculous.

Similarly unreal is the belief that only the mother's diet matters and then only after conception. I know of just two controlled experiments — one with dogs, one with human beings — both showing that the father's diet before conception matters as much as the mother's diet before and afterward. (It is fascinating to me that anyone who speculates on the possible importance of the man's nutrition to reproduction is likely to find himself ignored by orthodox nutritionists. True, there is not much evidence to support the theory, but there *is* some.) Weston Price recounts an experiment in which he mated a well-nourished male dog with four well-fed females, producing four litters of normal puppies. The same male was now fed an inadequate diet and remated with the well-fed females, with the result that a large percentage of all four litters were in some way deformed. The deformed males were then given good diets and mated with the same group of females — not their own mothers — the result was four normal litters. Despite the fact that medical men have used frogs to diagnose pregnancy and cats to measure the potency of digitalis, there will be those who will criticize this experiment on the grounds that one cannot leap from dog to man. That is, if they are aware of the experiment at all. Many nutritionists — particularly those of my school of thought — know of this research by Price, but I have yet to meet an obstetrician, internist, or orthodox dietician who is aware of his work.

Equal obscurity has been given to the research by Wilfred Shute, in which he demonstrated that nutritional treatment of fathers prior to conception resulted in a drop in the incidence of deformities in babies born to mothers with a previous record of bringing abnormal children into the world. Statistically speaking, mothers with a history of bearing deformed babies face a greater probability of such disasters in future pregnancies than do mothers whose previous babies were normal. Shute gave Vitamin E to the fathers of such deformed children, prior to the next conception. The result was a drop of approximately 84 percent in the anticipated number of abnormalities in the succeeding pregnancies. A type of research control was offered in two ways: Not only was there the record of a mother's previous reproductive disasters, but also in certain instances, the fathers subsequently discarded the Vitamin-E regime. In those cases, the incidence of deformity in succeeding pregnancies rose to its former level.

This experiment, too, has received less attention than it deserves. However, before you attribute this neglect — quite logically — to our excessive preoccupation with the mother's well-being and its relationship to the baby, you must remember that only recently has the ancient belief that there is an influence of prenatal diet upon the baby's structural normalcy or good health graduated from folklore to science. The "all or nothing" principle previously controlled the obstetricians' thinking. In other words, either the diet was good enough to support normal reproduction and result in a healthy baby, or it was bad enough to cause sterility — and there could be no result between these two extremes. Now even orthodox nutritionists and physicians are recognizing that there is a twilight zone of indifferent nutrition which allows the mother to conceive, permits the pregnancy to proceed, but engenders deficiencies that interfere with the baby's development and well-being. It may be that we'll move on to the realization that nutrition *before* conception in *both* sexes also has an influence on reproductive efficiency.

The girls of the pizza-pop generation are not our only concern; there is also a process of unnatural selection going on. The teen-age girl — marrying ever younger — is very likely to be the worst-fed member of the family; and one teen-age boy in every four is the victim of inadequate diet. If the two meet and are overcome by biological urge, we have the stage set for anything but healthy babies — with the responsibility equally divided between the mother and the father.

The responsibility for infertility is likewise evenly divided, although we hear more about the woman who cannot conceive than we do about the man who cannot contribute to conception. Masculine fears and ego prevent him from appearing for the examinations to which the woman will willingly subject herself in her effort to have a baby. It is estimated that one family in every ten in the United States is involuntarily barren, and that 16 percent of our young men, between the ages of sixteen and twenty-five, are at least intermittently infertile. The percentage rises as the age of the group increases. We know that 5 percent of our babies are premature, and consequently, more subject to imperfection, later learning difficulties, and other penalties for leaving the uterus too soon. We can expect that at least one baby in a hundred will be mentally retarded, and that one in two hundred will be deformed. When you think over statistics like these, it becomes doubly shocking to realize that the worth of a diet is usually estimated in part by the way in which it supports efficient reproduction. If the American dietary is measured by that standard, we are eating in a way we would not tolerate in thoroughbred horses or pedigreed dogs.

Were people as cynical about the platitudes of the orthodoxy in nutrition as they are about the spiel of door-to-door salesmen, the following paragraph would not be necessary. However, if you read the preceding remarks to a member of the American Dietetic Association, to a member of the faculty of nutrition at either the Harvard School of Public Health or at Rutgers, or to someone from the American Medical Association Council on Foods, you will probably be told that there is "*no* evidence" to support the thesis that our nutrition is responsible even partially for our dismal record in reproduction. Indeed, from such sources you will never learn that there is actual experimental evidence, derived from research with human beings as well as with dogs — that the male has preconceptual nutritional responsibilities as critical as those of the mother in pregnancy. (Were there no such evidence, this chapter would have been preceded with a brief statement concerning its theoretical basis.)

We have also been able to prove that administration of generous quantities of certain of the B vitamins reduces the tendency toward cleft palate and harelip in the babies of women whose previous record of bearing babies with such deformities promises a strong statistical chance of repetition. We have been able to demonstrate that sterility in the American family is more frequently based on inadequate nutrition that one would believe after listening to the eulogies of the "magnificent American diet." In fact, I was once introduced on the Mike Douglas television program as the "father of 227 children," a remark which Mike refused to explain. He left millions of women counting on their fingers until I volunteered the information that these represent children for whom I am nutritional godfather, since they were born to families whose diets we had improved, and whose successful reproduction had followed years of infertility. And to demonstrate the completeness of the indictment of our nutritional preparation for parenthood, consider the fact that a baby's chances to survive the first thirty days of life are better in twelve other countries than they are in the United States. Since the survival of the baby in the first month of life is affected most significantly by the mother's prenatal care, the infant mortality rate in this country also constitutes an appraisal of what we are feeding — and *not* feeding — our expectant mothers.

Some troubles derive from the naive belief — nonetheless promulgated by some obstetricians — that the first four months of pregnancy do not represent a critical period, since the baby is so small that its nutritional requirement must necessarily be satisfied. Actually, this is the period in which the "blueprints" of all the baby's organs are being laid down — the matrices on which the structures are built. The importance of the early stages of pregnancy is well demonstrated by the fact that thalidomide had its tragic effect on the baby's extremities when administered in the first 120 days of pregnancy, but had no impact when taken later. It is obvious that the diet in this period must bear some relationship to the incidence of premature birth too, for by careful supervision of the expectant mother's nutrition — preferably beginning before pregnancy — we have been able to reduce prematurity very significantly.

For many years it was customary for obstetricians to restrict the weight gain during pregnancy, as much as they could — to try to limit the expectant mother's weight gain to no more than eighteen pounds in the nine months. Obstetricians are backing off from this proposition now, on the grounds that it has yielded no real dividends in making deliveries easier, but in fact has contributed to the incidence of premature births. It is quite possible that the average pregnancy diet — mimeographed or printed, distributed uniformly to all patients as if all patients' nutritional needs were identical — might very well contribute to prematurity, particularly when such a diet is restricted in an effort to hold down weight gain. I should like to note that in the thirty years in which I have distributed *well-balanced* and *supplemented* pregnancy diets which have made an attempt to restrict weight gain, I have the distinct impression that such diets — in which the intake of nutrients is held at the level of the highest probable requirement — have not only contributed to reducing the incidence of prematurity, despite restriction of weight gain, but have yielded healthier babies. My personal standard for a healthier baby, incidentally, may include elimination of a characteristic of the newborn so universally present that it is considered normal. Virtually every textbook on pediatric nutrition assures the pediatrician and the mother that the newborn baby may be expected to lose one ounce for each pound of body weight in the first twenty-four hours or so, after which weight gain should normally begin. This would mean that a half-pound loss in an eight-pound baby would be considered normal. Actually, it is quite average, but it may not be acceptable. Being born is probably — other than death — the greatest stress to which we are subjected in the entire life span. If you consider what we go through — being taken from an environment where everything is provided and suddenly being forced to travel through the constricted birth canal — being required very suddenly to breathe on our own and to seek nourishment — and to suffer changes of temperature — you will realize that the name of birth is, in fact, stress. Stress, as you probably know, involves the production, among other hormones, of added amounts of corticosteroid adrenal hormones, similar to cortisone. You may recall that one of the side reactions of cortisone dosage in human beings is retention of fluid, with edema (swelling) of tissues. I have long considered that one of the dividends a baby earns from superior nutrition of the expectant mother is the ability to endure the rigors and stress of the birth process without the tissues filling with fluid. It is my educated guess that part of the weight loss of the newborn is simply a loss of retained fluid in the tissues, and as such, really not normal, merely average. To demonstrate the possible validity of the intuition, let me point to the fact that a number of babies born to mothers whose nutrition has been really optimal have managed to go through the first day or two of life with no weight loss at all, so that even experienced obstetricians tended to underguess their weight by a considerable amount.

The diet which follows is intended for use by both marital partners prior to conception. It is then followed by the mother during pregnancy. It may also be followed by the father during pregnancy, if only to help him withstand those pregnancy stresses that are, I think, infinitely harder on the man than they are on the woman. The same diet may be pursued during lactation. You may gather that I hope you will nurse your baby, for no bottle and no formula will substitute for the warmth of the maternal breast and the nutritious fluid produced by the mammary spheres.

DAILY INTAKE

One eight-ounce glass of fruit juice (orange or grapefruit), unstrained.
One serving of fresh fruit.
Two cups of cooked vegetables.
One cup of salad made with dark, leafy vegetables with a dressing of cottonseed oil, plus vinegar or any other condiments desired.
Three squares of butter or margarine. (Use both.)
One serving of oatmeal or whole-wheat or whole-grain cereal (without preservative).
Two eggs.
Six ounces of lean meat, fish or fowl — emphasis on liver, kidneys, sweetbreads, and tripe. (Cook rare, except pork.)
Four slices of whole-wheat bread.
Three glasses of milk. (Certified raw milk, if available.)
For dessert: Whole gelatin, junket, custard, stewed fruit or fruit whip.
No pastries, ice cream, nuts, or candy.
Not more than one-and-one-half tablespoons of potatoes, spaghetti, rice, corn, lima beans, or dried beans.

Not more than eight glasses of liquids of any kind in twenty-four hours.

Salt to be restricted, and salty foods minimized. (The use of salt substitutes is sometimes recommended by the physician when ankles swell during pregnancy.) Smoked brewer's yeast may be used to compensate for salt restrictions.

Brewer's yeast, wheat germ, dried skim milk, and soy flour can be added to appropriate recipes.

The supplements used with the diet consist of multiple vitamins, a natural source of Vitamin B Complex such as vacuum-dried liver tablets, a multiple mineral concentrate, powdered beef-bone tablets, concentrated Vitamin E, wheat-germ oil, bioflavonoids, and Vitamin C.

Some of these supplements overlap and with studied reason. Wheat-germ oil is used in addition to concentrated Vitamin E because it contains other factors which may help to prevent spontaneous abortion. The wheat-germ oil may be taken by the teaspoonful or can be added in appropriate quantities to the salad oil specified in the diet. A Vitamin-B-Complex source such as vacuum-dried liver tablets is used in addition to multiple vitamin capsules because the natural Vitamin B Complex contains factors not yet synthesized and, therefore, not yet adequately available in capsule form. A multiple mineral capsule is used to supply essential minerals, including iodine (which may be lacking when salt intake is restricted).

For those who prefer vitamin-mineral supplements of natural origin — for which a good case can be made, particularly when dealing with the supplementing of the pregnancy diet, there are available products of this type entirely derived from concentrates of natural substances, such as bone meal, brewer's yeast, desiccated liver, kelp, wheat-germ oil, rose hips, fish liver oil, organic iron, bioflavonoids, and similar sources. Some of these products also contain natural enzymes, derived from pancreatic tissue. A typical formula might provide, from such sources:

VITAMIN A: 12,500 units

VITAMIN D: 400 units

VITAMIN C: 100 mgs.

VITAMIN B₁: 3 mgs.

VITAMIN B₂: 6 mgs.

VITAMIN B₁₂: 12.5 micrograms

FOLIC ACID: 2.75 micrograms

NIACIN: 2 mgs.

PYRIDOXIN: 24 micrograms

VITAMIN E: 25 mgs.

RUTIN-HESPERIDIN-BIOFLAVO-
NOIDS COMPLEX: 10 mgs.

CALCIUM: 375 mgs.

PHOSPHORUS: 180 mgs.

IODINE: .075 mgs.

NATURAL ORGANIC IRON: 20 mgs.

PANCREATIC ENZYMES: 45 mgs.

If the diet and the use of supplements are instituted prior to pregnancy, the incidence of morning sickness may also be sharply diminished. If pregnancy nausea does appear, the obstetrician can add a substantial amount of Vitamin B_6 to the supplements. If excessive edema occurs, the obstetrician can increase the protein foods — eggs, meat, cheese, fish or fowl — and add supplements of bioflavonoids. When appetite is finicky in the presence of edema, strained baby meats may be stirred into the allotted milk and appropriately flavored.

The weight gain with this diet should aggregate about three to four pounds in the first three months, about ten pounds in the next three, and three to four pounds in the final three — a total of sixteen to eighteen pounds.

Conscientious newlyweds planning a family can adopt this diet with its supplements prior to conception. If weight is normal or below normal, the physician will probably want to increase the allotted portions.

Sometimes the benefits of good prenatal nutrition for the baby will simply not be recognized by the nonprofessional. The width of the palate, for instance, may be determined in part by the wisdom in which foods are selected in pregnancy. If you couldn't care less about the palate, it's time that you learned that the shape of a baby's mouth bears importantly on the level at which he will function throughout his lifetime. I have particular reference to the palate — the upper jaw, which, we frequently forget, is also the floor of the brain. Above it is the pituitary gland, formed from the same tissue and at the same time that the palate develops. Interference with the development of the palate may reflect interference with the development of the pituitary. The baby's palate tends to be compressed by three forces that operate on most babies. They are the pregnancy diet, the passage through the birth canal, and the use of bottles to replace the breast. It has been well established that undesirable diet in pregnancy will cause narrowing of the palate in both animals and human beings. We know that the passage through the birth canal misshapes the skull, but overlook the effect of these pressures on the shape of the upper jaw. Finally, the baby's use of his tongue in nursing from a bottle is a motion quite different from that which he uses on the breast, and it is one that tends both to push the front palate forward and to make it narrow. Associated with the narrow palate in women is a sense of inadequacy in facing the daily routine. A whole complex of symptoms develops, among them a tendency toward sore throats with pain radiating to the ears. These are maldiagnosed as strep throats. They are quickly cured by stimulation of the pituitary gland. Women with a narrow palate tend to have calloused soles and to have skin which is sensitive to the friction of woolen skirts, tight-fitting garments, garter belts, and garters. They sleep so deeply as to seem drugged or so lightly as to awaken with the slightest sound, but in either case they arise more tired than they were when they went to bed. Their premenstrual week is marked by retention of fluid, weight gain associated with it, irritability, hysteria, and a painful first day. Such women lean toward low blood sugar, and its anxiety, depersonalization, claustrophobia, and fatigability. In males, the deformed palate is most often associated with asocial behavior. Do not dismiss this information as academic — when we have imposed our diet on primitives, on whom it falls frequently as a blight, the impact includes a narrowing of the palate in the children conceived after the dietary change, plus many of these symptoms.

All the aforementioned is said to remind you of the real worth of the ounce of prevention. There are a handful of dentists and a number of osteopaths who have devised therapies aimed at stimulating the pituitary by widening the palate. There are nutritionists — again just a handful — who are familiar with the nutritional therapies that stimulate the pituitary function of those people with a narrow palate. The important point is that the ounce of prevention be valued for what it represents. We cannot do much about the passage through the birth canal and its influence on the shape of the palate, unless you are gaited for cesarean deliveries. There is a great deal we can do about diet in pregnancy, and this chapter I think has fully detailed that possibility. You certainly can nurse, rather than feed formula — even though you may have to fight your obstetrician, the nurses in the maternity hospital, and your pediatrician.

When nutrition is used successfully for therapy, keep in mind that it probably could have prevented the condition from *originally* occurring.

7.
NUTRITION VERSUS "MENTAL DISEASE"

The anguished parent of a schizophrenic teen-ager had addressed a query to psychiatrists at a major psychiatric hospital in New York City. "I've heard about vitamin treatments for schizophrenia," he said, "but you haven't mentioned them." One of the psychiatrists answered: "We do not recommend the vitamin therapy for schizophrenia — and we've never tried it." May I point out that if such a non sequitur were uttered by a layman, the psychiatrist would probably recommend remedial training in logic. How can one pass on the merits or deficits of a treatment with which one has absolutely no experience?

Without the slightest intention of being either cute or funny, I must demonstrate that the psychiatrist's negative attitude toward vitamin therapy is actually based on subconscious resistance. The average practitioner has spent tens of thousands of dollars on training based on the concept that mental disease *is* mental, and emotional disorders *are* emotional. If he is a psychoanalyst, he has also invested many thousands of dollars in a discipline based on the premise that the mind may affect the body, but that the reverse is not generally true. If you were to suggest to such a practitioner the possibility that a "mental" disease may be treated successfully with a few hundred vitamin pills, you would probably run into prejudice masquerading as professional judgment.

In the very next breath, however, the psychiatrist will admit that there is something physically wrong with the schizophrenic. He will know the story of orphaned twins who were adopted by two separate families, brought up in a sharply different environment, yet who developed schizophrenia in the same year and virtually in the same month. He is also aware that after receiving an injection of blood from a schizophrenic, a spider will spin an abnormal web with a distortion which is glimpsed in paintings by some schizophrenic artists. These facts, however, do not necessarily put the psychiatrist in the position of admitting that schizophrenia may represent mental and emotional disturbances caused by physical disease. It is at this point that the old argument arises: Which comes first — the disorder of the mind or the illness of the body?

Exactly the same kind of circular reasoning is employed when hypoglycemia (low blood sugar) is discussed. The one fact virtually no one disputes is a high incidence of low blood sugar in schizophrenia. The argument is old. Does schizophrenia cause hypoglycemia? Does hypoglycemia cause schizophrenia? All these debates waste time and deprive patients of possible benefits. If massive doses of the B-Complex Vitamins can quiet the inner voices that drive schizophrenics into asocial or homicidal behavior, if correction of low blood sugar can relieve some of the symptoms of schizophrenia or help the patient respond better to other forms of treatment, why should we tolerate any type of debate concerning these harmless treatments for a disease that fills more hospital beds than any other single sickness known to man?

It was in the early 1950s that Dr. A. Hoffer, a Canadian physician, began by trial and error to try to find a nutritional factor that might benefit schizophrenia. I believe that the first nutrient which he experimented with was niacinamide. This was a logical choice, for the action of niacinamide deficiency on the brain ranges from the loss of a sense of humor, to complete detachment from reality — delirium and psychosis.

In the twenty years in which Dr. Hoffer treated many thousands of schizophrenics with niacinamide, he had his share of therapeutic failures, but he also registered some striking successes. His research has received the irrational, hostile reception characteristic of the world of medicine when it is confronted with a new idea. I might pause here to remind you that the American Medical Association jeered at the concept of vitamin deficiency disease, and originally called the electroencephalograph electronic quackery which will not fool American medical men!

I have had the pleasure of meeting Dr. Hoffer, since we both gave papers at a medical meeting and, therefore, a part of what you read came to me firsthand. This physician, whose nutritional therapies for schizophrenia are now in use by hundreds of practitioners in the United States and Canada, does not report the treatment to be a panacea. He does point out that our record in the treatment of this disease is not one to which we can point with any sort of pride, and that the vitamin therapy has frequently elicited responses better than those achieved with shock therapy, psychoanalysis, or chemotherapy.* Mention of the last brings to mind an incident that emphasizes the irrationality of the opposition to Hoffer's concept. In a television interview, several psychiatrists attacking the vitamin therapy warned darkly about possible side effects of the megavitamin doses. Dr. Hoffer's response was simple. He admitted the possibility of side effects, although indicating that he had not encountered them with thousands of patients; and then pointed out that the tranquilizers, psychoenergizers, stimulants, and sedatives freely prescribed by psychiatrists are *known* to yield dangerous side effects.

It might be useful to document Dr. Hoffer's statement concerning the risks of the tranquilizers. Here, for instance, is a sampling of the warnings concerning a widely used tranquilizer, as exemplified in the package insert (rarely seen by the patient) with its warnings for the prescribing physician:

"Caution patient against hazardous occupations — driving, operating machinery. Use caution in administering to addiction-prone individuals. Withdrawal symptoms, including convulsions, have followed discontinuation of the drug. Paradoxical reactions such as excitement, stimulation, and acute rage have been reported. Use caution where suicidal tendencies may be present. Possible effects on blood coagulation have been reported. Drowsiness, ataxia (irregularity of muscle coordination), and confusion may occur especially in the debilitated and elderly. Occasionally encountered are skin eruptions, edema, nausea, constipation, changes in the electroencephalograph (the electro-activity of the brain), blood dyscrasias, and jaundice and liver dysfunction, the latter making periodic blood counts advisable during protracted treatment."

Under the circumstances, if it was Dr. Hoffer's intention to label his opponents as intellectually dishonest in using the specter of side reactions to vitamin therapy when they freely prescribe tranquilizers — I should say he had made a pretty good case.

In megavitamin therapy for schizophrenia, the psychiatrist or medical nutritionist may give 5,000 mgs. (5 gms.) of niacinamide daily; higher dosage is more common. Larger amounts are given of Vitamin C — as high as 40 gms. daily; with this vitamin, the schizophrenic shows a biochemical abnormality. When large doses of Vitamin C are given to a normal person, more than 90 percent of the dose will be

---

*In acute cases, megavitamin *and* shock therapies may be needed.

recovered in the urine, whereas in the schizophrenic, very little or none may be excreted. Whether his requirement is abnormally high, or whether something about his peculiar chemistry results in abnormal destruction of the vitamin, we do not yet know. High doses of Vitamin B_6 are also used. Not only is it known that this vitamin also has an effect on brain and nervous-system functions, but we are aware that large doses of niacinamide may cause a Vitamin-B_6 deficiency. The vitamin is often used in a ratio of 1 mg. of Vitamin B_6 for each 15 mgs. of niacinamide. Many psychiatrists will also administer Vitamin E, a typical amount being 1,000 units daily. The practitioner will usually give large amounts of the natural Vitamin B Complex with these factors.

Here we might pause to consider the implementation of this therapy on a typical schizophrenic. The patient was a young man who had become increasingly introverted in early puberty. Though he showed no signs of psychosis in his adolescence, by the time he was ready to leave for college he had built up a formidable and baseless hostility toward his parents.

At college he performed far below his potential and his level of accomplishment in high school, flunking two subjects. He now began experimenting with pot, speed, and LSD.

He dropped out of college, returned home, but finding it impossible to live with his parents, took up residence in a small cabin in an isolated area, supporting himself by teaching guitar. Experimentation with the various drugs had stopped, but the use of marijuana became more constant. After several years of this isolation, he again took up residence in his parents' home, but could not control his hostility against them. This finally led to a violent physical assault on his mother, after which he was briefly hospitalized in a psychiatric institution. On his discharge, he resumed his teaching activities, again living alone, until he was found, on a bitterly cold winter evening, running naked in the snow.

I saw him about a month after this episode, when he had recovered from frostbite. Asking for an explanation of his behavior, he quite coherently said that he had gone outdoors naked in subzero weather because three voices (two female, one male — the latter the voice of God) had commanded him to do so.

I asked him whether *I* could hear the voices, and whether he could answer them without moving his lips. He could not answer either question, thereby indicating his inability to distinguish between inner and outer realities.

It was then that megavitamin therapy was instituted, with Vitamin B Complex, niacinamide, Vitamin C, Vitamin B_6 and Vitamin E. The heavy doses of tranquilizers he had been taking were gradually tapered off over the next few weeks, a psychiatrist instructing him that he was to use a very minor dose of one of these medications if he felt "nervous." Two notes should be entered here: The tranquilizers had not at any time, at any dosage, quieted his inner voices. Also it is not uncommon in the first month on megavitamin therapy, whatever benefit may derive, for there to be one side effect, described by the patient simply as "feeling more nervous."

In the sixth week of megavitamin therapy I again saw the patient. Objectively, he seemed much less disturbed and did not mention the inner voices until asked the specific question. His response was: "The voices faded out about two weeks ago."

I asked: "Can you tell me now whether I could have heard these voices?"

He answered, "How could you? They were the voices of my own conscience."

He went on to explain that on one occasion when he ventured a walk in a large city, traffic trapped him in the middle of a crossing and the voices had briefly reawakened, because, he suggested, he was "nervous." I asked: "Were you startled when the voices disappeared?"

"No," he said. Then, with a sudden flash of insight, he remarked, "But, then — I wasn't startled when they first came." He then appeared to be briefly reviewing his own remark and added: "I guess that was pretty sick, wasn't it?"

I turned to the psychiatrist and questioned him. "This change took place in six weeks. How long might it have taken if you had continued the tranquilizers, used psychotherapy, or employed shock treatments?"

The psychiatrist replied, "A few weeks — a few months — a few years — or never!"

As I have reflected over this history — which is not unique in Dr. Hoffer's experience — I have been reminded of a comment by this psychiatrist who tested megavitamin versus conventional treatment and appraised the results by a simple measure: What percentage of hospitalized schizophrenics who recovered or at least improved to the point where they could be discharged from the hospital were subsequently forced to apply for readmission. Improvement in the megavitamin group was distinctly better sustained, but the psychiatrist nonetheless gave a gloomy forecast for the acceptance of this method of treatment by his peers. In the *Lancet*, a British medical journal, he wrote: "This treatment will never be popular.* It involves a vitamin — it is cheap — and it is widely available."

---

*His prophecy was unfulfilled: Hundreds of medical men now give this treatment.

Another thought that comes to mind, as I review the data on megavitamin therapy, is a remark made by a great scientist when I asked him how he thought posterity would review our present-day medicine and psychiatry. His reply was: "We shall be bitterly criticized — not for our ignorance, which is understandable and forgivable — but for our pretensions — which are neither!"

The emphasis upon niacinamide, Vitamin C, Vitamin B₆, and Vitamin E in megavitamin therapy for mental disease should not be permitted to obscure the demonstrated usefulness of other nutrients.

For example, in the 1950s a psychologist and chemist joined forces in administering to neurotics and psychotics doses of multiple nutrients — including many not considered to be essential in human nutrition.*

All the patients involved in this study were examined by psychiatrists, who established the diagnosis of neurosis or psychosis. In addition, other measuring devices were used to evaluate the pretreatment and posttreatment status of the patients. They included reexamination by the psychiatrist, administration of the Minnesota Multiphasic Personality Index, and evaluation by the family, teachers, and peers.

Many of the patients showed improvement with multinutrient therapy as the only treatment. The improvement ranged from slight to return to reality for several withdrawn individuals.

In subsequent research the experimenters were able to divide the patients into two groups, whom they termed "slow oxidizers" and "fast oxidizers." They were then able to tailor vitamin-mineral supplements specifically to meet the needs of each of these groups. The full study received healthful neglect by the entire profession — in fact, I have yet to meet a clinical psychologist or psychiatrist among the hundreds with whom I have conversed and corresponded who has been aware of the extent of this study.**

This neglect of the possible somatic base of "mental disease" is part of a persistent if ignoble tradition. The roles of hypoglycemia (low

---

*The phrase "not proved essential in human nutrition" does not mean what you think it does. The body manufactures certain nutrients from other nutrients. Choline, for instance, a B-Complex Vitamin, is manufactured from an amino acid, methionine. Therefore, the Food and Drug Administration requires that vitamin labels designate choline as "not proved essential in human nutrition." Choline is essential to life — but theoretically, it need not be present as such in the diet. Unfortunately, the labeling required by the Food and Drug Administration creates the impression that this particular nutrient is not needed and thereby need not be present in the *diet*. It would automatically follow that it need not be present in a vitamin supplement. This is the basis for the Food and Drug Administration to blast supplements that "deceive" the public by offering "unneeded" factors. Factually, choline has been a most useful supplement for persons with liver disease, gall-bladder syndrome, certain neuromuscular disorders, glaucoma, and lethargic nervous systems.

**A recent book by one of the experimenters has now made the study better known.

blood sugar) in simulating or aggravating the symptoms of neurosis and psychosis and in complicating the problems of the schizophrenic have been neglected. Even the early studies on Vitamin E in emotional disorders have received no attention, although more than twenty years ago the vitamin was reported to be useful for certain patients, and the German literature quietly accepted the findings, remarking: "It [the vitamin] dampens the transmission of anxiety impulses from the diencephalon to the cortex." Translation: Vitamin E does not wipe out anxiety, originating in the emotional brain, but reduces the transmission to the thinking brain.

In past years I have taught nutrition at a number of universities. A student in one of my classes sent this note to me:

"I am a schizophrenic. I have been through shock therapy, doses of all the tranquilizers, and years of other psychiatric therapy, the net result of which was that I could not hold a job, and I could not function in society. I am now being treated with ornithine. You can see the results — I am here — I am comprehending what you are teaching, and I shall be happy to let you look at my notebook, which is coherent."

Ornithine is not a nutrient. It is not required as such by the body. In fact, it might aptly be described as a laboratory curiosity. But such a description does not merit rejection, because niacinamide itself for some fifty years was also labeled as a "laboratory curiosity" — while hundreds of thousands of people for want of it died of pellagra.

Years ago a physician treating a patient with disturbances of the gums addressed a question to the "Queries and Minor Notes" department of the *Journal of the American Medical Association*. In his reply, the *Journal* expert answered: "The administration of 50 mgs. of niacinamide daily has been reported to improve the condition of a normal mouth." Make the dose larger, substitute the brain for the mouth, and might not the principle hold? After all, 50 mgs. of niacinamide daily is far beyond the amount of the vitamin "required," if one follows Food and Drug Administration tables of vitamin requirements. When the "normal" is improvable with supplements of a nutrient, it is obvious that we are underestimating the need for the vitamin or overestimating what is normal. Obviously, the same interpretation may be given of these reports on the response of neurotics and psychotics to superdoses of various vitamins and other nutrients. If an excessive dose of a vitamin can improve the normal, why not the abnormal?

It is interesting that alcoholics have been treated with all the new methods discussed in this chapter — megavitamin therapy, high-potency supplementing with many nutrients, and treatment of hypoglycemia. Predictably, practitioners in this field, where psychiatrists have had a virtual monopoly in deciding the therapeutic base of approach to alcoholics, have reacted exactly as their brethren who work with the neurotic and psychotic. They insist that the alcoholic is the victim of an ill-guided technique in escaping unpleasant reality, that the disease is purely emotional in origin, and that it is, therefore, to be approached on the purely psychological level, the modality ranging from psychoanalysis to deconditioning (sometime with drugs like Antabuse) to — once again — shock therapy. If, in fact, the alcoholic is escaping the stress of unpleasant reality, are we not entitled to request that the psychiatrist explain why the drinker has chosen such an unrewarding and self-punishing method of escape? In short: May not the excessive appetite for alcohol sometimes be constitutional, or at least on occasion an abnormal expression of some kind of constitutional aberration? Would you, the reader, see any parallel to this situation and that of the child from a family with a history of diabetes who craves and must eat large quantities of sugar, and, indeed, does not consider sweet a sugar solution which has been concentrated to such a point that a person without the diabetic gene finds it nauseating?

Let us demonstrate that there is more than a possibility that some percentage of the alcoholic population has a physical rather than an emotional disorder, on the simple grounds that the patient's problem is markedly relieved by purely nutritional treatment.

When you discuss hypoglycemia in alcoholics, when you point out that every agency that deals with alcoholic patients strongly emphasizes regular meals, those who command therapy for victims of alcoholism will invariably respond with: "Of course, we know that alcoholism causes low blood sugar." If you reply by stating that there is evidence in some alcoholics that the hypoglycemia comes *first* and causes, rather than is caused by, excessive drinking, the remark falls on unhearing ears. Yet, after some decades of watching alcoholics respond to treatment for hypoglycemia, I have been drawn inexorably to the conclusion that there *is* a sizable group of alcoholics who drink because they have low blood sugar; who make their hypoglycemia worse by substituting alcohol for food; and who, therefore, are caught in a vicious circle from which they can be rescued only by the cure of the underlying condition and not by conversation, the psychiatrist's couch, shock therapy, tranquilizers, willpower, discovery of the Almighty, or communal association with fellow sufferers.

Illustrative is the history of a woman who began to drink secretly after her only child was born (the stress of pregnancy frequently will trigger hypoglycemia in those who are susceptible by constitution and dietary history). She sought psychiatric care and underwent analysis for three years, with no improvement. Chancing upon a description of hypoglycemia as a possible pathway to anxiety, claustrophobia, insomnia, and alcoholism, she sought and obtained a six-hour test for low blood sugar, which confirmed her self-diagnosis. On the hypoglycemia diet her symptoms disappeared one by one, until she found herself able to take liquor or leave it, or take one drink and stop.

A similar demonstration of the effectiveness of nutrition in what may be another type of alcoholism has been given by Professor Roger Williams who, on the basis of animal experimentation, believed that there is one type of alcoholism which is the perverted expression of nutritional deficiencies based upon exaggerated requirements. With this type of alcoholism an individual on a "good" diet might not get adequate nutrition, and his excessive drinking would then reflect the inadequacy. If you are new to the field of nutrition, this theory might sound strange, but it is no stranger than the realization that a baby born with an exaggerated requirement for Vitamin B$_6$ may on an "adequate" diet (adequate for most babies) develop persistent convulsions resulting in brain damage (such cases are on record). Dr. Williams formulated his theory by observing the different appetites for alcohol in laboratory animals, which showed a spectrum of behavior similar to that of the human being — from the teetotaler to the constantly drunk. He was able to link these types of animal alcoholism to an inordinately high and unsatisfied nutritional requirement of the alcoholics, by dosing them with supplementary amounts of various vitamins and minerals. In some cases the alcoholics were able to stop drinking.

Dr. Williams' theoretical explanation of the basis on which certain animals become alcoholics has been challenged as has the interpretation of his results with human alcoholics. Of course, there is another possible explanation for the response of the human drinker. It is entirely possible, for instance, that the vitamin-mineral supplements and the appetite they may have stimulated may have helped the alcoholic to correct a hypoglycemia. At any rate, here is the second *and again unexplored* approach to a disorder which directly or indirectly involves millions of people and costs society billions of dollars.

As treatment for hypoglycemia has been used to help both schizophrenics and alcoholics, so have large doses of niacinamide helped both groups. A physician who gave megavitamin doses of niacinamide to alcoholics remarked: The vitamin shows marked ability to reduce the mood swings and insomnia common in alcoholics. It helps to stabilize behavior so that other treatment for alcoholism becomes more efficient, and it reduces or changes the effect of alcohol on the individual. Drinking becomes unrewarding when niacinamide is used. The vitamin also lessens the severity of the withdrawal symptoms. It is not a cure for the alcoholic, but rather it is an important addition to the traditional treatment. It is academic to debate whether alcoholics have an exaggerated need for niacinamide. Perhaps the effect of the vitamin is druglike.

There is some evidence in my research that certain "emotional" and "mental" symptoms actually do derive from an exaggerated need for niacinamide. On several occasions over a period of years I have been struck by a patient's description of his brain as "swimmy-headed." This is a phrase frequently used by individuals who are in the grip of a chronic deficiency of niacinamide and poor diet, who might later develop the classic symptoms of pellagra. When the "swimmy-headed-ness" is present, there are absolutely no physical signs of dietary deficiency — indeed, by most medical and government standards, these individuals would be labeled well nourished. Yet they do suffer the confusion or "swimmy-headedness," and it does leave when their intake of niacinamide and the Vitamin B Complex is raised. For nutrition aimed at a government-standardized "average American," there is unfortunately no room for these deviant individuals in the official scheme of things nutritional. I recall one patient who came back to her physician after five days of niacinamide treatment for "swimmy-headedness," a treatment she herself had suggested, and which he prescribed reluctantly. When she reported that for the first time in her life she was thinking clearly, he nodded in approval and said: "Fine — stop the dose."

I do not know how many counterparts of this woman there are in our 200,000,000 population. I do know that I have seen many instances of psychotics responding to nutritional therapy and to improvements in the diet. I have often quoted the reaction of an elderly woman to whom we gave vitamins and other supplements for a purpose unrelated to the emotions. Her comment was: "I don't know what you gave me — but it descended upon me like a blanket of peace."

There must be millions of people who would like shelter under that blanket, particularly when it may be gained by a handful of vitamins, some calcium, and a little lecithin.

It is unfortunate that the public thinks of Vitamin E as some kind of aphrodisiac, but this is understandable when one realizes that the professionals have also overemphasized the effect of this nutrient in reproduction. The nutritional term for Vitamin E — tocopherol — actually means "childbearing." However, among the many other actions of Vitamin E, there are some that bear directly on the problems of the mentally and emotionally disturbed. Approximately thirty years ago Vitamin E was found to be helpful in controlling some of the distressing symptoms of the menopause. In these reports emphasis was placed on the quieting effect of the vitamin on nervous, hysterical, menopausal women. Inspired by this, several medical researchers tested the vitamin in the treatment of severely neurotic and psychotic individuals. One of them remarked that Vitamin-E therapy is not as effective as shock treatment, but could be useful in cases where, for one reason or another, shock treatment could not be employed. One is inspired to wonder why a harmless vitamin therapy must be measured against the action of a treatment that actually causes small brain hemorrhages, but that is a question for another time and another book.

In the treatment of emotional and mental disorders with nutritional factors, individual differences again become very evident. One schizophrenic responds significantly, another, much less so or not at all. As a patient's history seen in this chapter indicates, a schizophrenic may show no reaction to vitamin therapy, yet may improve remarkably when given a protein substance.

Individual differences in responses to dosage also appear.* There are the mentally sick who respond gratifyingly to 20,000 mgs. of niacinamide daily, with no response at all to lesser dosages on which other patients improve.

It is possible, and the thought is not original with me, that what we are calling schizophrenia might be a dozen different diseases, including hypoglycemia, the effects of extraordinarily high unsatisfied requirements for nutrients, emotional stress, or a combination of these. It should not be assumed that mental disease caused purely by emotions will necessarily be unresponsive to nutritional therapy. If schizophrenia, in some cases, reflects the impact of an abnormal chemistry, even if that physical disability began with uncontrolled thinking and disordered emotions, nutritional treatment may still be helpful. This is simply the dignified, scientific way of saying that although you may have derived your stomach ulcer from your boss, mother-in-law, or your spouse, it is nonetheless a physical disease and thus may be treated on a physical level.

While there are cases of nervous disorders and mental disease that respond to nutritional therapies with what seems to be complete recovery, these are in the minority. The prime role of megavitamin and other nutritional treatments in these disorders is that of an adjunct — rendering the patient more cooperative and more amenable to other treatments. This statement could similarly be made for hypoglycemia.

*There is also individuality in the schizophrenic's response to individual foods as well as to diet. There is evidence that a sizable percentage of these patients have adverse reactions to milk and wheat, similar to those experienced by children with celiac disease and adults with malabsorption syndrome. Therefore, in addition to feeding the schizophrenic the hypoglycemia type of diet, it would sometimes be judicious to omit dairy products and wheat. A calcium supplement will replace milk products, and provided that the schizophrenic is able to tolerate other grains, rice as the least allergenic cereal may be substituted for wheat. (Rice bread and crackers are commercially available.)

There are times when all the symptoms believed to be neurotic or psychotic are caused by hypoglycemia and disappear when the underlying condition is competently treated. However, in genuine neurotics and psychotics who have hypoglycemia, perhaps secondary to their prime emotional or mental disorder, treatment of the low blood sugar renders the patient more amenable to psychiatric therapy.

One might ordinarily explain the unwillingness of the psychiatrist and the clinical psychologist to accept nutritional therapies for emotional and mental disorders on the basis that this is an exhibition of the resistance of an established profession to an innovation. One might also conjecture that practitioners who have been trained at great expense in the concept that emotional and mental disorders *are* emotional and mental in origin must necessarily be resistant to the idea that patients with such disorders may be helped by a dosage of this vitamin or that protein. However, that theory will not long stand when one reflects on the tide of prescriptions written by psychiatrists for mood-changing drugs, psychoenergizers, stimulants, sedatives, and tranquilizers. Perhaps we can best cope with the resistance of the professions that deal with the emotionally and mentally disturbed by reminding them that no one expects the medications to replace psychological treatment, and nutritional therapies are no exception. Seldom does such a therapy cure. More often it will make the patient more amenable to other needed treatments. Certainly the nutritional treatment should not be criticized because it is physiological and harmless!

However, the emphasis placed on nutritional therapy for neurosis and psychosis has tended to obscure some of the dividends that come to *normal* individuals whose nutrition is thus improved. Consider, for instance, the implications of a study conducted by a medical nutritionist with a group of professional men and their wives, all in excellent medical and physical health. Prior to the experiment their "psychological state" was evaluated by means of a standard test subsequent to which they were given doses of tryptophane — one of the amino acids that is a building block of protein and essential to the body. The same psychological evaluation was given again after a short period of tryptophane dosage. A large percentage of those participating in the experiment showed a significant improvement. As I have remarked previously, the improvement of a "normal mouth" following large doses of niacinamide certainly indicates that our concepts of a normal mouth and of the niacinamide requirement may require revision. In the case of tryptophane the same argument may be set forth. Doses in a magnitude of four times the "daily requirement" of the amino acid as set by the Food and Drug Administration have produced analogous improvement in the psychological state of healthy individuals. Question: Are the norms for "psychological state" accurate, or are they average? Question: Are we setting our requirements for tryptophane too low as we have set them too low for niacinamide?

It is of interest that tests of the administration of tryptophane in the treatment of endogenous depression (for which there is no justification in the life situation) yielded similar dividends. So did administration of the amino acid in the treatment of insomnia. This is orthomolecular psychiatry — meaning "the *right* molecule." It is apparent that when some of us achieve the intake of the molecule at the levels we need as individuals, we may respond by demonstrating that some of our troubles derive from diets that are "average" or even "well balanced" but which are obviously not well balanced for us as individuals.

If this information has in any way sounded academic, let me translate it in terms of the experience of people who found themselves in deep trouble which was labeled as "mental" and which derived from a vitamin need that in some cases may have been as much as 100,000 times the "average" or "normal" requirement. The vitamin we are dealing with is Vitamin B_{12}. Medical thinking concerning this vitamin is curiously channeled. If you mention it to a physician, he will tell you that this is the vitamin that treats or prevents pernicious anemia. If you press him for added functions of the vitamin, he will tell you that a deficiency of it can impair the functioning and degenerate the structure of the nervous system and the brain. At this point conversation tends to run dry, although Vitamin B_{12} is probably involved in the synthesis of RNA and DNA and plays a part in the body's management of food. However, the chief deficit in this description of the function of Vitamin B_{12} is the overemphasis on its role in pernicious anemia and the underemphasis on its action in protecting the nervous system and brain. For a number of years — and indeed to this very day — the blood has been regarded as being more sensitive to a deficiency of Vitamin B_{12} than any other tissue. This belief has turned out to be fallacious — tragically so. In some individuals a deficiency of the vitamin was subtly changing the function of brain and nervous tissue, with not a single sign in the blood to warn the physician of the source of the trouble.

Consider a story which H. L. Newbold, M.D., told at the American-Canadian-British Schizophrenia Association Conference in London on September 28, 1971. The patient was a thirty-three-year-old man, a PhD candidate at one of the country's major universities, who was being treated by a psychotherapist after having experienced a psychotic break with reality. Because the psychotherapy was not progressing well, the patient was referred to Dr. Newbold, who has experience in megavitamin therapy. At the time of his break with reality, the patient sat in his room and talked to himself for several days. He also encountered distortions of perception. Space had been greatly foreshortened — he felt like a midget, and the streets seemed extremely short. When he departed from reality he became frightened, left his home, and began running up and down the street, convinced that a blood vessel had, as he put it, broken in his head. After three days of totally psychotic behavior of this sort, he was hospitalized and placed on a tranquilizer which gradually brought the more overt aspects of his psychosis under control. Subsequent to discharge from the hospital, he took reduced doses of the tranquilizer. He was able to avoid rehospitalization, but he felt far from normal. He was very lethargic and could not work on his PhD dissertation. He was troubled by loneliness and insecurity, but at the same time could not interact with other people. His feelings of inadequacy and insecurity were reinforced when his wife left him. His head felt as if it were not clear and his emotions as if they were locked within him. He secretly harbored anger toward most people. It was difficult for him to drag himself to class, and there he found himself unable to participate actively. In addition to his depression, he was troubled that his memory and comprehension were poor, and he found it difficult to understand and remember what he read. At the time that Dr. Newbold interviewed him, the patient appeared to have vague paranoid feelings, but no evidence of any serious psychiatric disturbance. A number of chemical tests were performed, one of which revealed that the Vitamin-B_{12} levels in the blood serum were low. There was no evidence of pernicious anemia, but the patient was nonetheless given 1,000 micrograms of hydroxycobalamin, intramuscularly. Five days later the patient reported no change in his condition, and a second intramuscular injection of the vitamin was administered. When the patient returned eight days later, he reported a "remarkable improvement" of his condition, with memory and ability to learn restored virtually to normal. He was participating in class activities and had returned to work on his dissertation. Occasionally he still felt anger toward people. During the following five months the patient, taking injections of the vitamin twice weekly, maintained an excellent level of improvement on all except two occasions. Those occurred when the attempt was made to increase the interval between injections to ten days. This extension resulted in the patient becoming rapidly depressed and tired, and having difficulty concentrating. These symptoms were promptly relieved when the interval between injections was restored to the shorter period of seven days.

In the preceding case there *was* a low level of Vitamin B_{12} in the blood serum to warn the alert physician that extra supplies of the vitamin might be needed. In the next case history we learn that a normal Vitamin-B_{12} level in the blood serum is no guarantee that the brain and nervous system are receiving adequate quantities. The woman was thirty-eight years old with a long history of recurrent, severe depression and of disabling physical complaints. No clear diagnosis of the source of the physical illness had been made. She had been helped with her depressions by psychotherapy, but only temporarily. The B_{12} level in her blood serum was perfectly normal — 231 picograms per milliliter. Nonetheless, the doctor decided to try injections of Vitamin B_{12} for this patient. His decision was based on a thesis of Linus Pauling which points out that some genetically defective enzyme systems may function more effectively if vitamin levels — involving the vitamins which are part of the enzyme systems — are raised much higher than the accepted norms.*

When the Vitamin-B_{12} injections were started, the patient was taking several tranquilizers. This combination minimized some of her acute distress but did not allow her to function adequately as a housewife.

After the first injection of Vitamin B_{12} she reported an immediate increase in her energy reserves and in her feeling of well-being, but on returning to the doctor a week later, she indicated that the improvement had lasted only two and one-half days. Dr. Newbold points out that this is about the length of time one can expect high tissue levels of Vitamin B_{12} after an injection of the vitamin has been given intramuscularly. Therefore, instructions were given to her family doctor to repeat the injections every two and one-half days. At the time of the woman's next visit to Dr. Newbold, she was less depressed, her energy level was sharply improved, and her physical complaints were gradually disappearing.

The end of the story, with a year of injections — during which time the interval between the vitamin shots was gradually increased — is told in a simple sentence: The patient is now able not only to care for her large family, but also to work full time in a demanding position. It is Dr. Newbold's conclusion that this patient has an enzyme defect which requires larger than normal amounts of Vitamin B_{12}.

Many other stories could be told, but one last example of the impact of Vitamin-B_{12} deficiency on the personality will suffice. The patient was an elderly woman who had become paranoid; she had an elaborate persecution complex, much of it attributed to her husband. She had been hospitalized for shock therapy. The psychiatrist, however, had an uneasy hunch that he was dealing with a physical problem. No de-

*It is customary in science to indicate priority where it is due. The suggestion that a genetically defective enzyme system may be restored to something closer to normal function if a vitamin involved in the system is supplied in larger quantities was implied in the work of Roger Williams and explicitly stated by Helen Mitchell, in a communication to the *Journal of the American Medical Association* a number of years ago.

ficiency of Vitamin B_{12} in the blood appeared — but a test that examines the utilization of the vitamin indicated the possibility that the woman was developing pernicious anemia. Her bizarre behavior therefore represented degeneration of the brain and nervous system based upon inadequate tissue supplies of the vitamin. Injections of the vitamin supported the thesis, bringing complete normalcy to a patient who had hitherto been so "mentally" disturbed that when her husband brought the television set closer to her hospital bed for her comfort, she had accused him of trying to harm her with radiation.

In addition to the fact that the physician has been schooled to think of Vitamin-B_{12} deficiency as exhibiting itself in pernicious anemia first and in degeneration of brain and nervous system long afterward, there is another quirk of the physician's philosophy concerning this particular vitamin which bears importantly on his decision about using it. Dietary deficiency of Vitamin B_{12} — except in vegetarians — is extremely unlikely. The vitamin is supplied by most animal proteins, and most people have at least a modicum of these in the diet. Second, the average daily requirement is estimated to weigh about as much as a period made with a lead pencil. Under these circumstances, the physician believes that the only way in which an individual other than a vegetarian is likely to become deficient in Vitamin B_{12} would be through poor utilization. It *is* true that Vitamin B_{12} cannot be absorbed from the intestinal tract if the stomach is not manufacturing a "conveyer" which will take this large molecule through openings which are too small to permit it to pass. This "conveyer" is known as the intrinsic factor. The pathway to pernicious anemia is a deficiency in intrinsic factor rather than a deficiency of Vitamin B_{12}, unless, as I have remarked, one is a vegetarian.

Accordingly, when we talk to the physician about doses of Vitamin B_{12} 100,000 times the daily requirement, and when we talk in terms of psychosis caused by a deficiency in the vitamin which is not marked by pernicious anemia, you can see that we are asking the medical man to revise his thinking radically. If he happens to be a psychiatrist who has gone through his own psychoanalysis, and who is by training and therapy committed to the doctrine that the "mental" is "mental" in origin, then the difficulty obviously multiplies.

It is estimated that 1 percent of the old people now incarcerated in old-age homes and labeled as "senile dements" — suffering from second childhood, in the public's language — could be rescued with injections of Vitamin B_{12}. Newbold estimates that at least 1 percent of all patients seen in psychiatric practice might be markedly benefited, if not cured, by injections of Vitamin B_{12}. Add the considerable percentage of patients who are being treated for neurosis when they are actually suffering from hypoglycemia, or whose actual neurosis is being worsened by hypoglycemia. Now consider the considerable group of patients whose emotional disturbances are either initiated or aggravated by vitamin deficiencies. It has been known for nearly forty years that poor nutrition can be responsible for behavior perfectly simulating the neurotic or the psychotic — and this, sometimes, with no *physical* evidence of nutritional deficiency. It is less well appreciated that poor dietary habits frequently are born from emotional disturbances and feed back to them. It becomes evident that we are not talking about a small percentage of psychiatric patients. The patient who is being treated solely on a conversational level should arrive at such therapy only after he has been competently evaluated for the physical conditions that may simulate, initiate, or aggravate those disorders usually considered purely emotional or mental. Moreover, it is necessary that the evaluation should be made by a practitioner who is well aware that nutritional "norms" do not apply to everybody, and classical deficiency disorders are what we do not see.

In pellagra, a substance called "porphyrin" appears in the urine. While it is there in significant quantities, the patient shows the delirium of pellagra. When the dietary inadequacies are repaired, porphyrin disappears, and with it goes the delirium.

Less well-known is the role that porphyrin plays in the troubles of a group of patients who may find themselves mislabeled as psychotics. Prior to the appearance of the mental symptoms these patients may suffer from abdominal pain, which may be mistaken for a digestive disorder or a psychosomatic disease. In the urine of such patients a concentration of porphyrin was found, reflecting a metabolic disturbance that is responsible for both the mental and physical symptoms.

It has long been known that a marginally inadequate diet may produce the mental symptoms of pellagra, without the physical stigmata of the disease. To my knowledge, no one has tested such marginally deficient patients for porphyrinuria, which could, of course, be present and responsible for their neurotic or semipsychotic behavior. That thought led me to wonder why pellagra therapy has never been applied to patients suffering from porphyrinuria. I now have one case to report in which the patient was dosed with large amounts of niacin and Vitamin B Complex, and the abdominal pains and the psychotic behavior disappeared in less than two weeks.

This is not the only vitamin therapy successfully applied to this condition. While the publication, *Medical Letter*, has joined with the American Medical Association in discounting completely any claim for any usefulness of Vitamin E in the treatment of human disease, an

American Medical Association journal has reported that porphyria (abnormal porphyrin metabolism) is completely rectified by doses of Vitamin E. In fact, the paper indicated that there is some evidence that Vitamin-E deficiency may be responsible for the disturbance in the first place. Porphyria in alcoholics did not respond. The treatment certainly should be applied to the estimated 1 to 3 percent of the mental institute population believed to suffer from porphyria.

If you take the long perspective now, you will see that dogma concerning average nutritional requirements must no longer be allowed to interfere with the achievement of optimum nutrition for optimal health on the basis of individuality of requirement; nor can it be permitted to continue to block the application of nutritional therapies, however unconventional and in whatever unconventional doses. Only in this way will we arrive at effective treatment of some of the ills of the mind and the body to which we are so appallingly prone, and for which our methods of treatment are so appallingly inadequate.

In the treatment of psychotic children or children with learning disabilities, the diet employed is that for low blood sugar (see appendix).

For children weighing thirty-five pounds or more, niacinamide — one to two grams daily — is administered, accompanied by one to two grams of Vitamin C, 200 to 400 mg. of Vitamin B_6, and 400 to 600 mg. of calcium pantothenate daily. The smaller doses are for children under thirty-five pounds, but those may be increased after a two-week period if the child proves tolerant. For a child over forty-five pounds, Allan Cott reports the optimum daily maintenance level will be approximately three grams of niacinamide and three grams of Vitamin C. He also suggests riboflavin, thiamin, Vitamin E, folic acid, glutamic acid, and other nutrients. Use the vitamins listed above, plus 100 mgs. of Vitamin E, a multiple vitamin-mineral supplement, and the entire Vitamin B Complex from a natural source, such as liver. For children too young to swallow capsules, liquid preparations of multiple vitamins, multiple minerals, the natural B Complex, and Vitamin E are available. Niacinamide, Vitamin C, Vitamin B_6 and pantothenic acid can be made available in solution, but flavoring would be necessary for the potencies in which these vitamins are employed.

It should be emphasized that this approach may be helpful not only to psychotic children but to children with learning disabilities, those who are autistic, and those who are hyperactive.

By now, I anticipate that Dr. Linus Pauling will have published his new test for susceptibility to future mental disease in persons now considered normal. The test is based on the administration of very large doses of Vitamin C, Vitamin B_6, and niacin. Retention of more than half the dose of one vitamin increases the likelihood of schizophrenia, according to the description of the test which I have received, by a factor of two. If the person retains more than half the dose of two of the vitamins, the risk of schizophrenia is multiplied by a factor of eight. If more than half the dosage of all three vitamins is retained, the risk of development of schizophrenia in the future multiplies by a factor of forty. It is possible that the arithmetic is not stated correctly, since the communication to me was oral and secondhand.

A final word on senile dementia (second childhood): The principle on which the new hyperbaric (oxygen) treatment is based confirms the validity of the nutritional approach to the same problem. For, with administration of Vitamin E, high-potency B Complex, niacin, Vitamin C, bioflavonoids, accompanied by intramuscular injection of these factors and additional Vitamin B_{12}, together with the hypoglycemia-type diet, we were rescuing more than twenty years ago "psychotic" and "senile" men and women from "second childhood" which actually reflected metabolic derangements.

If you do not have access to hyperbaric therapy for your old people, they are still entitled to the benefit of the nutritional approach. And once again, nutrition may prevent what it mitigates or cures. The best time to take advantage of this help for old people is now — while they are still functioning.

And so, orthomolecular psychiatry is now used through the entire life span. It isn't *the* answer but it is *an* answer, and for many patients it is significantly helpful. As usual with every advance in the field of science, the majority of professional men remain skeptical at this point. When they finally accept orthomolecular psychiatry, it will no longer be new and therefore will be no cause for excitement.

8.

APPOINTMENT
IN DAMASCUS

There is the ancient story of the servant who shops for food for his master and returns to the household greatly agitated — Death has brushed against him in the marketplace. He pleads for a fast horse on which to escape to Damascus, and his master yields to his terror and permits his escape. But that afternoon Death visits the master, asks for the servant, and when told he has gone to Damascus, comments: "Good! I have an appointment with him there tonight!"

The inevitability of death is not likely to be challenged for many generations to come, although it is possible that increased understanding of microbiology and inevitable improvements in transplantation techniques mean that the useful life span may be fantastically extended. That, however, will not solve two philosophical problems we presently face. We are prisoners of time. It is a captivity made possible only because we surrender to the concept that there are certain disabilities and sicknesses that not only come *with* time but also are *caused* by it. So we allow the doctor to say: "Of course you have arthritis — you're sixty years old!" We allow the eye specialist to remark: "The cataract you have is a product of old age." We carry that philosophy into daily conversation: "Of course my hair is gray — after all, I am not getting any younger." We surrender to the idea that the ticking of the clock —

time itself — tears into our vitals and weakens our functions until death mercifully writes "Finis!" Consider, for instance, the implication of the old man's remark, "I still chase girls but I can't remember why."

As a result of this surrender to a negative philosophy, we find ourselves — or would, if we stopped to think about it — in a completely illogical position. Do not all these concepts mean that the sixty-year-old whose sexual functions are unimpaired, whose hair is not gray, whose eyes do not have cataracts, who has no "touch of arthritis," and whose teeth are not loose, is not only a physiological abnormality but actually, in the strange upside-down world this philosophy creates, some kind of a freak? The question is not really rhetorical. There is the celebrated story of the patient who is being queried by the nurse prior to an initial interview with the doctor. The nurse asks questions concerning previous illnesses, previous physicians, surgical history, dental record, and psychiatric history, if any. With the pat response that she has never been sick, nor suffered from tooth decay, nor had any surgery, the nurse puts down the pen and earnestly inquires: "What are you? Some kind of a health nut?"

If you stop permitting your concept of time to be a kind of mental hookworm, sucking at your vital fluids, help is available in resisting or mitigating to some degree the degenerative changes that come with time but are not caused by it.

The last sentence is not as innocent as it sounds. In order to adopt such a positive approach toward the infirmities of old age, you must accept the basic fact that aging itself is a sickness, and as such its effects may be prevented, modified, or at least mitigated. Of course, you will need to change more than your philosophy. It is one thing to accept calmly the inevitability of death; it is another to come to the realization that neither the clock nor the calendar can cause osteoarthritis, decalcification of the jaw bone and loosening of the teeth, graying of hair, wrinkling, or loss of zest for living.

It appears that there are several kinds of calendars built into our cells and an internal clock, too. For instance, no matter how much a woman lies about her age, her pituitary gland knows when menopause is due. That bespeaks some kind of glandular recognition of the passage of time. Built into the cells is another type of calendar — one which, oddly enough, has nothing to do with time or duration. This is the one that decides the total life span of individual species. Some such mechanism must be responsible for the fact that dogs live about twelve years, the monkey about twenty-five years, the tortoise about a century, and man and the African elephant somewhere around seventy years. This particular calendar may derive from the instructions that are inscribed in the protein of the cell from the first moment of life. It has been found that cells are programmed to reproduce about fifty times. This has no relationship to time for the fifty generations of cells may come to pass in a few years or many, but when the last generation of cells in an organ has lived its appointed term, that organ or tissue will die. What happens then is based on how essential the particular tissue or organ is. If it is the heart, this becomes your signal to exit this best of all impossible worlds. If it is the brain, you may linger with your capacities reduced. If it is the kidneys, you may wind up as an appendage to a dialysis machine.

It is possible for cells to die before they have reached the allotted fifty generations, and it is *that* eventuality with which we are concerned as we use nutrition to try to prolong the prime of life. There is no vitamin, and there are no diets that will give you the capacity for the fifty-first generation of cells. But whether you achieve the fiftieth — and the rate at which you will use up your cells — may be very much determined by the food you eat. Moreover, the evidence now shows that properly selected diet may help protect you against outside agents that silently are interfering both with cellular function and with the fifty-generation sequence to which you are normally entitled.

There are factors in our environment that cause cells to malfunction or to die prematurely. (Just so that you don't brush this fact off as something that will happen to George and not to you: In the last twenty years your heart volume has shrunk by approximately one-third of 1 percent because of premature death of cells.) Oddly enough, one of these appears to be oxygen, which is a requisite to life and a cause of premature aging. We do not know exactly what turns oxygen from friend to foe; we can only say that it is either cosmic radiation or something that acts like it. Radiation is inescapable — its energies are so great that ordinary matter is transparent to it, and coal miners a mile underground receive it as we do. The scientists who have been studying the phenomenon of aging believe that the process is at least accelerated, if not started, by such radiation or by something that has the same effect. They have good reasons for these conclusions: it is apparent that the cells are being subjected to something very similar to a tug-of-war, and that the battle among the opposing forces obviously interferes with the normal chemistry, function, and longevity of the cells. Let us say that the first force in this tug-of-war is either radiation or something closely resembling it. The second participant is the polyunsaturated fats in the cells on which this radiation action is exerted. The third group of forces is the protective factors derived from good diet. These help shield those fats from the destructive effects of the radiant energies.

The undesirable actions of radiant energy should not be compared to the effects of a Buck Rogers ray gun, melting tissues away. When ionizing radiation strikes polyunsaturated fat, a subtle and destructive chemical reaction begins that initially releases an atom of hydrogen. This in turn begins a process that allows oxygen to attack the unsaturated fat* in the cell. From these reactions comes the formation of a compound abnormal to the cell; its only function is destruction. You may picture the compound as a pool ball tossed on a pool table, striking other balls and setting them in random motion. Chaos is let loose within the cell. Beautifully balanced chemical processes are disturbed — to the point where the garbage-digesting mechanism of the cell may actually destroy its structure. When this biochemical anarchy is complete, the cell is then either prematurely senile, a "clinker," or dead.

The "clinker" stage requires some explanation. The cell may be viable and retain its potential capacity to function, but its chemical processes have been deranged by the abnormalities started by cosmic radiation. The cell can be compared to a piece of coal that is so thickly insulated by ashes that a normally functioning furnace could not make it burn.

Cells are built from protein and fats. About 17 percent of those fats are in the unsaturated form. Therefore anything that attacks those fats must have devastating effects on the architecture and the function of the cell. The proteins are also not immune. As part of the chaos created by radiant energies, there is a change in the ways in which proteins are linked. Cross linkages occur, creating abnormal compounds of protein nature never anticipated and for which there are no normal functions in the cell. When a cell has undergone this type of injury, a pigmentation appears. This has been long identified with the cells of aged animals and as a consequence, called "senile pigmentation." Only recently have we realized that this same pigmentation also appears in the cells of young and old animals when they are inadequately supplied with Vitamin E. The microbiologists came to a sudden realization: The

---

*The term "polyunsaturated" is applied to a fat whose molecules do not contain all the hydrogen that they could. Typical of fats that retain a capacity for adding hydrogen are most of the vegetable fats (with the exception of coconut oil). If you will picture an unsaturated fat as possessing hands that reach for and are eager for hydrogen, you can then visualize the saturated fat as having these hands filled. Fats of animal origin — lard, suet, butter — are examples of saturated fat. A hydrogenated fat is one in which man has introduced the extra hydrogen to fill the hands. In the process a liquid vegetable fat which is unsaturated is turned into a solid fat that is saturated with hydrogen. There are those who believe that the unsaturated fats are less likely to contribute to hardening of the arteries. Conversely, in this chapter you will learn that such fats are peculiarly vulnerable to cosmic radiation, which may cause them to release alien chemicals that induce premature aging of the cells.

cellular changes we have been calling "senile" — the peculiarities that mark the cell that has become a "clinker" — are accompanied by the peculiar pigmentation that had been considered to be one of the "normal" signs of old age; and yet every one of these phenomena could be initiated by a deficiency in Vitamin E.

It became obvious that one of the primary functions of Vitamin E in the body is protecting both structure and function of the cell against excessive exposure to the action of oxygen. Gradually, we began to understand that this vitamin is critically important in shielding the unsaturated fat from oxidation* initiated by cosmic radiation. Now "clinkers" and cells in which chemistries had become disorganized because of attack by oxygen could be looked upon as suffering from a chain of consequences resulting from lack of the natural antioxidants, among these Vitamin E.

But as Vitamin E is needed to help protect the unsaturated fats, so does the equation run in the opposite direction: The amount of Vitamin E we require is partially determined by the amount of unsaturated fat in the cell and, for that matter, in the diet. We have learned that eating large amounts of polyunsaturated fat may cause a Vitamin-E deficiency. This knowledge was gained the hard way, when a sick baby who was being fed intravenously died from Vitamin-E deficiency caused by overdosage with polyunsaturated fat that lacked the vitamin. Ultimately, a ratio was established — one of great importance to you if you are interested in helping keep yourself young. We need .6 mgs. of Vitamin E for every gram of unsaturated fat in the diet.

Knowledge of this interrelationship between the need for Vitamin E and the amount of polyunsaturated fat in the diet has been unforgivably slow in reaching both food processors and physicians. The techniques used in extracting vegetable oils, rather than those aimed at retention of Vitamin E, seem primarily directed at a bright, clear product that the American housewife considers the ultimate symbol of purity. (If she can read the label through the back of the bottle, all is well!) Dr. Phillip White, who at the time these lines are written is Chairman of the American Medical Association Council on Foods, confessed in a recent article in *Today's Health* that he is ignorant of any relationship between the intake of unsaturated fat and require-

*Oxidation refers merely to chemical reactions in which oxygen combines with other substances. Many such reactions are indispensable to life — the energy you are using to read these lines comes ultimately from the oxidation (burning) of sugar. But when oxidation is uncontrolled, we are in trouble. It is the difference between a cheerful fire in the fireplace and the fire that destroys a home. When oxygen combines with hemoglobin, it is supporting the flame of life. When excess oxygen combines with a fat, the fat becomes rancid. Rancidity for your cells is a pathway to premature old age.

ments for Vitamin E. Considering the influence the American Medical Association Council on Foods has on the attitudes of physicians, nurses, and dieticians, one may regret that the Association's accustomed cultural lag operates in the field of nutrition, too.

You must not conceive of the unsaturated fat in the cell as being stored there, inertly waiting withdrawal by the body. These fats are actually part of the membranes that enclose the cells and of certain structures within the cells themselves. There are also a number of cellular enzymes that are chemically similar to unsaturated fat and therefore equally vulnerable to attack by oxygen.

Lysosomes get rid of the waste materials of the cells. Their walls are made of protein and fat and are easy targets of attack by the abnormal chemicals created when the unsaturated fat is oxidized. Sometimes these chemicals actually puncture the wall of the lysosomes, releasing enzymes that ordinarily are solely engaged in destroying wastes. When such enzymes are at large in the main body of the cell, they proceed to destroy the lysosome itself and other cellular components. Indeed, it is for this reason that biologists have called the lysosomes the "suicide packs" of the cells.

By now it is evident that the sixteenth century alchemist Paracelsus displayed an ancient wisdom when he said: "Speak to me not of a poison, speak to me of a dose." He meant, of course, even water in sufficient amounts can kill. By the same token, it is obvious that the friendly oxygen that makes life possible can also — when released in the wrong place at the wrong time and in the wrong amount, without the safeguards nature has built into our foods — become an enemy, possibly threatening us with acceleration of the aging process.

With regard to the vitamin content of foods, it may be said that nature proposes and man disposes. It is enlightening to take a tour through a cornflakes factory and observe the care that is used to ensure that the Vitamin E of the corn does not reach the consumer of the cornflakes. Where does it go? Part is sent to the mink farms, since minks have cash value, and the breeder would not dream of depriving them of an essential nutrient. The remainder of the corn germ is sold to processors for extraction of corn oil. This sale would seem to guarantee that some of the Vitamin E as well as the unsaturated fat reaches the public — but that brings up the question of the type of processing to which corn oils and other oils are subjected.

The extraction of vegetable oils is technically a very complicated series of processes. The grain or the germ is treated with superheated steam, which makes it easier to extract the maximum amount of oil. (You use the same principle when you discover that oranges soaked in hot water will release more juice.) The oil is then extracted by pressure, which involves *more* heat. Afterward it is treated with alkalies to form soap. The soap is removed, and the residue is bleached, chilled, purged by filtration through activated charcoal, reheated, and filtered some fifty times. Exactly what happens to the original constituents of the oil and to the fatty acids themselves is anyone's guess — and do not dismiss this as academic. Not only may these techniques deprive you of a supply of Vitamin E in the proper ratio to the unsaturated fat and thus contribute to premature aging, but the mischief may go deeper. There is a minute amount of hormones in vegetable oils that may help protect man against heart failure. (According to Dr. Melvin E. Page, effective quantities may be as small as thousandths of a milligram.) That is if they survive the cold, the heat, the bleach, the lye, the charcoal, and the filter presses.

We can begin to set up requirements for Vitamin E, with three considerations in mind. We need enough of the vitamin to maintain the proper ratio to unsaturated fat, which is not easy to establish since we do not know how much unsaturated fat you are eating nor how much Vitamin E it contains. In addition, we are not sure how much you should be eating. After listening to medical eulogies of unsaturated fat as a means of escaping heart attacks associated with hardening of the arteries — an association, incidentally, which is not as frequent as it is made to seem — one would think that a sensible person would exclude all sources of saturated fat from his diet. Unfortunately, when a group of medical overenthusiasts excluded these, as I have noted elsewhere in this book, there was a gratifying decrease in heart attacks and an ungratifying increase in cancer, with the two balancing each other so that the death rate remained unchanged. Since it is more expensive to die of cancer than to die of heart disease, the choice would seem to be an easy one. One might exercise common sense, a rather rare seasoning in the thinking of some authorities in nutrition, to ascertain how much unsaturated fat man could possibly have had in his diet prior to the development of agriculture and the subsequent invention of machines for expressing the oil from grains and seeds. Such a calculation will lead immediately to one conclusion: Man at no time in his long history could have had a fat intake consisting entirely of the unsaturated varieties, unless he was positively "nuts about nuts." Even at the hunter's stage of his development, man had both saturated and unsaturated fat in his diet since animals are not made entirely of one or the other. If we must take an educated guess at the amount of unsaturated fat that should be in the diet, perhaps we might use the content in the cell as something of a guideline. This, you will recall, is about 17 percent. Taking into consideration this percent and other calculations which need not be retraced here, I long ago set a figure of about 20 percent unsaturated fat as a reasonable goal. It was then and it is now my feeling that venturing beyond this amount may be an uncharted journey into unknown dangers. I am in a better position to make statements in this area than most nutritionists, for I was recommending the incorporation of *some* unsaturated fat in the diet in 1941, when virtually everyone in the field of nutrition was agreed that it made no difference whether fat was taken in the saturated or unsaturated form. Having settled on 20 percent unsaturated fat in the diet, we are now left with another unknown: What percentage of your total diet is derived from fat? In the American diet this might be 40 percent, and there are authorities who would like to see it lowered to thirty percent or less. * At this point you may decide that since the Vitamin-E requirement is partially set by the amount of unsaturated fat you eat, and we don't know that figure, that we are left with nothing but question marks. However, the authorities, juggling all these considerations, have come up with an educated guess that intake of somewhere between 15 and 30 mgs. of Vitamin E daily should take care of all eventualities. It is possible, but there is also the likelihood that two factors that raise the Vitamin-E requirement may operate more frequently than the authorities realize. It has long been known that a continued deficiency of Vitamin E in the body is the slowest of nutritional conditions to respond to treatment. The effects of four months of a diet lacking in the vitamin may not be overcome by a year of large doses of the factor. Therefore, if the person taking supplements of Vitamin E has previously eaten the average American diet with this factor removed from virtually all the breads and cereals, it may require a very long time to replenish reserves depleted by twenty or thirty years of attenuated gastronomic suicide.

At this point we have considered the need for Vitamin E as it is affected by the amount of unsaturated fat in the diet, and the length of time during which the individual has been eating a diet inadequately supplied with the vitamin. There is also the matter of giving the cells maximum protection against the oxidation processes we have been discussing. If you want to raise your Vitamin-E intake to a level that will achieve all these objectives, you will not be able to do it with food alone. You will have to use a supplement, one supplying at least 100 mgs. of Vitamin E per dose.

*On the other hand, there are thoughtful physicians and nutritionists who are aware that one way to encourage gall-bladder syndrome and gall stones is a low-fat diet. This doesn't explain why medical treatment for gall-bladder syndrome is almost invariably based on a low-fat diet, but that in turn does explain why diets restricted for gastrointestinal diseases have been termed irrational by an ad hoc committee of the American Medical Association.

Unfortunately, supplements have their own complexities. The form in which Vitamin E appears in nature is called "mixed tocopherols." Although each of these (alpha-, beta-, gamma-, and delta-tocopherol) is a form of Vitamin E, it is the alpha variety that is the most active in the human body. Current belief is that the other forms of Vitamin E are expendable, serving to protect alpha-tocopherol from oxidation. We can therefore conclude that a Vitamin-E supplement ideally should be in the form of a mixture of all these tocopherols, but that the potency should be expressed in terms of the alpha variety since that is the most active.*

A label might read: "Two hundred mgs. of mixed tocopherol, yielding the activity of 100 mgs. of alpha-tocopherol."

The figures given are illustrative.

When you survey the Vitamin-E shelf in the drug or health-food store, you will discover that mixed tocopherols come in several different forms. There is the oily and the nonoily. Alternately the nonoily may be called "dry" or "nonfatty." In lieu of these terms, you may encounter "mixed-tocopherol emulsion." If you are below the age of forty, in good health, and have no disorder that interferes with fat utilization, nor any sign of fat intolerance, the ordinary oily form of mixed tocopherols, with the potency expressed in alpha-tocopherol content, will be a suitable choice.

However, if you are over forty, your ability to manage fats has already begun to diminish. The sixty-year-old requires many hours to clear the fat content of a meal from the blood; the thirty-year-old metabolizes it in a fraction of the time. The fat-soluble vitamins — A, D, and E particularly — should be taken in the "nonfatty" ("dry" or "nonoily"), "emulsified" or water-dispersible forms when question marks surround the efficiency of the utilization of fatty substances, whether created by fat intolerance or gall-bladder syndrome, or arising as a concomitant of the aging process.

A parenthetical note of interest: A tablespoon of lecithin crystals or granules, or the equivalent in capsule form — perhaps some four or five 9-grain capsules daily — will often help the utilization not only of the fat-soluble vitamins, but of fats in general. In fact, a nutritionist may use lecithin to aid the person with gall-bladder syndrome or fat intolerance.

Since Vitamin E is only one of four dietary factors that might be

---

*It may be of interest to note that the Food and Drug Administration when calculating the amount of Vitamin E available in staple foods in the American diet, almost invariably has grouped all the forms of tocopherols together, which of course creates the impression that all the forms of Vitamin E are equally useful to the human body. It is a technique that makes the "average Vitamin-E intake" appear more adequate than it is.

labeled "antiaging," it would seem that we are devoting a disproportionate amount of this discussion to it. However, there are numerous controversies centering about Vitamin E, and an equal number of misunderstandings arising from them. It has been said that those who have searched in vain for Vitamin-E deficiency in the human being have been looking for very gross and easily observed disturbances in the function of the body. In other words, people who look for signs of nutritional deficiency in cracked lips, bowed legs, or bleeding gums could not use such standards to search for an inadequacy in Vitamin E, since an insufficient supply of this vitamin might — from what you have just read — exhibit itself only in a speeding up in the aging process. So it is that a deficiency of this vitamin might be to man what salt water is to a deep-sea fish — high on the list of phenomena unlikely to be discovered.

There are many reasons why this vitamin has occupied a blank spot in the professional eye for so many years. The problem began with the name for the vitamin, tocopherol, which delimited it to a role in reproduction. Second, there was the illusion deliberately created by the Food and Drug Administration that Vitamin E was not proved to be essential in human nutrition, although there was considerable evidence to the contrary. This in turn obscured the fact that this vitamin is removed from the foods that contribute 50 percent of the calories to the American diet. This is another way of saying that half our diet, in terms of calories, is derived from starches and sugars — and over 90 percent of these have been subjected to processing, which removes both the polyunsaturated fat (which we need) and the Vitamin E (the need is related to our intake of unsaturated fat). When the pressure of the evidence forced the government agency to recognize that Vitamin E is indeed essential to human beings, it promptly proceeded to deny the possibility of an inadequate supply of the vitamin in the human diet, despite the toll of processing.* Similarly, when evidence accumulated to show that a deficiency of Vitamin E induces some type of heart disturbance — ranging from dysfunction to heart failure and death — in every mammalian species, the Food and Drug Administration insisted that man was the sole mammal in which this deficiency had no such effect.

Actually, every survey of the American diet in any population group

*The value of Food and Drug Administration dogma about the adequacy of the American diet can be appraised by pondering the implications of a recent statement by the commissioner of that agency, who urged that we find out exactly what is the human requirement for Vitamin E. This plea was uttered some fifteen years after the agency had assured the public that no one could possibly be deficient in the vitamin.

at any income level has shown a sizable percentage of unsatisfactory intake of Vitamin E, however measured. Actual assays of heart tissues in patients who have died of heart disease have revealed strikingly low values for this vitamin as well as for certain others. These are facts that should provide food for thought in a country where cardiac disease is the number-one killer.

What you are reading in this book is documented, and, very often, that documentation is buttressed by my own observations of the responses of the sick and the ailing to certain vitamins or to nutritional therapy. I pose this background against a recent announcement by the *Medical Letter*, a technical publication for physicians, finding Vitamin E to be useless in the treatment of many disorders in which the public believes the vitamin to be effective. One would never know from the manner in which this pronouncement was delivered that the therapeutic effectiveness of Vitamin E in many disorders has been established in hundreds of medical papers published in virtually every country in the world, reflecting research performed by competent investigators, and reported in medical journals regarded as reliable sources of scientific information. Nor would one gather from the quotations in the announcement that it is merely an expression of opinion — plainly so labeled in the original text, but not so labeled in the story as it was carried by many newspapers. Thus the opinions expressed in the *Medical Letter* will have the force of fact in the eyes of physicians and the public. Yet these are nothing more than value judgments, and erroneous judgments at that.

You might remember that the authorities who are now telling you that you need not worry about Vitamin E are the same authorities who misinformed you concerning the importance of taking part of your fat in the unsaturated form, and are — likewise — the same authorities who assured you that since starches are converted into sugar in the body, it does not matter in which form you take your carbohydrate. History proved them wrong, and they admitted that their dogmatic advice about diet was invalid and contributed to the rising incidence of heart attacks. It would be a good investment therefore to follow the instructions for supplementing the diet with Vitamin E, as outlined in this chapter, and it might also be very wise to return to sanity by using wheat germ, whole grain, wheat-germ oil, and other foods rich in Vitamin E. Then, you will have taken care of the first requirement in the front line of defense against premature aging.

Vitamin E is the fat-soluble antioxidant for the body, and Vitamin C is the water-soluble antioxidant that works with Vitamin E. The technical term for their interaction is "synergism" — it is believed that the two vitamins have additive effects greater than the sum of their individual actions. Vitamin C also helps keep the permeability of cell membranes normal, an action it shares with adrenal hormones and with Vitamin B_{12}. And it reacts with the protein called glutathione, a scavenger that picks up the abnormal type of compound likely to be formed when ionizing radiation attacks the polyunsaturated fat in the cells. This activity, of course, suggests that a high intake of Vitamin C might be very important in slowing the rate of cellular aging. Moreover, it casts a new light on research that has indicated that higher levels of blood Vitamin C are compatible with survival. In other words, those with lower levels tend to die younger.

There are other protein factors that act as scavengers of abnormal compounds in the cell. These include some of the sulphur-containing compounds and an amino (protein) acid. Such a list should give cause for thought to those who have tried to prolong life by avoiding eggs, which are among the richest sources of the sulphur-containing amino acids. (Eggs are also a good source of lecithin, whose helpfulness has already been discussed. Arbitrary restrictions on the diet — however worthy the purpose — often become two-edged weapons, do they not?) Therefore, an adequate intake of these protein factors should help slow down aging.

There is a mineral that may be synergistic with Vitamin E and that certainly acts in a manner similar to that of the vitamin. This is selenium, which is both an antioxidant for fats and a water-soluble scavenger of these abnormal cellular compounds. What we don't know about selenium could fill a number of books. It is a touchy substance: Excess amounts are dangerous, our quantitative need has not been determined, and deficiencies may interfere with the action of Vitamin E. There appears to be a fair supply of selenium in a wide variety of foods, and we have already noted that in brewer's yeast there is a selenium-containing compound that is known to help the action of Vitamin E. This compound is known as "Factor 3." Its existence was discovered when brewer's yeast, containing it, proved helpful in the nutritional rehabilitation of malnourished children in Biafra, where torula yeast, lacking this factor, was ineffective.

Suffice it to say, we know of numerous nutrients that help protect the body from radiation, including certain vitamin and protein compounds. However incomplete our knowledge is, it at least contributes to the conclusion that the rate at which we age is partly determined by heredity, in part by cosmic radiation or something like it, and in part by the diet we eat. It may be that a genetic tendency toward accelerated aging is simply a corollary to a more constructive equation: Such genes dictate a heightened need for certain nutrients to offset that proclivity for premature aging. These nutrients you now know. It is apparent that the person who eats whole grains, citrus fruits, wheat germ, wheat-germ oil, and a high-protein diet, and who supplements his diet with Vitamin E, Vitamin C, the B Complex, and the bioflavonoids may be giving himself more protection than the authorities are willing to grant.

There is a fascinating vitamin that undoubtedly could play an important role in mitigating some of the degenerative changes that come with time. This is para-aminobenzoic acid, known to the chemist as "PABA." Since the individual vitamins and their actions are described elsewhere, I do not intend to tell the story of PABA here. But I do wish to point out that any factor that interacts with many hormones — including some of those produced by the pituitary, the adrenals, and the ovaries — and that in so doing tends to slow down or even to reverse loss of muscle tone, wrinkling, and graying of the hair, is worthy of mention in a discussion of dietary safeguards against premature aging. There are several methods of introducing PABA into one's diet, including eating the good foods that contain it, such as the whole grains, brewer's yeast, liver, and the organ meats. All foods and concentrates that supply the natural Vitamin B complex will automatically supply PABA. The so-called "enriched" carbohydrate food generally does not retain any significant amount, nor is the vitamin included in the enrichment program. So you who have eaten whole-wheat bread have had your PABA; you who have consumed cornflakes and puffed rice have diminished your supply.

Another way to obtain PABA is to see that it is included in any vitamin supplements you use. The quantity provided by the manufacturer is limited, in accordance with a long-standing policy of the Food and Drug Administration, which promptly puts quantitative limitations on any vitamin that threatens to benefit the public. At any rate, PABA is available both in multiple-vitamin supplements and in Vitamin-B-complex concentrates as well as in natural sources of the latter.

There are two other ways in which this vitamin may be used. Advertised in the medical journals is the potassium salt of para-aminobenzoic acid. The advertisements recommend this form of PABA in the treatment of arthritic and rheumatic disorders, which is interesting when one remembers that the Arthritis Foundation has insisted that no vitamin helps arthritis. It is necessary, however, to obtain a prescription in order to purchase this form.

For many years another form of para-aminobenzoic acid has been employed in research with large groups of aged people. In Romania, Dr. Anna Aslan has been giving the vitamin in the form of procaine — a local anesthetic, which is most widely known to American doctors and dentists under the trade name of "Novocain." As might have been predicted, Dr. Aslan's research has been greeted with jeers and catcalls by the American medical community. Not only did our medical people fail to realize that the claims made for Novocain injections by the European researchers largely overlap the findings of American doctors who have experimented with PABA, but very few physicians, in my experience, are aware that this vitamin is synergistic with estrogenic hormone, the corticosteroid hormones (the cortisone type), and insulin — to name just a few. Any nutritional factor with such a variety of interactions with hormones must have the potential to help preserve the effectiveness of glandular chemistries intimately related to our resistance to the aging process. The result of the American medical cynicism concerning the administration of PABA via injections of procaine was to create a black market for oral preparations of this vitamin, smuggled in from Europe and heralded as replacing injections of procaine as an aid to prolongation of the prime of life. Of course, these supplements had been vastly overpriced. Even worse, their effectiveness has been greatly overrated. This is not to say that doses of PABA by mouth do not have favorable effects, but rather that the procaine injections are more effective for some individuals and have actions beyond those that can be achieved by oral dosage.

When I became interested in Dr. Aslan's research with procaine, I asked a physician, a consultant to my staff, who was bound for Europe, to stop in at Dr. Aslan's institution in Romania and give me firsthand observations of the responses of her patients. We had heard that Dr. Aslan had started her research with a small group of aged people, that she was injecting procaine in large amounts, two or three times weekly, and that her results indicated not only a prolongation of the prime of life, but an actual reversal of the aging process. This physician — with whom I later wrote my book on low blood sugar — not only visited Dr. Aslan in accordance with my request, but also returned to her institution several times at intervals of three or four or five years. Thus, he was able to observe the long-term responses to procaine therapy of a group of people who were old at the time Dr. Aslan's research began.

The physician reported that he could not evaluate the subjective benefits claimed by the patients. He did see some instances where gray hair appeared to have darkened — an observation which I have made in response to vitamin therapies; he also noted that people who were at least sixty years old on the occasion of his first visit, and who then appeared to be vegetating in a fashion similar to those who live in old-age homes, were working in the library, the laboratory, or the office on his third or fourth visit, some ten years later.

I do not propose to detail all his observations, but it will suffice to note that procaine therapy became a part of this doctor's own standard treatment for older people.

American medical men promptly announced their cynicism. "Why," they asked, "should a local anesthetic display an action such as we might expect from a vitamin?" This type of query — which was also voiced by the medical editor of *Time* magazine — indicated that the cynical had not paused to look up the formula for procaine. It actually consists of a vitamin (PABA) linked with a solvent. Moreover, it is the vitamin for which similar claims of prolonging the prime of life have been made by the researchers in this country. I know this vitamin as a pituitary stimulant, with a marked influence on infertility in women and with an occasional aphrodisiac effect on men. I have personally watched administration of PABA recolor gray hair. I have seen it contribute to a therapeutic response to rheumatoid arthritis. I have seen a rise in estrogen activity in women who had been treated with this vitamin for various conditions caused by an undersupply of that hormone.

From the administration of procaine injections, I have seen similar responses. Indeed, the action on muscle tone in some subjects has been most remarkable, resulting in a change in the face or figure of some women that inspired their friends, who had not seen them in some time, to ask whether they had had plastic surgery. Perhaps the keenest memory of responses to procaine hovers about a venerable lady deep in her eighties, who was a patient of the physician who investigated Dr. Aslan's work. At the time that he first saw her, she was bedded, semi-conscious, and appeared to be terminal, with no particular disease to indict as the potential cause of death. He began the administration of the procaine injections, returning approximately three times a week to administer them. In the seventh or eighth week of his visits, he was told that the lady no longer required his services — she had gone for a walk in the park!

The procaine injections then — particularly if they are started early enough — may be an important contribution to retention of the characteristics of youth or prolongation of the prime of life. For those who do not wish to have the injections and who do not wish to pay the exorbitant sums asked for the European oral version of this therapy, there are supplements of PABA available, or a physician can prescribe the potassium salt of para-aminobenzoic acid.

I leave the topic of the procaine injections with the story of a dentist who rose at one of his profession's conventions and said that dentists give injections of procaine as a local anesthetic; therefore patients should, if Dr. Aslan's research is actually valid, be a little younger after each visit to a dentist's office. This public admission of ignorance was painful to hear. The dentist administers a small quantity of procaine, accompanied by a hormone to keep the injection from spreading in the tissue. The injection is obviously given infrequently. When Dr. Aslan or an American practitioner using procaine therapy administers the drug, it is given in large amounts, five cc's three times weekly, by deep intramuscular injection over a period of many weeks. The usual course of treatment is about eighteen or twenty weeks, with a four-to-six-week rest period and then a resumption of the injections.

Whether administered in the form of the procaine injections or in the form of PABA itself, this treatment is ideally calculated to help post-menopause women retain youth a little longer. By its interaction with whatever estrogen production remains in the body after menopause, PABA contributes to keeping the complexion from drying excessively. This action would be fortified by folic acid. I am aware as I write this that folic acid is regarded by most physicians as a vitamin used solely for the purpose of treating anemia. However, folic acid does contain PABA as part of its molecule and does exert some of the actions that we attribute to PABA itself. I use both in my work because I believe that folic acid may have other useful effects. You should be reminded here that since folic acid and PABA are members of the Vitamin B complex, the rest of the Vitamin B complex should always be taken simultaneously. This combination would bring in Vitamin B_{12}, which is important not only because it exerts certain actions that may help in the prolongation of the prime of life, but also because the administration of folic acid may hide an anemia resulting from a lack of B_{12}. The two vitamins should therefore always be taken together. Furthermore, it is never rational to use B-Complex vitamins one at a time, or for that matter, two at a time. There are interrelationships among the B vitamins; they work better together; and they are called a complex because they often appear in food together, making deficiency in just one or two of these factors rather unlikely.

The calcium intake is another part of the story of the prolongation of the characteristics of youth. Elsewhere in this book I have pointed out that calcium requirements may vary by a factor of four. Since you do not know what your requirement is, it is safer to assume that you require more rather than less. If you do not tolerate milk and do not eat sufficient cheese, it would be wise to use a calcium supplement. It may be taken in the form of dolomite, which also supplies magnesium, or as bone meal or dicalcium phosphate, or in forms ranging from powdered egg shell to powdered limestone and oyster shells. Contrary to cultist opinions, calcium is well utilized whether it is taken in the organic or inorganic form. Those who cannot tolerate milk are at something of a disadvantage, for milk sugar provides the acid medium in which calcium is better utilized. * I have already indicated that a gram of calcium is an amount that will cover virtually every conceivable level of requirement.

I shall not pause here, since the discussion will be found elsewhere in this book, to delineate the roles of other nutrients in helping one to look and feel younger longer than the calendar normally permits. A chapter could be written on the actions of Vitamin B_6 alone. Prolongation of the prime of life by supernutrition was reported by H. C. Sherman, of Columbia University decades ago. The truths of his observations remain unchallenged. Some Establishment nutritionists tend to fault Sherman's work on the grounds that his observations were made on laboratory animals. Such criticisms come with a singular lack of grace from a medical profession that has long used cats to evaluate the potency of digitalis. Assuming all other factors are equal, we can collectively (not personally) make a promise to the public: If you use vitamins intelligently, if you take the procaine injections or use the equivalent oral dose of PABA and folic acid, and if you follow faithfully the tenets of diet as they are outlined in this and other texts by competent authors, there is every reason to expect that you will avoid, mitigate, or delay many of the changes that take the fun out of living and that are regarded as an inevitable toll of time itself. The average multiple or Vitamin-B-complex supplement will supply about 20 mgs. of PABA. This intake might be adequate for a young person who is using vitamins preventively, but for those who want to explore its usefulness in slowing down or reversing accelerated aging, PABA is available as a single vitamin in tablet form, in potencies up to 100 mgs. Recommended

---

*There are many who are allergic to milk, and others who consider themselves to be so because consumption of milk is followed by cramps, flatulence, and diarrhea. Actually, these symptoms may be caused by lack of an enzyme, lactase, which is needed for splitting lactose (milk sugar). When milk sugar is allowed to remain in the digestive tract "unprocessed" for lack of the enzyme, fermentation takes place, yielding these unpleasant symptoms. This is an interesting example of an individual difference, and one which, incidentally, is more frequent in black people than in other races. For such individuals, milk and cheese cannot be used as sources of calcium. Since dairy products are about the only staple foods rich in the mineral, individuals so disadvantaged must use calcium supplements. The only food that contains calcium in high concentrations and that is not of dairy origin is Tahini, a kind of sesame seed butter used as a spread on bread. Consumption of this is unlikely to be great enough to supply calcium in adequate amounts daily, however.

quantities of folic acid and calcium have already been outlined, although it is possible that for some aging individuals intake of these factors should be raised too.

Some of my readers may be concerned with glaring omissions in this chapter. What of exercise? Frankly, I have no expertise on which to base judgment, nor any desire to acquire it. It is possible to assemble evidence that exercise shortens life and equally impressive evidence that it lengthens it. The psychologically oriented will ask about emotional factors in aging. I have perhaps a better vantage point in this area and will remark merely that the outwardly turned mind tends to be self-healing and to remain younger. But what is more important than any of these observations is the one fundamental truth, operative whether you are discussing nutrition, exercise, or the emotional environment versus the aging process: You must remember that time of itself is not toxic, and the calendar of itself does not determine your age.

9.
SHELF LIFE OR YOUR LIFE

In the mid 1960s I came into a violent collision with the Establishment on the subject of food additives, one in particular, which is an ingredient of hundreds of popular foods — butylhydroxytoluene.

I had been watching with growing uneasiness the increasing use of antioxidants in food products, especially those with a large fat content. Sometimes the label merely stated "freshness preserver." Sometimes it read "antistaleness ingredient." Other labels announced the presence of "BHT," which turned out to be chemical shorthand for butylhydroxytoluene. Other labels read "BHA," the initials for butylhydroxyanisole. Another popular preserver was "propyl gallate."

Questions arose concerning these and other additives. Who, for instance, is benefited by their presence? The public? The manufacturer? How safe are these preservatives? On the basis of what kind of research was their safety established? Was it with mice or men?

I did not realize that the search for the answers to these questions would embroil me in a running battle with the chemical industry, the food industry, and those who believe that preservatives are innocent until proved guilty, such as Stare of Harvard, and the Food and Drug Administration.

I selected BHT as the first subject of investigation. What I learned was disquieting — so much so that to this very day I will not permit foods preserved with this antioxidant in my home. Over the years in which I pursued this investigation, I learned that the World Health Organization of the United Nations had labeled BHT as the most suspect of all antistaleness food additives. The *Australian Medical Journal* had published a paper reporting the administration of BHT to pregnant mice had resulted in the birth of 15 percent of the young without eyes. The British Ministry of Food had considered banning the chemical completely (and, incidentally, still has it under consideration), but had compromised in the interim by restricting its use to cooking oils and limiting the amount to one-half the level permitted by the United States Food and Drug Administration. West Germany banned the use of this preservative with one exception — it can be added to emergency rations for use by the army, where a long "shelf life" is obviously more a service to the military than to the food manufacturers. Sweden and Romania banned BHT completely. Yet here it was in what appeared to be a thousand American foods, ranging from breakfast cereal to salad oil, from luncheon meats to chewing gum.

The next step was to ascertain on what basis the United States Food and Drug Administration had decided that its counterparts in the German, Swedish, Romanian and British governments were wrong, and that Americans could safely swallow many common foods seasoned with a chemical that began its career as an antioxidant used solely to preserve the colors in motion-picture film.

The United States Food and Drug Administration proved singularly reluctant to release any information on the research that demonstrated to its apparent satisfaction that butylhydroxytoluene was a safe preservative to feed to several hundred million Americans. Despite the Freedom of Information Act and despite inquiries by several members of the Congress, the agency dragged its feet until great pressure was brought by Consumers' Union. Then the Food and Drug Administration reluctantly released the papers. The reason for official procrastination quickly became apparent: There were only two meaningful papers, and both of them had been written by manufacturers of BHT. I am not trying to earn a reputation as a cynic, but let it be recognized that research by the staff that synthesizes the chemical very seldom finds it unfit for sale.

I then decided to bring this information to the attention of the public on my ABC network broadcasts. This was easier said than done, for the network censors found the story to be virtually incredible, and I had to submit detailed documentation for every statement — which I did. When the public heard the story of butylhydroxytoluene, they reacted by writing thousands of letters to me, announcing that they would no longer buy breakfast cereal, luncheon meat, or anything that contained BHT.

I returned to the subject in a succeeding broadcast and pointed out that such a boycott would be completely meaningless unless the manufacturers were advised and told the reason for it. The concrete example I used was a major cereal company, which sells 324 million dollars worth of largely foodless cereals yearly. I remarked that even 10,000 boycotters would make no significant dent on the gargantuan sales of such a company. Their absence would not be noted. But, I told the public, if those of you who stop buying the cereal write to the manufacturer and indicate why, you may be astonished to find that it does not require hundreds of thousands or even tens of thousands of such letters to provoke a prompt and constructive reaction. The example I gave to affirm this truth was the capitulation of a television network when *eleven* letters were received, objecting to identification of all of the gangsters in the "Untouchables" as being Italian. The result was that the writers were instructed to make indefinite the ethnic background of the criminals in future episodes!

The public acted upon this suggestion, and hundreds of letters came to a substantial number of manufacturers of food products ranging from breakfast cereal to spices, from macaroni to luncheon meats. The spice manufacturer was the first to react. He responded to these letters by announcing that his chemists had reviewed the formulation of the particular product in which BHT was an ingredient and had come to the conclusion that the preservative was actually not necessary. (I should like to meet the salesman who sold the idea of the antistaleness ingredient to them!) A large cereal company responded with a letter indicating that its customers should not listen to crackpots on the radio. A major manufacturer of cookies and crackers wrote a rather snide letter, which suggested that matters like these are best left in the hands of the men with the white jackets — which was to say, I concluded, that we idiots should certainly be willing to accept and to swallow uncomplainingly and uncritically whatever scientists decide we should. For several years a spaghetti manufacturer responded to all letters by announcing that he was "investigating Dr. Fredericks' research." Since I had not claimed to have performed any research with BHT, it was remarkable that the company thought this statement seemed an adequate reply from a major manufacturer to anxious customers.

There are two endings to this story. Twenty-seven major manufacturers discarded the use of butylhydroxytoluene as their final response to communications from my radio listeners. But, don't mistake me! Most of them did it only temporarily, waiting for the end of the broadcast series, well aware that the public would lapse back into apathy. A few, however, did not restore the objectionable ingredient. A major soup company, for instance, in its final responses to complaining customers, remarked: "We do not for a moment believe that butylhydroxytoluene presents any danger, but we do not wish to contribute to the anxieties of our customers!" Another by-product of those broadcasts — which you must remember were delivered at a time when anyone who displayed anxiety about the American food supply or the additives used in it was automatically excommunicated from the world of science as some kind of crackpot — was a sudden outburst from the American Chemical Society, of which I was a member for many years. In a monograph on the subject of food additives, the Society wrote: "Carlton Fredericks, the controversial broadcaster, conducted a crusade against butylhydroxytoluene." I wrote to the Society to indicate that I had not in fact conducted a crusade. I had made it plain that the decision — whether or not to swallow BHT — remained with the listener. I merely wanted to be sure that he knew exactly what he was swallowing. A paragraph from my letter to the American Chemical Society, which in the spirit of fair play they were perfectly willing to print and did, read: "I am a controversial broadcaster, I believe, because my remarks on butylhydroxytoluene derive from statements by the World Health Organization, the British Ministry of Food, the *Medical Journal of Australia*, and similar sources. Had I chosen instead to quote the statements of the chemical industry that manufactures butylhydroxytoluene, I should assume that I would be a respectable member of the Establishment." I added the suggestion that members of the Society remember the old story of the woman at a cocktail party who told her husband that he had too much to drink and must stop. Indignantly, he asked her how she knew he had had more than enough. To this she responded: "Because your face is getting all blurred." (The Society published that story, too.)

As the concepts of ecology and pollution have become popular, those who worry about internal pollution via food additives are no longer labeled controversial, or crackpots and hypochondriacs. Food processors have reacted to this new awareness in a predictable way. No longer able to insist that anyone who is worried about food additives is automatically off his rocker, they warn us instead that without these preservatives, the industry will simply not be able to meet the growing food needs of humanity's billions.

You may recall that the response to Rachel Carson's *Silent Spring* was identical. We were first told that Rachel Carson had no business expressing opinions about DDT — she was only a marine biologist and therefore "writing outside of the area of her competence." When this appeal did not prove persuasive, we were then told that banning of DDT would give us a "starvation spring."

The fact that many of these food additives have nothing to do with preserving food prevents the industry from defending them solely on the grounds that our victuals will turn to inedible and unnutritious garbage if they are outlawed. Manufacturers therefore have adopted a second line of attack which, in the words of the numerous writers whose living depends on the goodwill of the food and food-additive industries, says: "After all, food itself is nothing but a handful of chemicals. Food additives are all chemicals. If you swallow the first, why should you be apprehensive about swallowing the second?" It is my considered opinion that anyone who urges this specious doctrine is at best incompetent or, at worst, a compliant tool of the oligarchy who control food processing, additive manufacturing, and distribution of much of the information and misinformation about nutrition, which reaches us in our newspapers, women's magazines, children's textbooks, and other mass media.

To urge the acceptance of food additives on the grounds that they are simply chemicals, exactly as food is an aggregation of chemicals, requires blindness to the obvious fact that the body has had millions of years in which to adapt to food chemicals. The vast majority of the additives have no counterpart in nature; therefore the body has no physiological experience with them, and the results of their continued ingestion must be learned the hard way.

The potent food industry and its sycophant writers espouse another doctrine of which the public is apparently completely unaware. It is obviously their point of view that food additives should be considered innocent until use by the public demonstrates that they are not safe. At least one newspaper, appalled by this philosophy, recently dropped a column originating with the heavily subsidized Harvard Nutrition Department, on the specific grounds that testing of additives on the public does not provide the kind of "protection" of the public with which the newspaper would wish to be identified. The presence of BHT in foodless cereals, chewing gum, or candy cannot be justified on the grounds of preserving nutritional values. In fact, if candy, chewing gum, and most sticky cereals disappeared from the market, any conscientious dentist would applaud. Moreover, the addition of BHT to chewing gum is an additional insùlt, for the composition of this American confection is already so dubious that chewing it becomes an adventure into the unknown. Even the term "gum base," which manufacturers of chewing gum are permitted to use, hides a surprising number of strange ingredients.

The story of BHA lets the nutritionist rest no easier. Its application to the skin of animals has routinely resulted in skin cancer. When informed of this report, an officer of the Food and Drug Administration dismissed it contemptuously. "That," he snorted, "is *British* research."

Manufacturers of the foodless cereals will justify the use of BHA and BHT on the grounds that they help to preserve the "nutritional values" of the products. Aside from the fact that most of the nutritional values claimed for these cereals come from the milk that we add to them, one wonders what was in the cornflakes in 1935 when this alphabet soup of additives had not been invented, yet these cereals were advertised as veritable bonanzas of good nutrition. Which is to say, there is no question that there is misrepresentation; it is only its date that remains in question.

It is at this point that some readers may join the school of "It's going to happen to George — not to me." and ask: "Of the 2,500 substances that are now being used as food additives, how many have ever been demonstrated to be harmful to a single person?" This is, of course, begging the question. The origin of the cancer that kills you is seldom established. But cancer authorities will tell you that there is no doubt that twenty or thirty years may elapse between the physiological insult and the advent of cancer. Despite repeated assurances that the proper use of pesticides carries no danger for the public, a Mayo Clinic physician has had no hesitation in flatly charging certain pesticides with the responsibility for causing certain cases of leukemia. If minute quantities of these unphysiological chemicals can cause an allergy, there is the possibility that they likewise can touch off sickness. Idiosyncrasy of reaction need not be expressed only as hives or asthma, which means that there are individual differences in tolerances to these chemicals exactly as there are to foodstuffs themselves. (Dr. Theron Randolph tells the story of a patient who had a violent allergic reaction that was traced to an antifungus chemical sprayed on oranges that had been brought into her home, sealed in a paper bag, and stored several rooms away from her.)

It is estimated that more than 2,500 chemicals are presently added to our food supply for the purposes of preserving, dyeing, and flavoring, as well as for various other purposes. We have already learned through hard experience that agents considered to be safe, because they have been used without apparent harm for decades, may not necessarily be innocuous. Numerous coal-tar dyes labeled safe even ten years ago have since been demonstrated to be capable of causing cancer in animals and as a consequence, have been taken off the market. A vanilla substitute was found capable of causing tumors after we used it in our food supply for some thirty years. The safety of saccharin has recently been questioned, and yet it has been marketed to diabetics and others for more than a half century. An ingredient used to make root beer and other types of soda foam — safrole — was discovered to be tumor producing and forced off the market. Red #4, used to tint maraschino cherries and drug tablets, was withdrawn when a carcinogenic effect on dogs was demonstrated. However, the pharmaceutical manufacturers succeeded in prolonging the use of this questionable dye by taking advantage of a loophole in the law that permits hearings to drag out. Red #2, used in so many foods that sales of the dye aggregated some ten million dollars a year, and responsible for the tint in some ten *billion* dollars worth of food and beverages yearly, was recently discovered to reduce fertility. A plasticizer that makes food wrap flexible has also been used to soften the plastic bags containing blood transfusions. In its latter use, it has been accused of causing some deaths. This observation was made in Vietnam, but subsequently the plasticizer has been detected in the blood of civilians who never had blood transfusions. "Shock lung," the condition caused by the plasticizer, has been on the increase in the United States. Is the plasticizer responsible? If so, which source of it is the significant one? Are we getting an overdose from the large quantity of the material in the vinyl upholstery in our cars, or is it being transferred from the food wrap to the food itself? Do plastic disposable gloves, from which the plastic can transfer to the foods being handled, contribute to the problem? And what is the significance of the fact that the Food and Drug Administration labeled as low in toxicity the very plasticizer now being subjected to this searching investigation by a group at Johns Hopkins University?

It must be obvious that certification of a food additive by the Food and Drug Administration may be meaningful or meaningless. It is apparent that the label "generally regarded as safe," which is an official classification of many additives, constitutes again no guarantee of safety. It is also apparent that the consumer must ultimately come to grips with this problem — either decide to swallow unhesitatingly whatever the men in the white jackets choose to add to food; or go to the other extreme, rejecting all ingredients he cannot pronounce; or take the middle-of-the-road position, which is that of the author, avoiding additives that serve no useful purpose for the consumer himself. The latter position is not hard to define — we are all aware that cherry soda is red by virtue of artificial color, and the cherry flavor is likewise artificial. Flavoring agents generally have not been found guilty of toxicity, but food colors are a very suspect group. If you must drink soda — and the wisdom of drinking such concoctions is itself questionable — would it not be reasonable to insist that the sin of artificial flavor not be compounded with the risk of artificial color? Of course, one may ask why you don't drink fruit juice, instead?

Additives are used for many purposes: They are anticaking agents, preservatives, nutrients and dietary supplements, emulsifying agents, sequestrants, stabilizers, flavoring agents, dyes, flavor enhancers, and sweetening agents. Apart from amino acids, vitamins, and minerals, a list of the additives "generally regarded as safe" by the Food and Drug Administration is a formidable one:

SYNTHETIC FLAVORING SUBSTANCES

Acetaldehyde
Acetoin
Aconitic acid
Anethole
Benzaldehyde
N-butyric acid
d- or l-carvone
Cinnamaldehyde
Citral
Decanal
Diacetyl
Ethyl acetate
Ethyl butyrate

Ethyl vanillin
Eugenol
Geraniol
Geranyl acetate
Glycerol tributyrate
Limonene
Linalool
Linalyl acetate
1-malic acid
Methyl anthranilate
3-Methyl-3-phenyl glycidic acid
    ethyl ester
Piperonal

Vanillin

CHEMICAL PRESERVATIVES

Ascorbic acid
Ascorbyl palmitate
Benzoic acid

Butylated hydroxyanisole
Butylated hydroxytoluene
Calcium ascorbate

Calcium propionate
Calcium sorbate
Caprylic acid
Dilauryl thiodipropionate
Erythorbic acid
Gum guaiac
Methylparaben
Potassium bisulfite
Potassium metabisulfite
Potassium sorbate
Propionic acid
Propyl gallate

Propylparaben
Sodium ascorbate
Sodium benzoate
Sodium bisulfite
Sodium metabisulfite
Sodium propionate
Sodium sorbate
Sodium sulfite
Sorbic acid
Stannous chloride
Sulfur dioxide
Thiodipropionic acid

Tocopherols

ANTICAKING AGENTS

Aluminum calcium silicate
Calcium silicate
Magnesium silicate

Sodium aluminosilicate
Sodium calcium aluminosilicate
Tricalcium silicate

STABILIZERS

Acacia (gum arabic)
Agar-agar
Ammonium alginate
Calcium alginate
Carob bean gum
Chondrus extract

Ghatti gum
Guar gum
Potassium alginate
Sodium alginate
Sterculia (or karaya) gum
Tragacanth

SEQUESTRANTS

Calcium acetate
Calcium chloride
Calcium citrate
Calcium diacetate
Calcium gluconate
Calcium hexametaphosphate
Calcium phosphate, monobasic
Calcium phytate
Citric acid
Dipotassium phosphate

Disodium phosphate
Isopropyl citrate
Monoisopropyl citrate
Potassium citrate
Sodium acid phosphate
Sodium citrate
Sodium diacetate
Sodium gluconate
Sodium hexametaphosphate
Sodium metaphosphate

Sodium phosphate
Sodium potassium tartrate
Sodium pyrophosphate
Sodium pyrophosphate, tetra

Sodium tartrate
Sodium thiosulfate
Sodium tripolyphosphate
Stearyl citrate

Tartaric acid

EMULSIFYING AGENTS

Cholic acid
Desoxycholic acid
Diacetyl tartaric acid esters of mono- and diglycerides
Glycocholic acid

Mono- and diglycerides
Monosodium phosphate derivatives of above
Propylene glycol
Ox bile extract

Taurocholic acid

MISCELLANEOUS ADDITIVES

Acetic acid
Adipic acid
Aluminum ammonium sulfate
Aluminum potassium sulfate
Aluminum sodium sulfate
Aluminum sulfate
Ammonium bicarbonate
Ammonium carbonate
Ammonium hydroxide
Ammonium phosphate
Ammonium sulfate
Beeswax
Bentonite
Butane
Caffeine
Calcium carbonate
Calcium chloride
Calcium citrate
Calcium gluconate
Calcium hydroxide
Calcium lactate
Calcium oxide
Calcium phosphate
Caramel
Carbon dioxide

Carnauba wax
Citric acid
Dextrans
Ethyl formate
Glutamic acid
Glutamic acid hydrochloride
Glycerin
Glyceryl monostearate
Helium
Hydrochloric acid
Hydrogen peroxide
Lactic acid
Lecithin
Magnesium carbonate
Magnesium hydroxide
Magnesium oxide
Magnesium stearate
Malic acid
Methylcellulose
Monoammonium glutamate
Monopotassium glutamate
Nitrogen
Nitrous oxide
Papain
Phosphoric acid

Potassium acid tartrate
Potassium bicarbonate
Potassium carbonate
Potassium citrate
Potassium hydroxide
Potassium sulfate
Propane
Propylene glycol
Rennet
Silica aerogel
Sodium acetate
Sodium acid pyrophosphate
Sodium aluminum phosphate
Sodium bicarbonate
Sodium carbonate

Sodium citrate
Sodium carboxymethylcellulose
Sodium caseinate
Sodium citrate
Sodium hydroxide
Sodium pectinate
Sodium phosphate
Sodium potassium tartrate
Sodium sesquicarbonate
Sodium tripolyphosphate
Succinic acid
Sulfuric acid
Tartaric acid
Triacetin
Triethyl citrate

In addition to additives "generally regarded as safe" that sometimes turn out not to be, there are also hundreds of chemicals that must be demonstrated to be safe before their addition to food is permitted. Some unusual loopholes have opened for manufacturers hastening to place these products on the market. At the time these notes were gathered, it was possible for a manufacturer unilaterally to make the decision that his particular additive was "generally regarded as safe," which obviously incorporated the proposition that the additive would be considered innocent until proved guilty. Loopholes like these have generally been closed, but additives are proliferating, and the expense of testing is so great that even the task of reexamining the safety of long-accepted flavors constitutes a capital investment which may be well beyond the financial capability of private industry.

There are two extremely disturbing elements in this situation, besides the sheer arithmetic of the hundreds of additives not yet tested for safety that we are swallowing. One is that the tests for additives are made individually, although we know that there are situations where one and one do not make two, but four — which means that the interaction between two chemicals very often is unpredictable. Innocuous substances may combine to produce cancer-producing agents, for instance. An example of this is the interaction among the nitrites and nitrates, and the meats to which they are added. The resulting reaction may produce a member of the most active cancer-producing chemical family yet discovered. In addition, there is also the matter of pesticide residues. Certainly the average person has no concept of the variety of pesticides that legally may be applied to fruits and vegetables. There *are* restrictions on quantity, and certain rules that govern the use of more than one pesticide at a time. Pesticides in the same chemical family, for instance, must be used in such a way that the combined quantity does not exceed the allowance for residue that would be allocated to *one* of the chemicals. Pesticides that share a common ingredient must also comply with such regulation. The following lists give a somewhat exaggerated view of the scope of the problem — but there is no exaggeration in this observation:

1. We are swallowing a fearful number of chemicals that come to us as food additives or as by-products of pesticide usage.

2. Some of these agents are unbelievably toxic. A pair of jeans, for example, had been stained with an insecticide permitted for use on apples (legal residue one part per million). Though the stain was dry, the wearer of the jeans landed in the hospital. This is not surprising, for the pesticide is chemically related to the nerve gases considered too horrible for the American military to store, much less use. Some of these agents are also known to be cancer-producing.

3. The fact that limits are set on the residues of pesticides that may be present on a crop is not reassuring when the Food and Drug Administration has repeatedly complained that it does not have the manpower to inspect more than 1 percent of the fresh produce that enters the market. It ought to be noted here that this agency seems to have an inexhaustible supply of inspectors to implement its effort to stamp out the vitamin and health-food industries. In fact, during the week when the agency was complaining that it did not have the available manpower to inspect the Bon Vivant plant so that the botulism tragedy might have been prevented, numerous seizures were made in health-food stores across the country. If you are curious concerning this imbalance in the allocation of manpower and the motives behind it, you will find the full story in the appendix.

The following is a list of some common fruits and vegetables, accompanied by lists of the insecticides that may be legally applied to them (regulations at the time the book was written, subject to change), and the residues that may be left upon them as they come to market, subject to the rules concerning chemicals of the same family or composition, previously cited.

APPLES

Aldrin — 0.25 ppm

Bacillus Thuringiensis Berliner — exemption

Benzene Hexachloride — 5 ppm

2-(p-tert-Butylphenoxy) — Isopropyl-2-Chloroethyl Sulfite — zero

Captan — 100 ppm

Chlorbenside — 3 ppm (including its sulfoxide and sulfone oxidation products)

Chlordane — 0.3 ppm

p-Chlorophenyl Phenyl Sulfone — 8 ppm

1,1-bis (p-Chlorophenyl)-2,2,2-Trichloroethanol — 5 ppm

S-(p-Chlorophenylthiomethyl) 0,0,-Diethyl Phosphorodithioate — 0.8 ppm

DDT — 7 ppm

Demeton — 0.75 ppm

Diazinon — 0.75 ppm

Dichlone — 3 ppm

2,4-Dichlorophenoxy Acetic Acid — 5 ppm

Dicyclohexylamine Salt of Dinitro-o-Cyclohexylphenol — 1 ppm

Dieldrin — 0.25 ppm

0,0-Dimethyl S - (4-oxo-1,2,3-Benzotriazin-3 (4H) Ylmethyl) Phosphorodithioate — 2 ppm

Dodine — 5 ppm

EPN — 3 ppm

Ethion — 1 ppm

Ethoxyquin — 3 ppm

Ethyl 4,4'-Dichlorobenzilate — 5 ppm

Ethylene — exemption

Ferbam — 7 ppm

Glyodin — 5 ppm

Heptachlor and Heptachlor Epoxide — zero

6,7,8,9,10,10-Hexachloro-1,5,5a,6,9,9a;Hexahydro-6,9-Methano-2,4,3-Benzodioxathiepin-3-oxide — 2 ppm

Lead Arsenate — 7 ppm

Lindane — 10 ppm

Malathion — 8 ppm*

Maneb — 7 ppm

Maganous Dimethyldithiocarbamate — 7 ppm

Mercaptobenzothiazole — 0.1 ppm

1-Methoxycarbonyl-1-propen -2-yl Dimethyl Phosphate and its Beta Isomer — 0.5 ppm

---

*I am reminded here that pesticides considered to be nontoxic to warm-blooded creatures or to have very limited toxicity to organisms other than insects are not always what they seem. I recall reading a statement that Malathion, dumped on the orange groves of Florida in an effort to stamp out the fruit fly, would have virtually no effect on fish, save perhaps on fingerlings (very young fish). I read the story on the patio at my Miami Beach home, which is backed by Indian Creek — and as I read, floating down the creek came hundreds of fish, some of them over two feet in length, belly side up and very dead.

Methoxyclor — 14 ppm
Methyl Bromide as inorganic Bromide — 5 ppm
Naphthalene Acetic Acid — 1 ppm
Nicotine-containing compounds — 2 ppm
Ovex — 3 ppm
Parathion — 1 ppm
Phenothiazine — 7 ppm
Sodium 2,2-Dichloropropionate — 3 ppm
Sodium o-Phenylphenate — 25 ppm
TDE — 7 ppm
Thiram — 7 ppm
Toxaphene — 7 ppm
Zineb — 7 ppm
Ziram — 7 ppm

APRICOTS

Aldrin — 0.25 ppm
Benzene Hexachloride — 5 ppm
Captan — 100 ppm
Chlordane — 0.3 ppm
1,1-bis (p-Chlorophenyl)-2,2,2-Trichloroethanol — 10 ppm
S-(p-Chlorophenylthiomethyl) 0,0-Diethyl Phosphorodithioate — 0.8 ppm
DDT — 7 ppm
Demeton — 0.75 ppm
Diazinon — 0.75 ppm
Dicyclohexylamine Salt of Dinitro-o-Cyclohexylphenol — 1 ppm
Dieldrin — 0.1 ppm
0,0-Dimethyl S-(4-oxo-1,2,3-Benzotriazin-3(4H) Ylmethyl) Phosphorodithioate — 2 ppm
EPN — 3 ppm
Ferbam — 7 ppm

6,7,8,9,10,10-Hexachloro-1,5,5a,6,9,9a-Hexahydro-6,9-Methano-2,4,3-Benzodioxathiepin-3-oxide — 2 ppm
Lead Arsenate — 7 ppm
Lindane — 10 ppm
Malathion — 8 ppm
Maneb — 10 ppm
Methoxychlor — 14 ppm
Methyl Bromide as inorganic Bromide — 20 ppm
Nicotine-containing compounds — 2 ppm
Parathion — 1 ppm
Sodium 2,2-Dichloropropionate — 1 ppm
TDE — 7 ppm
Toxaphene — 7 ppm
Zineb — 7 ppm
Ziram — 7 ppm

ASPARAGUS

Aldrin — 0.1 ppm
Benzene Hexachloride — 5 ppm
Calcium Arsenate — 3.5 ppm
DDT — 7 ppm
Dieldrin — 0.1 ppm
Ethylene Dibromide as inorganic Bromide — 10 ppm
Ferbam — 7 ppm
Lead Arsenate — 7 ppm
Lindane — 10 ppm
Malathion — 8 ppm
Methoxychlor — 14 ppm
Nicotine-containing compounds — 2 ppm
Sodium 2,4-Dichlorophenoxyacetate — 5 ppm

Sodium 2,2-Dichloropropionate —
 30 ppm
Sesone — 2 ppm

BARLEY GRAIN

Aldrin — 0.1 ppm
Dieldrin — 0.1 ppm
*Ethylene Dibromide as inorganic
 Bromide* — 50 ppm
Heptachlor and Heptachlor Epoxide —
 zero
Malathion — 8 ppm

BEETS (GARDEN)

Aldrin — 0.25 ppm
Captan — 100 ppm
Chlordane — 0.3 ppm
*S-(p-Chlorophenylthiomethyl)
 0,0-Diethyl Phosphorodithioate*
 — 0.8 ppm
DDT — 7 ppm
Diazinon — 0.75 ppm
Dieldrin — 0.25 ppm
EPN — 3 ppm
Ferbam — 7 ppm
Heptachlor and Heptachlor Epoxide —
 zero
Malathion — 8 ppm
Methoxychlor — 14 ppm
Methyl Bromide as inorganic Bromide
 — 30 ppm
Nicotine-containing compounds —
 2 ppm
Parathion — 1 ppm
Zineb — 7 ppm
Ziram — 7 ppm

BEETS (SUGAR)

Aldrin — 0.1 ppm
Captan — 100 ppm
*S-(p-Chlorophenylthiomethyl)
 0,0-Diethyl Phosphorodithioate*
 — 5 ppm
Demeton — 5 ppm
*0,0,-Diethyl S-2-(Ethylthio) Ethyl
 Phosphorodithioate* — 2 ppm
Endrin — zero
Heptachlor and Heptachlor Epoxide —
 0.1 ppm
Methyl Bromide as inorganic Bromide
 — 30 ppm
Sodium 2,2-Dichloropropionate —
 5 ppm

BROCCOLI

Aldrin — 0.25 ppm
Benzene Hexachloride — 5 ppm
Calcium Arsenate — 3.5 ppm of
 combined As_2O_3
Captan — 100 ppm
Chlordane — 0.3 ppm
DDT — 7 ppm
Demeton — 0.75 ppm
Diazinon — 0.75 ppm
*1,1-Dichloro-2,2-bis
 (p-Ethylphenyl)
 Ethane* — 15 ppm
Dieldrin — 0.25 ppm
*0,0-Dimethyl S-(4-oxo-1,2,3-
 Benzotriazin-3 (4H) Ylmethyl)
 Phosphorodithioate* — 2 ppm
*Ethylene Dibromide as inorganic
 Bromide* — 75 ppm
Ferbam — 7 ppm
Lindane — 10 ppm

Malathion — 8 ppm
Maneb — 10 ppm
1-Methoxycarbonyl-1-Propen-2-yl Dimethyl Phosphate and its Beta Isomer — 1 ppm
Methoxychlor — 14 ppm
Parathion — 1 ppm
TDE — 7 ppm
Toxaphene — 7 ppm
Zineb — 7 ppm
Ziram — 7 ppm

BRUSSELS SPROUTS

Aldrin — 0.25 ppm
Benzene Hexachloride — 5 ppm
Calcium Arsenate — 3.5 ppm of combined As_2O_3
Captan — 100 ppm
Chlordane — 0.3 ppm
Copper Arsenate — 3.5 ppm of combined As_2O_3
DDT — 7 ppm
Demeton — 0.75 ppm
1,1-Dichloro-2,2-bis (p-Ethylphenyl) Ethane — 15 ppm
Dieldrin — 0.25 ppm
Ferbam — 7 ppm
Heptachlor and Heptachlor Epoxide — zero
Lindane — 10 ppm
Malathion — 8 ppm
Maneb — 10 ppm
1-Methoxycarbonyl-1-Propen-2-yl Dimethyl Phosphate and its Beta Isomer — 1 ppm
Methoxychlor — 100 ppm
Nicotine-containing compounds — 2 ppm
Parathion — 1 ppm

TDE — 7 ppm
Toxaphene — 7 ppm
Zineb — 7 ppm
Ziram — 7 ppm

CABBAGE

Aldrin — 0.25 ppm
Benzene Hexachloride — 5 ppm
Calcium Arsenate — 3.5 ppm of combined As_2O_3
Captan — 100 ppm
Chlordane — 0.3 ppm
Copper Arsenate — 3.5 ppm of combined As_2O_3
DDT — 7 ppm
Demeton — 0.75 ppm
Diazinon — 0.75 ppm
1,1-Dichloro-2,2-bis (p-Ethylphenyl) Ethane — 15 ppm
Dieldrin — 0.25 ppm
0,0-Diethyl S-2-(Ethylthio) Ethyl Phosphorodithioate — 0.75 ppm
0,0-Dimethyl S-(4-oxo-1,2,3-Benzotriazin-3 (4H) Ylmethyl) Phosphorodithioate — 2 ppm
Endrin — zero
Ferbam — 7 ppm
Heptachlor and Heptachlor Epoxide — 0.1 ppm
Lindane — 10 ppm
Malathion — 8 ppm
Maneb — 10 ppm
1-Methoxycarbonyl-1-Propen-2-yl Dimethyl Phosphate and its Beta Isomer — 1 ppm
Methoxychlor — 14 ppm
Nicotine-containing compounds — 2 ppm

Parathion — 1 ppm
TDE — 7 ppm
Toxaphene — 7 ppm
Zineb — 7 ppm
Ziram — 7 ppm

CANTALOUPE

Aldrin — 0.1 ppm
*2-(p-tert-Butylphenoxy)-
Isopropyl-2-Chloroethyl
Sulfite* — zero
Captan — 100 ppm
*1,1-bis (p-Chlorophenyl)-2,2,2-
Trichloroethanol* — 5 ppm
*S-(p-Chlorophenylthiomethyl)
0,0-Diethyl Phosphorodithioate*
— 0.8 ppm
Diazinon — 0.75 ppm
Dieldrin — zero
Ethyl 4,4-Dichlorobenzilate —
5 ppm
*Ethylene Dibromide as inorganic
Bromide* — 10 ppm
*1-Methoxycarbonyl-1-propen-
2-yl Dimethyl Phosphate and
its Beta Isomer* — 0.5 ppm
Methoxychlor — 14 ppm
Methyl Bromide as inorganic Bromide
— 20 ppm
Sodium o-Phenylphenate — 125 ppm
(of which no more than 10 ppm
shall be in the edible portion)

CARROTS

Aldrin — 0.25 ppm
Calcium Arsenate — 3.5 ppm of
combined As_2O_3
Captan — 100 ppm

Chlordane — 0.3 ppm
Copper Arsenate — 3.5 ppm of
combined As_2O_3
DDT — 7 ppm
Diazinon — 0.75 ppm
Dieldrin — 0.1 ppm
*Ethylene Dibromide as inorganic
Bromide* — 75 ppm
Ferbam — 7 ppm
Heptachlor and Heptachlor Epoxide —
zero
Malathion — 8 ppm
Maneb — 7 ppm
*1-Methoxycarbonyl-1-Propen-
2-yl Dimethyl Phosphate and
its Beta Isomer* — 0.25 ppm
Methoxychlor — 14 ppm
Methyl Bromide as inorganic Bromide
— 30 ppm
Parathion — 1 ppm
TDE — 7 ppm
Toxaphene — 7 ppm
Zineb — 7 ppm
Ziram — 7 ppm

CAULIFLOWER

Aldrin — 0.25 ppm
Benzene Hexachloride — 5 ppm
Calcium Arsenate — 3.5 ppm of
combined As_2O_3
Captan — 100 ppm
Chlordane — 0.3 ppm
Copper Arsenate — 3.5 ppm of
combined As_2O_3
DDT — 7 ppm
Demeton — 0.75 ppm
Diazinon — 0.75 ppm
*1,1-Dichloro-2,2-bis
(p-Ethylphenyl) Ethane* —
15 ppm

Dieldrin — 0.25 ppm
0,0-Dimethyl S-(4-oxo-1,2,3-
    Benzotriazin-*3 (4H) Ylmethyl)*
    Phosphorodithioate — 2 ppm
Ethylene Dibromide as inorganic
    Bromide — 10 ppm
Ferbam — 7 ppm
Heptachlor and Heptachlor Epoxide —
    zero
Lindane — 10 ppm
Malathion — 8 ppm
Maneb — 10 ppm
1-Methoxycarbonyl-1-Propen-
    2-yl Dimethyl Phosphate and
    its Beta Isomer — 1 ppm
Methoxychlor — 14 ppm
Nicotine-containing compounds —
    2 ppm
Parathion — 1 ppm
TDE — 7 ppm
Toxaphene — 7 ppm
Zineb — 7 ppm
Ziram — 7 ppm

CELERY

Aldrin — 0.1 ppm
Benzene Hexachloride — 5 ppm
Calcium Arsenate — 3.5 ppm
Captan — 100 ppm
Chlordane — 0.3 ppm
DDT — 7 ppm
Demeton — 0.75 ppm
Diazinon — 0.75 ppm
Dichlone — 3 ppm
2,4,-Dichloro-6-o-Chloroanilino-s-
    Triazine — 10 ppm
Dicyclohexylamine Salt of
    Dinitro-o-Cyclohexylphenol —
    1 ppm
Dieldrin — 0.25 ppm

Ferbam — 7 ppm
Lead Arsenate — 7 ppm
Lindane — 10 ppm
Malathion — 8 ppm
Maneb — 10 ppm
1-Methoxcarbonyl-1-Propen-
    2-yl Dimethyl Phosphate and
    its Beta Isomer — 1 ppm
Nicotine-containing compounds —
    2 ppm
Parathion — 1 ppm
Thiram — 7 ppm
Toxaphene — 7 ppm
Zineb — 7 ppm
Ziram — 7 ppm

CHERRIES

Aldrin — 0.1 ppm
Benzene Hexachloride — 5 ppm
Captan — 100 ppm
Chlordane — 0.3 ppm
1,1-bis (p-Chlorophenyl)-2,2,2-
    Trichloroethanol — 5 ppm
S-(p-Chlorophenylthiomethyl)
    0,0-Diethyl Phosphorodithioate
    — 0.8 ppm
DDT — 7 ppm
Diazinon — 0.75 ppm
Dichlone — 3 ppm
1,1-Dichloro-2,3-bis
    (p-Ethylphenyl) Ethane —
    15 ppm
Dicyclohexylamine Salt of Dinitro-o-
    Cyclohexylphenol — 1 ppm
Dieldrin — 0.25 ppm
0,0-Dimethyl S-(4-oxo-1,2,3-
    Benzotriazin-*3 (4H) Ylmethyl)*
    Phosphorodithioate — 2 ppm
EPN — 3 ppm

Ethylene Dibromide as total combined Bromide — 25 ppm
Ferbam — 7 ppm
Glyodin — 5 ppm
Heptachlor and Heptachlor Epoxide — zero
Lead Arsenate — 7 ppm
Lindane — 10 ppm
Malathion — 8 ppm
1(Methoxycarbonyl-1-Propen-2-yl Dimethyl Phosphate and its Beta Isomer — 1 ppm
Methoxychlor — 14 ppm
Methyl Bromide as inorganic Bromide — 20 ppm
Nicotine-containing compounds — 2 ppm
Parathion — 1 ppm
Sodium O-Phenylphenate — 5 ppm
TDE — 7 ppm
Zineb — 7 ppm
Ziram — 7 ppm

COLLARDS

Aldrin — 0.25 ppm
Benzene Hexachloride — 5 ppm
Calcium Arsenate — 3.5 ppm of combined As_2O_3
Captan — 100 ppm
Chlordane — 0.3 ppm
DDT — 7 ppm
Diazinon — 0.75 ppm
Dieldrin — 0.25 ppm
Ferbam — 7 ppm
Lindane — 10 ppm
Malathion — 8 ppm
Maneb — 10 ppm
1-Methoxycarbonyl-1-Propen-2-yl Dimethyl Phosphate and its Beta Isomer — 1 ppm

Methoxychlor — 14 ppm
Nicotine-containing compounds — 2 ppm
Parathion — 1 ppm
Toxaphene — 7 ppm
Zineb — 25 ppm
Ziram — 7 ppm

CRANBERRIES

Aldrin — 0.1 ppm
Captan — 100 ppm
DDT — 7 ppm
Diazinon — 0.75 ppm
Dieldrin — 0.1 ppm
Ferbam — 7 ppm
Lead Arsenate — 7 ppm
Malathion — 8 ppm
Maneb — 7 ppm
Methoxychlor — 14 ppm
Nicotine-containing compounds — 2 ppm
Parathion — 1 ppm
Toxaphene — 7 ppm
Zineb — 7 ppm
Ziram — 7 ppm

CUCUMBERS

Aldrin — 0.25 ppm
Benzene Hexachloride — 5 ppm
2-(p-tert-Butylphenoxy)-Isopropyl-2-Chloroethyl Sulfite — zero
Calcium Arsenate — 3.5 ppm of combined As_2O_3
Captan — 100 ppm
Chlordane — 0.3 ppm
1,1-bis (p-Chlorophenyl)- 2,2,2-Trichloroethanol — 5 ppm

S-(p-Chlorophenylthiomethyl)
0,0-Diethyl
Phosphorodithioate — 0.8 ppm
DDT — 7 ppm
Diazinon — 0.75 ppm
Dieldrin — 0.25 ppm
Endrin — zero
Ethylene Dibromide as inorganic
Bromide — 30 ppm
Ferbam — 7 ppm
Lindane — 10 ppm
Malathion — 8 ppm
Maneb — 7 ppm
1-Methoxycarbonyl-1-Propen-
2-yl Dimethyl Phosphate and
its Beta Isomer — 0.25 ppm
Methoxychlor — 14 ppm
Methyl Bromide as inorganic Bromide
— 30 ppm
Nicotine-containing compounds —
2 ppm
Parathion — 1 ppm
TDE — 7 ppm
Toxaphene — 7 ppm
Zineb — 7 ppm
Ziram — 7 ppm

ENDIVE

Aldrin — 0.25 ppm
Captan — 100 ppm
DDT — 7 ppm
Diazinon — 0.75 ppm
Dieldrin — 0.25 ppm
Malathion — 8 ppm
Maneb — 10 ppm
Parathion — 1 ppm
Zineb — 25 ppm

GARLIC

Aldrin — 0.25 ppm
Captan — 100 ppm
2,4-Dichloro(6-o-Chloroanilino-s-
Triazine — 1 ppm
Malathion — 8 ppm
Methyl Bromide as inorganic Bromide
— 50 ppm
Parathion — 1 ppm

GRAPEFRUIT

Aldrin — 0.25 ppm
Biphenyl — 110 ppm
2-(p-tert-Butylphenoxy)-
Isopropyl-2-
Chloroethyl Sulfite — zero
Captan — 100 ppm
S-(p-Chlorophenylthiomethyl)
0,0-Diethyl Phosphorodithioate
— 2 ppm
Demeton — 0.75 ppm
Dieldrin — 0.25 ppm
2,3-p-Dioxanedithiol S,S-bis
(0,0-Diethyl
Phosphorodithioate) —
2.8 ppm
Diphenyl — 110 ppm
Ethion — 1 ppm
Ethyl 4,4'-Dichlorobenzilate —
5 ppm
Malathion — 8 ppm
Monuron — 1 ppm
Ovex — 5 ppm
Sodium 2,2-Dichloropropionate —
5 ppm
Sodium o-Phenylphenate — 10 ppm

It is obvious that we are swallowing an enormous number of chemicals with which our bodies have not had previous experience. If your reaction to what you have read is like that of my college students, you will presently be reassuring yourself that the government has wisely limited the amount of chlordane on your apples to 0.3 parts per million — a ceiling so low that obviously the material is highly toxic. But don't be of good cheer. In order to keep pesticide residues from mounting too high, growers must obviously exercise two precautions: Spraying must not be excessive, and the use of pesticides must be stopped at a decent interval before the harvest. In response to this optimistic thought, let me voice my own cynicism, for which I have good reason. The use of diethylstilbestrol in fattening cattle has recently been brought under fresh scrutiny. Cancer has developed in some of the daughters of women who were dosed with the hormone twenty years ago. The response of the regulatory agencies was to lengthen the interval between the last administration of the hormone and the date of the slaughter of the cattle. But, as one livestock breeder remarked to me, "What do you do if you have just finished feeding the hormone to your steers, and a buyer comes in who wants to pick up $50,000 worth of meat, not tomorrow, the next day, or next week — but right at that very moment? Do you let him go his way, to some other fellow who is going to fracture the regulation, or do you fracture it yourself?" *

Indeed, it is this very possibility that was the "justification" for the most rank censorship of my radio broadcasts that I have encountered in some thirty years on the air. My program was literally forced off the air in Connecticut because I was discussing insecticide residue on apples. Joining in the assault on freedom of the press was one of the state agricultural experiment stations as well as representatives of the growers. The insurance company that owned the radio station promptly capitulated. If this shocks you, don't let it — Connecticut is also, as far as I know, the only state that published a list of "books not recommended for reading" — an expurgatory index, published by the State Health Department at the taxpayers' expense, and listing first, above all books not to be recommended, *Silent Spring* by Rachel Carson. This action, on the grounds that the book might cast suspicion on the Connecticut apple growers, who — as everyone but a cynical New Yorker

---

*As we go to press, the use of diethylstilbestrol in cattle feed has again been made legal.

might know — would never dream of using any insecticide in any way contrary to federal or state regulations!

Occasionally, attempts are made to reassure the housewife that much of the pesticide residue is removed in the household preparation of foods. Sometimes, a sizable amount of the residue is removed. If the material is soluble, two-thirds of it may be removed. Often, the percentage is less. In any case, it is never 100 percent, and there are undoubtedly millions of careless housewives who will serve apples and other fruit without the benefit of the most superficial washing.

When you consider the long list of additives and pesticides and realize that the testing for toxicity and carcinogenicity is individual — not on the composite witch's brew that we are swallowing — it will be perfectly understandable if you make the same decision that I have made for my own family. Given a choice between a food with no additives and the same with one additive, I'll choose none. Sometimes it requires searching, but the search can be rewarding. American dried potato products appear to contain more chemicals than potatoes. Yet there is a German product that contains nothing but potato and salt. There are imported cereals, available in both the supermarket and health-food store, which not only contain no additives and have not been contaminated with spray residues, but also are infinitely more nutritious than the confetti optimistically labeled as cereal by American manufacturers. And do not argue that they cost more. They are infinitely cheaper than liver disease or terminal cancer.

Given a choice between the food with one additive and the food with two additives, I'll choose the single additive. I go to the health-food store to avoid additives as much as possible. Although peeling of fruits is a poor practice nutritionally, it is a good practice in terms of pesticide residue — and I practice it. Even though there are no solvents or detergents that will remove all residues, I thoroughly wash all foods that are consumed raw. Although freezing destroys Vitamin K and blanching causes a loss of trace minerals and Vitamin C, the major freezers and the canners will maintain quality-control departments, in which a determined effort is made to exclude crops that contain illegal quantities of pesticide residues. While the Food and Drug Administration is totally unable to muster the manpower to inspect fresh produce, it is comparatively easy for them to keep a more watchful eye on the major canners and freezers. Therefore the use of frozen and canned foods offers a measure of protection, achieved at the loss of some nutritional values.

When memory fails me, as it must when I am trying to determine if a given additive is safe or not, I give my family the benefit of the doubt by not buying the product until I have written to the manufacturer. I not only inquire about the tests for safety — and ask for detail beyond the usual letter of general assurance or the usual remark "this has been approved by the government," which to me is meaningless — but I also inquire about the purpose for which the additive is used. As insane as the indiscriminate use of pesticides, which has simply created resistant insects or given an edge to one predator over another, is the use of additives which serve the manufacturer but do nothing for the public. I often have an uneasy feeling about the trend, remembering the story of the farmer who remarked: "I began by putting 1 percent sawdust in the cattle feed. I raised it 1 percent a week and got along fine, and just when I reached 99 percent sawdust, the damn fool critters upped and died!"

Years ago Professor Ernest Hooten, Harvard anthropologist, remarked that we should establish an institute of clinical anthropology, dedicated to the study of man as he was before there were physicians. Then we could determine how modern man should look after doctors are through with him. Perhaps we should expand the concept and hastily study man before he has too many years of exposure to additives and pesticides. Otherwise we may exterminate him before we realize that adaptation to a new system of diet may be catastrophically unsuccessful.

10.

DIETARY SUPPLEMENTS

If you believe that the American market basket, as befitting our cornucopia of plenty, is richly laden with vitamins, minerals, and protein, then you will probably accept the corollary: Anyone who takes vitamins is at the very least a food faddist, and at the worst wasting money on supplements because he is an easy target for propaganda or because he is a hypochondriac.

The truth often lies between the extremes of an argument, but in this case, it resides in the statements of the vitamin industry. By the time that food has been subjected to improper fertilization, been exposed to air, light, and heat in transportation and storage, been overprocessed and overcooked, it is entirely possible that the estimated vitamin content is nowhere near the reality.

Some years ago, this thesis was put to the test when a researcher analysed the vitamin content of meals actually taken from an average American dining table. He found 40 percent less potency of certain of the vitamins than the food charts would lead us to anticipate. There are few everyday diets in this country that can stand a 40 percent depreciation in vitamin values without jeopardizing the health of the individual — we just don't have that much vitamin margin in the average diet. This is written with no consideration of the possibility that the individual might have extraordinarily high requirements for vitamins and other nutrients. If this fact is taken into account, and certain ostensible vitamin values of the food discounted 40 percent, the result must be a marginal diet that cannot support well-being. Unfortunately, such borderline deficiency is the most vicious type of malnutrition. This does not cause the beriberi, scurvy, pellagra, rickets, xerophthalmia, or sprue we classically identify as the penalty for diets that grossly fail to meet the needs of the body. In the early stages of borderline deficiencies, we find ourselves in a kind of twilight zone — the diet is neither truly good nor truly bad, with the result that the person is neither truly well nor truly sick. Most of the complaints tend to be functional: The person with a borderline deficiency in Vitamin B Complex does not develop a magenta tongue or cracks at the corners of the mouth, but complains of fatigue, irritability, a tendency toward overemphasis of minor deviations from health — symptoms, in short, that are much more likely to invite a prescription for tranquilizers or psychiatric attention than reference to a nutritionist for repair of the diet.

After many years of existing in the twilight zone, individuals will finally develop a physical disease — often a degenerative disorder, such as arthritis, diabetes, disorders of the heart or blood vessels — and when such a disorder appears, as it does in 36 percent of those who survive to the age of sixty — it is then misinterpreted as the penalty for living a little too long. (Some forty-five years ago, the American physician Langstroth found dietary deficiencies to be uniformly present in older people with degenerative diseases and just as uniformly absent in healthy people of the same age.) The relationship between cause and effect goes unrecognized, because the physical penalties for poor nutrition take twenty years to make their appearance, and the classical phrase becomes: "I have arthritis, I must be growing old."

One of the reasons twilight-zone deficiencies are not recognized for what they are rests in a misconception created by misstatements by government agencies and medical societies. If you query such agencies about the incidence of nutritional deficiencies in this country, you will be told that except for alcoholics and the very poor, we have very, very few people who eat so badly that they develop beriberi or pellagra or scurvy. The philosophy underlying this statement can be spelled out in these terms: "A dietary deficiency takes you overnight from a state of good health to a life-threatening deficiency disease." In other words, there is no discernible penalty for an inadequate diet up to the point at which it causes serious and life-threatening diseases. This is patently untrue; to demonstrate, consider the following sequence in the development of a dietary deficiency.

The first stage of a dietary deficiency occurs when there is failure of supply — either because food is mishandled, the diet is poorly selected, or the individual, for one of many reasons we shall discuss, has increased his needs. Failure of supply may also be initiated or aggravated by difficulties in the digestion, the absorption, or transport of nutrients within the body. Other difficulties may be created by a breakdown in enzyme systems.

Once supply has failed for any of these reasons, there will be a drop in the blood levels of the nutrient. The blood now draws upon the tissues and when that process comes to an end, it borrows from the organ reserves. Note: Although you are well on your way toward trouble at this point, the blood levels of nutrients reveal nothing abnormal, because of the borrowing the body initiates to achieve more equitable distribution of an inadequate supply.

Then functional disability begins — indigestion, nervousness, irritability, a tendency to weep without provocation, a shortening of the memory and attention spans, difficulty in concentration, insomnia, and bad dreams — for which the doctor's X ray, blood tests, urine analysis, stethoscope, and blood-pressure instruments will find no physical justification. What are your chances of being told: "It's all in your mind"? What are the chances that you will be labeled a hypochondriac? What are the odds in favor of your leaving that medical office with a prescription for tranquilizers or psychoenergizers or sleeping capsules?

Your troubles are obviously not over, since your diet has not been repaired. You have progressed from inadequate supply to drop in blood levels to depletion of tissue and organ reserves and to functional disabilities.

If missing nutrients are not supplied now, the next penalty is physical but invisible, both to you and the doctor. It consists of microscopic changes in tissues, a degenerative process visible only under the microscope. Shortly thereafter will follow the last stage: Macroscopic breakdown in the tissues. Now, at long last, you have earned your medical spurs. The physician will perceive your purple, shining tongue, your very rapid or abnormally slow heartbeat, or the fat you are excreting undigested and will finally grant: "You are suffering from a dietary deficiency."

It would be logical for you to wonder why the physician seems to have a blind spot about the signs of minor dietary deficiencies, or, to use the language I have previously employed, why he seems so totally unaware of the twilight zone of nutritional deficiency. Part of his myopia derives from lack of training in the field of nutrition. Seventy-two percent of

American medical schools do not offer a course in this subject as a part of the medical curriculum. In the 28 percent of the schools that do offer such a course, the longest one given is some five hours of nutritional training in 1,000 hours of medical education. This time is scarcely enough to qualify a physician to comment competently on diet for healthy people, much less on the complicated nutritional problems of the sick. In addition, the physician has been subjected to indoctrination that has him believing that he is warranted in looking for impacts of nutritional inadequacy only in alcoholics and in Appalachia.* There is also the matter of the physician's concept of "normal health." He is prepared to accept and to label as well-being dozens of disorders that limit our potential, and for the management of which our medicine chests are crowded with palliatives of one kind or another. He has not yet come to grips with the realization that good health is more than the mere absence of major disease; that it should represent a state of positive well-being. If he accepted that definition, he would then be driven, literally, to a search for optimal diet for optimal performance.

Your own unwillingness to recognize the possibility that you yourself are a victim of dietetic inadequacy derives again from a lack of training and from indoctrination. It is perfectly possible for you to take a Ph.D., Ed.D., M.D., or D.D.S. degree and not to have had five minutes of instruction in selecting foods to meet the needs of your body. What is even worse is the possibility that you did receive some instruction, but that a large part of it was pure propaganda on the part of the manufacturers of highly processed foods. Speaking from personal observation, there are many textbooks in use in our school systems that inform a child that he needs sugar for energy, and neither child nor teacher will pause long enough to realize that the caveman survived long enough to sire our forebears and had energy enough to escape the saber-toothed tiger, yet never saw a sugar bowl. Helping to perpetuate

*From the experience of Dr. Tom Spies, the physician who was honored by the American Medical Association for his pioneering research in the twilight-zone deficiencies that group now refuses to recognize, we gain insight into the physician's inability to realize that dietary deficiencies do not always produce the "classical" symptoms, and that they are common rather than rare. Dr. Spies was an honored guest at a major Chicago teaching hospital, where he was invited to accompany the physicians on their rounds. After the chief of the medical staff had completed the tour, he turned to Dr. Spies and said: "Of course, we physicians in the North do not see the nutritional deficiencies you and your staff encounter in Alabama." He obviously referred to pellagra and beriberi, reflecting, thereby, his definition of what constitutes the effects of nutritional deficiencies. Dr. Spies' reply was, "Let us make the rounds again." His host physician agreed and did not long remain puzzled by the request. Dr. Spies stopped at one bed after another pointing out clear-cut symptoms of nutritional deficiency and naming the dietary inadequacies that caused them. It has been said that the physician does not find what he is not looking for. He is even less likely to find it when he has been persuaded that it doesn't exist.

the ignorance or protect the indoctrination is the belief that so many of us hold — that we who have eaten three times a day for thirty, forty or fifty years could not possibly be doing it wrong. It is assumed that eating is learned intuitively as are breathing or walking. Unfortunately, there are people who do not walk properly and must wear special shoes; there are people who faint because they do not breathe properly; and there are people whose eating habits are based on habits colored by prejudice, molded by allergy, dictated by seasonable availability of food, budget, or medical prohibitions on food selection — and none of these is likely to lead to a balanced diet.

In addition to popularizing foods unknown in man's history, our culture has forced upon us a pattern of food selection that in itself creates problems. It is sometimes difficult to appreciate the technical trap we have created for ourselves in a mechanized civilization addicted to highly processed foods. The net effect of processing is to increase the concentration of calories and deplete the vitamin-mineral values. Meanwhile, because of labor-saving devices in our culture, our need for calories has declined while our need for vitamins and other essential nutrients has not. To make this fact clearer, consider a calorie ceiling over the diet and a calorie floor under the diet The ceiling is there because if one overeats, he gains undesirable excess weight. The floor is there because no selection of foods, however intelligent, will form the basis of an adequate diet if we aren't eating enough food. This problem was best understood by my university students when we were studying thiamin (Vitamin B_1), and one of my students asked what intake of Vitamin B_1 would I recommend. I said, with due consideration for those whose requirements might be high, that 2 mgs. of Vitamin B_1 daily should keep a majority of the public well supplied. Her second question was: "What food is richest in the vitamin?" When I indicated that whole-wheat bread, among staple foods, was the best source of the vitamin, the next question became inevitable. "How much whole-wheat bread would I have to eat daily to obtain 2 mgs. of Vitamin B_1?"

I replied that one is not likely to rely on just one food for the vitamin, but that 2 mgs. of thiamin are supplied by approximately one loaf of whole-wheat bread. Again her response was to be anticipated. She protested, "I couldn't eat that much bread — I'd gain too much weight."

It is a mark of the food faddist to eat wheat germ — but 400 calories from this excellent food gives 50 percent more Vitamin B_1 than an entire one-pound loaf of bread, with 1,200 calories. In a culture that keeps an anxious eye on its waistline, which food is better gaited to meet the needs of a sedentary public: the bread (consumption of which brings no social disapproval) or the wheat germ (which must be eaten surreptitiously if one does not wish to reap the wrath of the community)?

So it is that vitamin supplements and special-purpose foods* fulfill an important function for those who do not want to pay too great a price in calories for an optimal intake of other needed nutrients.

Much of this seems to be contaminated by common sense. Yet, at least until recent years, those who patronize health-food stores, where such concentrates and foods were sold, have been considered to be cranks. Various university nutrition departments criticize "venal" vitamin manufacturers who milk the public, and their "gullible food-faddist" customers. The leading agency in bringing down the wrath of the community on vitamin and health-food purveyors has been the United States Food and Drug Administration. This agency has attempted to regulate the vitamin supplements out of existence — save for those that might occasionally be prescribed by a physician; it has done its best to harrass the health-food manufacturers, distributors, and retailers into closing their doors; and with all the public-relation pressure a giant and well-financed government agency can bring to bear, it has done its best to destroy those nutritionists whose judgments in nutrition, vis-à-vis the inadequacy of the American diet, and the usefulness of special-purpose foods and vitamins, differ from those of the government agency.

We now have one excellent example of the services rendered to us by vitamin supplements, food concentrates, or specially prepared foods such as brewer's yeast, wheat germ, liver, rice polishings, and nonfat milk. Their ratio of nutrients to calories is favorable.

Years ago — and the situation has not changed since — H. C. Sherman of Columbia University remarked if two people ate the same meals, selected on the basis of the same household criteria, one might achieve nutritional adequacy and the other might not. So the "diet insurance" of these concentrates and foods tends to offset not only the variations in nutrient values normal to biological products like food, but those others that are caused by poor soil, improper fertilization, long transportation, improper storage or display in the retail establishment, excessive processing, and improper cooking. *Don't* discount these influences on the adequacy of your diet. There are nutritionists (and I am one) who will tell you that excessive cooking of protein in foods

---

*Special-purpose foods are wheat germ, brewer's yeast, nonfat milk, liver, rice polishings, and certain soy products that provide high concentrations of important nutrients and are therefore used to reinforce dietary values in such factors.

eaten during pregnancy may impair for a lifetime the ability of a baby to bear stress.

What has been written to this point does not take into consideration the possibility to which this book is largely devoted: That you, as an individual, may have unusually high requirements for this nutrient or that, so high that even a diet consisting of well-selected foods that have not been abused may still be inadequate to meet your needs. This is not theory, and a very good example can be found in an everyday mineral — iron. Here we are not dealing with a high requirement that arises out of the individual chemistry of a person; instead, we are faced with a problem created by an idiosyncrasy of an entire sex. The iron requirement in women has been set by the Establishment at 18 mgs. daily. This is a much higher figure than the requirement for men, largely because of the menstrual loss of iron, which may be as high as 50 mgs. of the mineral. You may eat eggs, Boston brown bread, liver, meat, apricots, and molasses — all the foods labeled as "rich in iron" — and yet fall short of the 18 mgs. of iron daily. The problem has been expressed in these terms: An assortment of staple foods will convey about 6 mgs. of iron for each 1,000 calories. This is the kind of mathematics that will elicit a cry from women who do not want to be too curved. Can you not hear a woman responding: "If that means I must eat 3,000 calories a day to get 18 mgs. of iron, you're giving me a choice between anemia and wearing girdles in the gee-whiz and holy mackerel sizes — and I'd rather be anemic!" So far, we are dealing with the logic of science and arithmetic, *but*, let a nutritionist yield to science, logic, and arithmetic by suggesting that it would be a good investment for our young girls to form the habit of using an iron supplement and he will find himself stigmatized as a food faddist.

Do not discount the possibility that you may be unknowingly restricting your functions by failing to recognize and satisfy an unusually high nutritional requirement. In considering such requirements, I have examined many possible causes. There are individuals whose enzyme chemistry is in some way abnormal — the spectrum ranging from no production of an enzyme to inadequate manufacture. Usually, there is no way for us to supply a missing enzyme to our body. Many enzymes are not available and, except for those that are active in the stomach, the rest would not be likely to survive the journey through the stomach to the lower digestive tract, for, being protein substances, they would be digested. The few enzymes that *are* available from animal or vegetable sources and *are* active in the lower digestive tract must either be given in tremendous doses, so that some part will survive to reach the intestine, or must be taken in a special tablet form to protect against the digestive process in the stomach.* Therefore, our only treatment that offers any hope of effectiveness in enzyme deficiency is the administration of super amounts of the building materials from which the body manufactures the enzyme. In many cases, these materials include vitamins and minerals, whose intake may solve a problem created by inadequate manufacture arising from some peculiarity in the individual's biochemistry. This explains response to concentrated vitamins in some "well-fed" people. It is not the complete explanation, because, as you will see later in this chapter, difficulties with enzyme reactions are not the only cause of heightened requirement for vitamins. What has just been written collides head on with a doctrine that has been widely publicized as absolute scientific fact. This doctrine says that "doses of vitamins beyond your requirements" are at best wasted, and at worst, toxic. The fact is that there are individuals who profit from vitamin concentrates in doses "beyond their requirements" because their requirements are high, or because their enzyme chemistries are disturbed, or because they do not absorb well — true of many older people — or because of a fundamental law of chemistry, the "law of mass action." Without entering into the complexities, the law of mass action states that when two liquids are separated by a membrane, a chemical dissolved in the liquid on one side of the membrane will, by osmosis, penetrate the barrier until the concentration of the chemical on the two sides is equal. A second aspect of the law says simply that the speed and efficiency of the transfer of the chemical are related to its concentration. In other words, a very concentrated solution of the chemical will be transferred more efficiently and more rapidly until equilibrium is reached. For the liquid on one side substitute blood. For the membrane substitute the wall of a blood vessel — which is a membrane. Let the interior of the body serve as the liquid on the other side. Let the chemical in the blood be a vitamin, and apply the law of mass action: The greater the concentration of the vitamin, the more efficient and the faster the transfer. That there has been virtually an attempt to repeal this law in terms of vitamin chemistry does not mean that medical men are not acquainted with it. The law of mass action is in use in medicine every day and governs responses to certain types of prescriptions, but medical propaganda and government agencies bent on protecting the nutritional status quo find it convenient

---

*The fragility of enzymes from food reminds me of a fallacy some authors have voiced as fact. Certain books describe foods as "dead" when their enzymes have been destroyed in cooking. The emphasis is therefore on the desirability of raw foods and raw vegetable juices — living foods — because of their enzyme content. The fact is that virtually all enzymes in food are simply nuisances. If you have watched a sliced apple turn brown, you have seen an enzyme at work — certainly no boon to people who like apples!

to forget that concentrations alter the properties of certain substances, and that vitamins are not immune.*

Requirements may also vary because of the peculiarities of an individual's glandular chemistry. For instance, an overactive thyroid will raise vitamin requirements. Similarly, when a physician administers thyroid tablets, he is increasing your requirement for the B Vitamins. A parallel effect is caused if, because of the glands you inherited, you produce unusually high levels of estrogen (female hormone). (Production of estrogen may differ among women by a factor of five.) To control the activity of this hormone, excess of which can cause serious disturbances and disease, requires generous intake of Vitamin B Complex and protein. But the heightened need for these factors created by excess female hormone production is not recognized in the table of "minimum daily vitamin requirements."

If you dismiss as academic the fact that you need more protein and Vitamin B because you produce more estrogen or because you are taking the birth-control pill, you should know that you are playing a kind of nutritional Russian roulette. If you hit upon the loaded chamber and pull the nutritional trigger by not eating as you should to meet your requirements, the excess hormone activity may be registered in side effects ranging from stroke to cancer.

Not all women have problems with water retention and weight gain in the premenstrual week. Those who do may be paying the price for failing to gear their nutrition to their glandular activity, but they often compound the error by using diuretics to cope with the excess fluid in the tissues. The diuretics may remove the water, but they will also remove water-soluble nutrients — including some of the ones needed to keep the estrogen from contributing to the water retention. The treatment is symptomatic — it does nothing to offset the cause.

Similarly, the patient with congestive heart failure who takes diuretics may wash out of his system quantities of vitamins and minerals needed by his failing heart. These examples are given merely to show factors that raise vitamin requirements. There are many such forces that operate — without our knowledge — to determine our vitamin requirements.

---

*In the case of vitamins, it is more than their physical properties that are altered by concentrations. Their biochemical effects are also quite different. For instance, small concentrations of Vitamin C do not display an antihistaminic effect in the body, but high concentrations do — some allergic individuals are completely relieved of their symptoms with high Vitamin C dosages. Vitamin A in nutritional amounts will not show the action that it does in large doses — 250,000 units taken daily at the first sign of a cold can completely check the symptoms and eliminate the infection if the dosage is continued for four or five days. Ordinary dietary levels of niacin do not help a schizophrenic, but megavitamin doses frequently do.

The list that follows is partial, but it should make you aware of some of the conditions that raise vitamin-mineral requirements:

I. *Interference with Food Intake*
Gastro-intestinal diseases
    Acute gastro-enteritis
    Gallbladder disease
    Peptic ulcer
    Diarrheal diseases
    Food allergy
Mental disorders
    Neurasthenia
    Psychoneurosis
Operations and anesthesia
Loss of teeth
Infectious diseases associated with lack of appetite
Heart failure (nausea, vomiting)
Pulmonary disease (vomiting due to cough)
Toxemia of pregnancy (nausea and vomiting)
Visceral pain (as in renal colic, and angina that produces nausea and vomiting)
Neurologic disorders that interfere with self-feeding
Migraine

II. *Interference with Absorption*
Diarrheal disease
    Ulcerative and mucous colitis
    Intestinal parasites
    Intestinal tuberculosis
    Sprue
Gastro-intestinal fistulas
Diseases of liver and gallbladder
Lack of hydrochloric acid

III. *Interference with Utilization*
Liver disease
Diabetes mellitus
Chronic alcoholism
Functional hypoglycemia (low blood sugar)

IV. *Increased Requirements*
Abnormal activity as associated with prolonged, strenuous physical exertion, with lack of sufficient sleep or rest

Fever
Hyperthyroidism or other instances of high-glandular activity
Pregnancy and lactation

V. *Increased Excretion*
   Biliary or gastro-intestinal fistula
   Perspiration
   Loss of protein in nephritis and nephrosis
   Long-continued excessive fluid intake as in urinary tract infections

VI. *Therapeutic Measures*
   Therapeutic diets
      Sippy regimen (for peptic ulcer)
      Gallbladder disease
      Antiobesity diets
   Antacids
      Mineral oil
      Diuretics
      Medicinal charcoal
      Birth-control pills
      Antiepilepsy drugs

At least two factors are not listed in the preceding table, and both contribute importantly to vitamin-mineral deficiencies. It has been said that each physician, as he learns his profession, fills a small graveyard. There is some measure of truth in this statement. Medically prescribed bed rest — which the profession is discarding — is probably the most frequent and deadly error. The human organism functions like the Red Queen in *Through the Looking-Glass* who, if you remember, had to run like mad to stay in one place. Resting, she would of course lose ground. Similarly, the human organism achieves balance in the midst of forces of anarchy only by remaining in motion — as the astronauts learned when weightlessness caused loss of calcium from their bones and protein from their tissues, losses that could not be prevented even by ideal nutrition. So, similarly, patients who are bedded over long periods will develop osteoporosis or other bone diseases, as calcium is excreted faster than it can be replenished, and nitrogen is lost in amounts greater than intake. Studies have not been made, to my knowledge, of vitamin excretion under such circumstances, but it is unlikely that the negative balance would occur only in protein and calcium.

Another (and likewise neglected) cause of vitamin-mineral deficiency is emotional stress. In human beings, calcium metabolism alone has been studied under circumstances of emotional pressure, and once again — regardless of the level of intake — excretion becomes greater than dietary supply. This means that the difference is being taken from the bones.

As for vitamins, it has been established that symptoms of nutritional deficiencies will reappear when emotional pressures, such as acute anxiety, are exerted on patients — even when they are receiving massive doses of the vitamins and other factors that originally cured the lesions.

The situations with which we are dealing have a common denominator. They all induce at least mild dietary deficiencies in the presence of what may appear to be good or even optimal nutrition. If the deficiencies are mild and last long enough, symptoms will arise that will not be clearly referable to good nutrition but which might masquerade as hypochondriasis, neurosis, or any one of a number of physical diseases. Obviously, the time must come when we are no longer insensitive to the subtleties of poor nutrition. It is apparent from what you have read, that the term "nutritional deficiency" can very well be all things to all people. The medical establishment says that dietary deficiency is rare. The nutritionist is aware of the extreme subtlety of the disturbances created by chronic deficiencies of a lesser degree. He also knows that the early stages of severe deficiency produce a galaxy of disturbances that may look more like neurosis than the price of indiscriminate selection of foods.

When a hen is fed a diet with less than the required amount of Vitamin E, the chicks that hatch from her eggs may turn backward somersaults. The human being who has less than the ideal amount of Vitamin E may, as the only visible consequence, age more rapidly. The unwary veterinarian might well ascribe the peculiar behavior of the chicks to an infection not uncommon in fowl — encephalitis. The physician may very well fall into the trap of considering the aging process normal when, in fact, the evidence now accumulating indicates it is a sickness, and in part due to improper diet. In short, if the yardsticks by which we gauge the adequacy of the diet were scientifically more accurate, there would be a concerted drive to prod millions of Americans into seeking nutritional help. Beriberi is rare; nervousness or irritability from poor diet is not. Scurvy is rare; more frequent colds from inadequate intake of Vitamin C are common. Rickets is rare, but the type of nutritional error in diet that may produce, twenty years later, the "constitutionally inadequate woman" is at this moment at work, subtly affecting the unborn babies of thousands of expectant mothers. Sterility from Vitamin-E deficiency is rare, but premature or accelerated aging from want of this vitamin may be common.

There is another error in the American diet, posing a problem apart from those with which we have dealt. We have been concerned with people whose nutrition is inadequate to the point where it causes mild chronic deficiencies or acute deficiencies. These problems, we have learned, may not only originate from biological insanity in the *choice* of foods, but can arise in the presence of a normally good diet when nutritional requirements have been raised too high by genetic or environmental factors.* We have not, however, confronted a problem of deficiencies that are even more subtle, where the diet appears to be normal and needs are not exaggerated, but our standards of normality in diet and well-being do not permit achievement of *optimal* health and performance.

Consider, for instance, the implication of innumerable animal experiments in which administration of liver or wheat-germ oil, *supplementing a well-balanced diet*, have allowed the animals to exhibit greatly increased resistance to fatigue. Before the supplements were added to the diets, the rats would have been described by any laboratory worker as being well fed — yet when they were forced to swim to the point of exhaustion, the rats on the supplemented diet remained afloat twice as long as those on the diet alone. Their nutrition was adequate without the liver and the wheat-germ oil, but it certainly didn't allow for optimal performance.

How do you know that you are not in the position of the rats on the stock diet? How do you know that your diet does not fall short of letting you reach maximum performance physically or emotionally? The Establishment, looking at you, would say that you are "well nourished," but they would also say that of the rats on the stock diet. May not your diet be like that of those professional men and their wives previously discussed who were considered healthy and well fed, but responded to a rise in the intake of tryptophane with an improvement in their psychological well-being?

Question: What aspects of your mental or emotional well-being are being altered without your knowledge by a set of menus that meets the Food and Drug Administration's standards, or complies with *your* concept of the nutritional requirements of your body, but falls short of meeting your actual needs?

You have a possible potential for dividends from improved nutrition. That likelihood grows stronger as you grow older. Although physiologists well know that the aging organism loses efficiency in absorbing and

---

*Among the environmental factors may be the total composition of the diet. For instance, an intake of thiamin (Vitamin B₁) that ordinarily would be adequate would be rendered inadequate by too high an intake of sugar. This sets up a "relative deficiency." Despite the comfort the sufferer may find in the term "relative," the effects are just as devastating as a direct deficiency.

utilizing food and its factors, the official doctrine states that the diet on which you have grown old is so successful that no changes in food selection and no use of food supplements are indicated. But the risk of malnourishment grows as age increases. The older organism extracts less from its food and needs, if anything, more.

This is a process that can become a vicious cycle, for as the utilization of food becomes increasingly impaired by processes concomittant with aging, the rate of aging and the impact of these processes will tend to increase. Indeed, standard texts on endocrinology will indicate that dietary deficiencies can impair function of the pituitary gland, but usually do not indicate that this becomes a vicious circle, since impaired pituitary function can in turn interfere with proper digestion and absorption of nutrients.

From the deep well of misinformation accumulated from propaganda and advertising, we are likely to dredge up some beliefs that will dilute your receptivity to what you are reading. For instance, when I suggest that you use wheat germ as a supplemental special-purpose food, you may ask: "But white bread is enriched — doesn't that take care of its deficiencies?" That is precisely what the baking industry wants you to think. The American Baking Association has published propaganda, showing the favorable comparison between the vitamin content of enriched white flour and the content of whole wheat in the same vitamins. Frederick Stare, the cornflakes professor from Harvard, performs prestidigitation with perhaps as much effrontery as any other spokesman for those highly processed foods. In one of his books, he makes enriched white bread and whole-wheat bread nutritionally equivalent by comparing their thiamin, riboflavin, and niacin content. The comparison, of course, stops there. It does not go on to Vitamin B_6 — in which whole-wheat is four times as rich as white flour. And it does not mention Vitamin E, the content of which in white flour is virtually wiped out. Neither vitamin is restored in enrichment. That is an understatement, for at least twenty-three factors are depleted in the processing of white flour, and at best, some six are restored.

We have now established that you have been ingesting propaganda, and we hope you are persuaded that it might be much more sensible to swallow some supplements. That brings us to the questions: What, how much, and in what forms? There is the question of natural versus synthetic vitamins. It is not sensible to propose a chemical difference between the natural and the synthetic vitamins. After all, the synthetic factor must be a compound that matches the natural, atom for atom and molecule for molecule. Otherwise it would fail to live up to the definition of a vitamin. Synthetic Vitamin B_1 must cure all symptoms caused by a deficiency of natural Vitamin B_1. To that point, it can be said that there is no distinction between the two, but if we stop there we are guilty of oversimplification. There are obviously differences between a natural and a synthetic vitamin that we encounter more or less frequently — for instance, some people are allergic to one and not to the other. We must begin to speculate on chemical distinctions that are beyond our present knowledge, if not in the structure of the vitamin, then perhaps in the factors that normally accompany it in foods. These would include minerals, enzymes, and possible cofactors, or unknown nutrients. There is also evidence — if not of a distinction between the synthetic and natural vitamin, at least of helpful actions by these natural cofactors. Besides such interaction, what will satisfactorily explain our occasional ability to heal gingivitis with orange juice more effectively than with doses of synthetic Vitamin C? Perhaps the synthetic and natural ascorbic acid are identical to the last decimal point, but the orange juice, we know, provides the bioflavonoids that help to make Vitamin C more effective and is a source of potassium, folic acid, zinc, and other factors known and unknown that may well account for the difference.

What I have just written sounds like a condemnation of the use of synthetic vitamins. It isn't. It merely means that our knowledge of the constituents in food is far from complete. Therefore, supplements should not be used as substitutes for proper eating. A fire-insurance policy does not license you to play with matches or to build a hazardous house. Once a supplement is employed as a kind of dietary insurance policy, the diet to which it is added should be nutritionally as optimal as you can make it. In this way, you supply yourself with significant amounts of the unknowns that are not in synthetic vitamin supplements. Natural vitamin supplements would of course contain many of these unknown factors, but ordinarily cannot be concentrated enough to yield high potencies of the known vitamins. Thus, generally speaking, natural vitamin supplements are preferable when modest amounts of vitamin protection are wanted. When you need very high intake, either because of high or therapeutic requirements, the use of synthetic vitamins is inescapable — there is no way to concentrate the natural factor that much.

Unless you know your natural vitamins, be sure that you are dealing with a reputable firm. I have seen vitamin products labeled as natural which could not possibly be. For instance, when the label informs you that there are 60 mgs. of thiamin in each capsule, among other vitamins, you should immediately know that this must be the synthetic vitamin. The richest natural source of thiamin that is used in supplements is a concentrated brewer's yeast, of which we must use 200 mgs. to obtain 1 mg. of Vitamin B_1. A little arithmetic will show you that twelve grams (nearly one-half ounce) of the concentrated yeast will yield 60 mgs. of the vitamin. The capsule containing it and the other vitamins would choke a horse.

Whether you use a natural or synthetic multiple-vitamin concentrate, it is very desirable that you accompany it with a concentrate of a natural source of the Vitamin B Complex — for it is within this group of factors that many unknowns still await discovery. If you have a logical mind, you will now ask how we can definitely know that an unknown exists, if in fact it is unknown. The evidence is not hard to find. Earlier in this book, you learned that the liver has the capability of inactivating estrogenic hormone. This action is based upon a well-fed liver. The biochemist's reasoning at this point will tell him that in liver there is an enzyme that breaks down estrogens. It has never (to my knowledge) been isolated; and we therefore do not know its composition.

I have already mentioned high resistance to fatigue from the use of supplements of liver. That action cannot be achieved with dosages of any of the vitamins known to be contained in liver. Therefore, we can say that there is an unknown factor in liver, which in some way we do not understand, increases resistance to being tired — yet it remains, in terms of its chemical identity, unknown.

Intelligent use of supplements will result in your taking several capsules and pills. This can be done at a cost ranging from slight to considerable. It is a matter of some interest that the professional agitators against vitamin supplements dwell upon cost, but fail to point out that the public spends far more on the gastronomical insult of snack foods and the toxic effects of liquor and smoking. In any case, the supplements for a year will cost considerably less than the medical care and prescriptions for any significant illness — and may help to prevent or mitigate some of these as well as to increase the response to medication when needed. Note that people who eat properly and use vitamin supplements still do get sick. I am weary of those who seem to believe that for the well fed there are no physical problems. I sometimes receive this remark from readers: "I did everything you said I should — and still came down with the whatsis!"

Perhaps the most vivid explanation of this type of thinking appeared in a remark made to me by a radio listener, who came to the studio after a broadcast and opened the question and answer period by asking: "Are you Dr. Fredericks?" When I assured her that I was, she responded disbelievingly: "*You wear glasses!*"

Although I have behind me thirty years of observation of the dividends from vitamins and other food supplements so that I may say dogmatically that the majority of people who live in our civilization will experience dividends from the use of these concentrates, I must confess that I am weary of some of the extravagant claims made by the manufacturers and purveyors of these products. There is one producer who has a monopoly on the correct ratio of the various vitamins, which, he insists, must parallel the amounts of the nutrients found in the human tissues. This of course is highly dubious. Human tissue, like all meat, will show vitamin concentrations that vary greatly from individual to individual, depending upon the vagaries of food selection and the chemistry of the body. Some of my fellow nutritionists differ with me and among themselves about recommended ratios of vitamins in supplements on the grounds that an oversupply of one vitamin can conceivably aggravate a deficiency in another. This is a valid point of view when we are dealing with very high doses, as in schizophrenia where megavitamin dosages of niacinamide may induce a Vitamin B_6 deficiency if the latter factor is not given in sufficient amounts. But ratios are simply not that critical when we are dealing with the concentrates of vitamins used for protection of the diet by people who are not sick.

Particularly objectionable are both the claims and the prices of some of the supplements that are sold by door-to-door salesmen. These salesmen work on commission, operating under an endless hierarchy of wholesalers, distributors, and sales managers who likewise participate in commissions — a financial scheme that has resulted in the public's paying $25.00 per month's supply of supplements for one person. This amount is "justified" on the grounds of the presence in the supplement of an insignificant amount of alfalfa, liver, or more esoteric ingredients, none of which can make any worthwhile contribution unless the dosage is raised to a level that is physically impossible to swallow in capsule form. In addition, such products can be purchased from reputable manufacturers at an expense of $4.00 for a month's supply. While I am naturally concerned that you do not overpay for dietary supplements, let me reject the proposal that these concentrates are expensive at any price. When the public spends more than sixty billion dollars a year on health care — or more accurately, sickness care — it does not seem to me that a few dollars a month spent on something that might prevent or mitigate sickness, or help in response to needed medications should be counted as an extravagance.

From the research of Dr. Tom Spies I learned the proper way to use supplements. In his work with the malnourished, he set up a procedure in therapeutic nutrition that I modified for preventive use more than twenty-five years ago. Dr. Spies started his treatment with a well-balanced, high-protein, high-vitamin diet, supplying as much as 4,000 calories a day. I spare you the calories but endorse the point that good nutrition begins with a diet as good as you can possibly make it.

To this, Dr. Spies added:

1. Doses by mouth of all high-potency vitamins available. This he called "therapeutic formula."*
2. Four ounces of brewer's yeast daily.
3. High-potency injections of Vitamin C and Vitamin C Complex.
4. Four ounces of desiccated liver daily.

Dr. Spies used these doses and potencies because he was *treating* sick people. We are dedicated to the ounce of prevention. We therefore need not insist on a 4,000-calorie diet, but can legitimately suggest that you do your best to eat intelligently, with the accent on protein and on the foods that are rich in vitamins and minerals. Similarly, we do not need a quarter of a pound of brewer's yeast and one-quarter pound of dried liver daily. Since unknown factors of the Vitamin B Complex are concealed within these rich sources, and we cannot incorporate a significant amount of yeast or liver in a capsule or two, it *is* desirable to use a reasonable amount of liver or yeast daily — preferably both. If you are going to choose one of the two, make it dried liver. Although both are rich in the Vitamin B Complex, liver contains all the vitamins supplied by yeast and also concentrates certain unknown factors that are known not to be in yeast. (Liver, for instance, will frequently prove more beneficial to gingivitis than will yeast.) On the other hand, brewer's yeast is rich in an unsaturated fat emphasized in control of blood cholesterol.

Before considering the list of factors that should be in supplements, we should pause to examine the types of liver and of yeast that are available.

Brewer's yeast should be distinguished from baker's yeast. The latter

*The pharmaceutical houses reached into this list and pulled out a plum: The therapeutic vitamin capsule. Not only did this capsule represent an unwarranted fractionation of Dr. Spies' treatment, but the overemphasis on a therapeutic vitamin capsule neatly exploited the physician's ignorance of nutrition at large, and Dr. Spies' research in particular. The medical man who prescribed or recommended the therapeutic capsule now had the misconception that he solved all the patient's nutritional problems with this pill. When such nutritional therapy failed — as it frequently must have — the physician's cynicism about the claims made for vitamins and other nutritional therapies was reinforced. Medical ignorance of nutrition also allows the physician to believe that it doesn't matter what brand of vitamin supplement you take. In other words, if vitamins are pep pills or placebos, why should he care if a supplement contains a given vitamin or what potencies of other vitamins are supplied?

when dried or in the cake form is a living organism that helps in the leavening of bread and baked products. It is better than baking powder, for it contributes nutritional values, whereas baking powder actually destroys vitamins. However, baker's yeast is not a good choice as a supplement. Should it survive the digestive process as a living organism, it will take vitamins from its host.

Brewer's yeast, as the name suggests, was originally grown to help in the fermentation of beer and other alcoholic beverages. For over a century, the spent (dead) yeast, redolent and bitter with salt and hops, has been used as a dietary supplement. Ultimately we succeeded in removing the salt and hops, thus making the yeast more palatable. However, the brewers are not interested in the vitamin content of the yeast, but rather in its aid to fermentation. Therefore, the secondary use of yeast was neglected until growing interest in its nutritional values stimulated research that showed that strains of yeast could be grown that are richer sources of vitamins than the variety used for brewing. There are now on the market varieties of brewer's yeast enormously rich in vitamin value, some containing vitamins not normally found in yeast — as a result of culturing the organism in special nutrient broths. Moreover, some have a pleasant taste. There is another type of yeast available called torula that is grown on the waste liquors of the paper industry. Research with the starving children of Biafra and other African areas revealed that torula yeast lacks "Factor 3." This is a selenium-containing nutrient that appears to be essential to proper utilization of Vitamin E. In the American diet there are probably other sources of Factor 3, but to play safe, I have always preferred brewer's yeast.

The technique of growing brewer's yeast in special broths has given us yeast with higher potencies of certain vitamins — such as pantothenic acid and pyridoxin — and has even supplied a Vitamin B_{12} content ordinarily missing in this food. Not only has the technique been used to increase the protein content of the yeast as much as 60 percent, but also to make the yeast a significant source of the sulphur-containing amino acids not normally supplied by vegetable foods. A collateral dividend has been a great improvement in the taste of some of these yeasts.

As there are varieties of yeast, so are there varieties of liver concentrates. There are two types you should never use. One is fractionated liver — portions remaining after extraction of this or that nutrient. Fortunately, there is little of this type commercially available. The second is liver that has been heat dried without benefit of vacuum. This requires enough exposure to heat and air to cause a loss of vitamins, seriously denaturing the high-quality protein in liver.

The quantity of brewer's yeast needed to make a significant contribution to enriching the diet with B Complex vitamins would be about two tablespoonsful daily — perhaps an ounce. I carefully note that no food is indispensable, however desirable it may be, so that I may not receive the comment that has come to me from earnest, dedicated individuals who remark: "Brewer's yeast gives me indigestion — what shall I do?" The obvious answer is: "Don't use it." Intolerance may occur to any food or, for that matter, to any vitamin — and if it cannot be overcome by lowering the dose, then you must resort to other measures.

Since the purpose of supplements is that of protecting yourself against deficiency and assuring the supply of nutrients adequate to meet even a high requirement, it will be better if the yeast is taken in several installments, rather than in one dose. When we wish a pharmacological or drug effect from a nutrient, we use it in very high single doses. When we are supplementing the diet with such factors, we prefer to avoid the spilling (in the urine) that follows ingestion of large amounts. We accomplish this by spacing out the intake.

After making sure that the liver product one chooses represents whole liver — not a fraction of it remaining after removal of a factor for some other purpose — one must then make a distinction between liver that has been dried under ordinary atmospheric pressure, and that dried in a vacuum. Vacuum drying, of course, makes it possible to utilize much less heat; in fact, many vacuum-dried whole-liver supplements are actually prepared at room temperature. There is also on the market liver dried by treatment with solvents. This liver is satisfactory since its nutrients have not been harmed by excessive heat, but the solvent will obviously remove a substantial part, if not all, of the liver fat — and in the fat there may very well be nutrients, identity unknown at the present time. On the other hand, the removal of the fat also means removal of cholesterol and while I certainly do not share the conventional viewpoint concerning cholesterol as being a universal problem (it *is* for *some* people), there are physicians who would like to keep their patients on a low-cholesterol regime.

Popular magazines have discouraged the public from eating liver or using it as a supplement on the grounds that DDT and other insecticides concentrate in liver fat. This is a gross exaggeration. The fat-soluble insecticides do concentrate in body fat — but that fat is distributed throughout the entire body and certainly is not confined to the liver alone. In addition, the detoxification processes of the body depend upon adequate liver function, and to support this, there is no better food than liver itself. If you insist upon being concerned by the DDT content of liver, it should be reassuring for you to know that there is at least one brand of vacuum-dried liver on the market derived from Argentine steers, raised on the pampas where no spraying takes place, and with much fat removed.

If you are curious about the nutritional contribution made by these good foods, we might pause to list some of them for you. In taking liver and yeast, you are enriching your diet with high-quality protein, containing all the amino acids by which the body profits, plus thiamin (vitamin B_1), riboflavin (vitamin B_2), niacinamide (miscalled vitamin B_3), pyridoxin (vitamin B_6), folic acid, pantothenic acid, para-amino-benzoic acid, inositol, choline, cobalamin (vitamin B_{12}), and, in the quantities of liver and yeast recommended, amounts that may be significant of the "unknown factors."

The rest of the vitamin-supplementing procedure would consist of multiple vitamins and multiple minerals. As you read the following table of suggested amounts of supplementary vitamins and minerals, you will note that the potencies recommended are perhaps higher than those you have read elsewhere. You will also note that there are some factors included that are labeled "need in human nutrition not established." The potencies recommended are easily justified — you are reading a book that has great respect for individual variations in human needs for nutrients. When one is dealing with the public at large, rather than with an individual, the path of safety lies in the assumption that *everyone* has a requirement at the upper end of the spectrum. Only in this way will everyone be safe. With regard to the inclusion of nutrients not demonstrated to be essential in human nutrition, an explanation of this familiar legend appearing on the labels of many vitamin supplements in accordance with a Food and Drug Administration regulation has partially been given. Let us expand upon that explanation here. This phrase does not mean that the nutrient is not essential in the human body. It means it is not essential to obtain it from the diet. The nutrient is actually needed in the body, but ordinarily can be manufactured from other nutritional factors. Thus, there are amino acids the body is able to manufacture from other amino acids; there is choline, a vitamin the body constructs by breaking down methionine, which is one of the essential amino acids from protein foods. There is niacin, which the body manufactures from the essential amino acid tryptophane. Thus, if the statement required by the Food and Drug Administration were really to be made explicit it would read: "This substance is manufactured in the body from other dietary factors. Therefore, it is not necessary that the diets supply this nutrient as such." Of course, this statement implies that the ability of our cells to manufacture choline, amino acids, or niacin differs not at all from one person to another — which is ridiculous. Actually, some of the responses I have seen to the administration of choline and other factors "not essential to human nutrition" in the concentrated form argue for inadequate manufacture of such factors by some individuals. The responses I have seen to doses of glutamic acid are another case in point. Here is an amino acid manufactured by the body, generously conveyed by several protein foods — including milk — and yet as little as 9 grams daily has produced improvements in mental alertness and in the personality of epileptic and retarded children and adults. Elsewhere, I have recorded the response of "neurotics" to doses of factors legally considered to be unneeded in human nutrition. So it is that such nutrients are included in the list of supplementary factors I suggest on the simple basis that a dietary insurance policy should be broad in its scope.

In the suggested potencies of the supplement described in the following table, you will note that there are trace minerals recommended, as well as vitamins which, any "expert" will tell you, are so widely provided in our foods that supplements of these factors become a testimonial to the suggestibility of a hypochondriac. I must pause here to comment on that belief. Many years ago, I was director of education for a laboratory headed by Dr. Casimir Funk, the originator of the name "vitamin." That laboratory's first product was America's first nationally distributed vitamin-mineral supplement. In that supplement was a content of zinc — perhaps some four to five mgs. I remember being assured by a Food and Drug Administration inspector that supplements of zinc were simply not needed and might be dangerous. I responded that the mills that make white flour and white sugar extract a considerable amount of zinc from these highly processed foods, and that the diet is replete in foods similarly abused. Furthermore, any case involving toxicity from zinc would have to take into consideration at least one very popularly used remedy for indigestion that contains much larger quantities of zinc than we'd ever thought of incorporating into a supplement. Today, two and one-half decades later, we find in the papers of Air Force researchers, indications that supplements of zinc — among other dividends — speed the healing of wounds even in purportedly well-nourished individuals.

With that preface, consider the following suggestions for the formulation of a supplement.

VITAMINS

Vitamin A

Theoretically, obtaining an adequate supply of Vitamin A from food should be easy. Vegetables and fruits contain carotene, a precursor of Vitamin A, which the body is able to convert into the finished form. In fact, there is even a dividend — because one part of carotene yields two parts of Vitamin A. However, diabetics fail at this conversion — a fact that seems to be unknown to the dieticians who prepare diabetic diets, in which heavy reliance is placed on vegetables as a source of the precursor of Vitamin A. (Because of the diabetic's deranged fat metabolism and elevated blood cholesterol, the physician frequently taboos or minimizes the use of eggs, milk, butter, and liver — every one of which happens to be an important source of Vitamin A in the finished form. The result may be that the diabetic develops a Vitamin A deficiency. This is particularly threatening to a diabetic, for the disease brings with it a heightened susceptibility to cancer, and Vitamin A has been shown to protect against at least one type of cancer.) Likewise, people who have gall-bladder syndrome or some other form of fat intolerance may have difficulty in utilizing Vitamin A, since the vitamin is soluble in fat, which is its normal vehicle in the body. Some attention must be paid, too, to the fact that as we age, utilization of fat becomes less and less efficient, and this must have its impact on the efficiency of utilization of fat-soluble vitamins as well. For all these reasons, not only is the use of a Vitamin-A supplement justified, but a generous amount is also in order. Let us not forget that the dean of all nutritionists — H. C. Sherman of Columbia University — learned from his animal experiments that generous supplies of certain nutrients, with emphasis upon Vitamin A, prolonged the prime of life of his animals. The exact figure was 10 percent — a dividend devoutly to be wished.

On the basis of the preceding thinking, Vitamin A in the form of a fish-liver concentrate is a fine supplement for most people under the age of forty-five. Past that age, it might be wiser to use Vitamin A in a water-dispersible form. In this form, the vitamin particles are broken down, so that they are more efficiently absorbed The water-dispersible form will also be useful to those who are intolerant of fats, or who have disorders in which fat utilization is not normal.

The amount of Vitamin A recommended for adults is 10,000 units daily.

Vitamin D

For many years pediatricians have been persuaded that a child's need for supplements of Vitamin D tends to disappear when he enters school, and physicians generally have pursued that philosphy by assuring adults that there is no need for Vitamin D in the mature human organism. Many of us in nutrition have severely doubted the validity of both doctrines, and at least one paper has strengthened our convictions by citing previously unrecognized rickets in a shocking percentage of hospitalized children. Recently, the Estabishment has begun to toy with the idea that Vitamin D is likewise important to adults. This reversal of attitude should be received wryly by those women (and, for that matter, men) who, suffering from such bone diseases as osteoporosis, have been treated with Vitamin D.

At any rate, Vitamin D in 500-unit dosages is a safe amount to take.

Vitamin C

It is perhaps with this vitamin that we encounter our greatest difficulty setting a requirement. The minimum amount of Vitamin C I suggest for an adult is 250 mgs. daily. The orthodox dietician and the physician will assure you that estimates of the amount of Vitamin C needed to prevent scurvy never range beyond 35 mgs., and that estimates as low as 10 mgs. daily are on record. Why do I offer 250 mgs. as a proposed yardstick for daily intake, and why do I believe there are those who will require a great deal more?

For one thing, I do not believe that the function of a vitamin is restricted to prevention of the deficiency disease that occurs in its absence. Vitamin C has many functions in the body besides its role in prevention of scurvy. As I write this, I think with amusement of a British physician who decided to test an antibiotic in the treatment of a common cold. In these days of pervasive psychiatric indoctrination, we must always, in properly controlled studies, have a group of people who believe that they are taking the medication being tested, but who are actually being given something innocuous — a placebo. For this purpose, as his placebo, the British physician chose Vitamin C. This choice indicated, of course, that he discounted entirely the "folklore" attributing to Vitamin C any effect in checking colds. In the conclusion of his paper, he came to face to face with the realization that there is a basis for this folk legend. He said he did not understand why, but the group on the placebo fared better than those who were given antibiotics. He indicated his amazement that Vitamin C appeared to have a more profound antiviral effect than did the drugs created for that purpose.

It is pertinent here to remark that the range of requirements for vitamins in guinea pigs can be so great that an intake completely satisfactory for one animal may fail to keep another animal *alive!*

So it is that in recommending 250 mgs. of Vitamin C daily, I know that the gap between this level and that which is optimal for some people will be longer than for any other vitamin. (A good case in point is that of people who have avoided operations for slipped disc by taking large doses of Vitamin C. Those who say that doses of vitamins beyond our requirement are wasted have been careful to ignore this finding, which was reported by the Baylor University School of Medicine, and chronicled in *Reader's Digest*.) One must really experiment with Vitamin C to determine the daily dosage that will help most in preventing colds or, for that matter, in breaking them. Incidentally, I do not understand the excitement about Dr. Linus Pauling's remarks about Vitamin C and the common cold. That information was brought to the public in 1943, in my first book — from which the public stayed away in droves.

Vitamin B$_1$

I have set 2 mgs. of vitamin B$_1$ as a fair compromise for a daily supplementary amount. I am aware that there are individuals whose tendency to headaches has been reduced or eliminated by quantities of thiamin beyond this level, and I have already called your attention to the possibility that some speech impediments might yield to treatment with larger amounts of thiamin. However, I have the impression that for a large majority of the public, this quantity of vitamin B$_1$ will suffice. Again, there is no law against experimenting to determine if a higher level will give you dividends. It is always possible to add amounts of a single vitamin to the basic supplementing procedure.

Riboflavin

I do not know why the need for this factor is not as critical as the requirement for others. It *is* necessary to life, but over the years it seems to me that responses to large doses of riboflavin have been rather rare. Perhaps its greatest usefulness is in building resistance to fungus infections, such as athlete's foot. In some people an unsatisfied and elevated requirement for riboflavin will cause sensitivity to glare, particularly when facing bright sunlight on snow. Vision in dim light might likewise be impaired. At any rate, 4 mgs. of riboflavin daily would be a good investment.

Vitamin B₆

Pyridoxin is a vitamin of great importance to the brain and nervous system, muscles, skin, and the utilization of fat and protein. But it is a vitamin in short supply in the American diet. This shortage is partially due to the overprocessing of our flour, bread, and cereals. A loaf of white bread has about one-sixth the amount of Vitamin B_6 that is contained in whole-wheat bread. Although every reason that led to the enrichment of bread with Vitamin B_1 exists with Vitamin B_6, the bread industry now insists — since enrichment did not prove to be a bonanza in added sales and profits — that man does not live by bread alone, and that Vitamin B_6 can be obtained elsewhere in the food supply. This is, of course, the same industry that alternates in praising bread as the staff of life.

Four mgs. of pyridoxin daily should be a good basic intake. This amount may be increased in adolescence, when there are problems with the skin; in pregnancy, when utilization of the vitamin appears to be disturbed in most women; and in old age, when the effect of the vitamin in increasing the retention of nitrogen (protein) may help offset the negative nitrogen balance that causes wasting of aged tissues.

Niacinamide

This vitamin — miscalled Vitamin B_3 — is officially labeled as the prime antipellagra factor. Again, we are dealing with the very early stages of deficiency. However, niacinamide has profound effects on functioning of the brain and nervous system, and on the health of the soft tissues — as in the mouth. Dentists do not seem to know that a generous intake of niacinamide will sometimes reduce the deposits of tartar. Evidence exists that emphasizes a larger need for niacinamide than the amount officially set. I suggest 50 mgs.; I find that this benefits people who do not respond dramatically to the comparatively small amount recommended in the official tables.

Pantothenate

Pantothenic acid, calcium pantothenate, panthenol are all varieties of this vitamin. The quantity found in human tissues — particularly the muscles — and the relatively large amounts found in human milk as compared to other forms of milk suggest a need for pantothenate that goes far beyond the level suggested in the official tables of vitamin requirements. I therefore set pantothenate intake at about 20 mgs. It might help keep the male uric acid levels in the blood lower, thus possibly helping prevent gout or heart attack; and it might aid in preserving the functions of the adrenal glands, therefore serving to keep the hair from turning gray.

Vitamin B$_{12}$

Vitamin B$_{12}$ or cobalamin is an odd vitamin in several respects. Deficiency in it is unlikely, unless you are a vegetarian who avoids not only meat, fish, and fowl, but milk, dairy products, and eggs. However, failure of absorption is more common with Vitamin B$_{12}$; it usually is identified with the process that leads to pernicious anemia. This vitamin is actually too large a molecule to pass through any of the openings in the digestive tract, and manages the entry only by linking with a carrier, a kind of shuttle that acts to convey the Vitamin B$_{12}$ into the interior of the body. This shuttle is called the "intrinsic factor," (Vitamin B$_{12}$ was once called the "extrinsic factor." Therefore, when there is any question of proper utilization of Vitamin B$_{12}$, increasing the dose is not likely to solve the problem as it may for other vitamins. (The problem of inducing proper absorption of Vitamin B$_{12}$ explains the physician's frequent use of injections of the vitamin. This method of course bypasses the digestive tract and the difficulties.) Instead, doses of the vitamin would have to be accompanied by a supply of the intrinsic factor, obtained most conveniently from stomach tissue dried under vacuum (which *is* commercially available).

Ten micrograms of vitamin B$_{12}$ daily is a useful goal.

Vitamin E

There are four forms of Vitamin E that appear in food together. Collectively they are called the tocopherols. Of these, the one most fully active in the human body is the alpha form. It is believed, however, that the beta, gamma and delta forms of tocopherols serve to protect the alpha form from destruction in the body. For this reason, Vitamin E is best used — and incidentally, is least expensive — in the form of nonesterified mixed tocopherols, with the potency measured in terms of the most active form, alpha-tocopherol.* A supplement of 50 mgs. per day is adequate for the person who has eaten whole grains routinely over a period of years; 100 mgs. a day will be needed for the person who has eaten like the average Amer-

---

*There are some people in the field of nutrition who believe that the tocopherols are likely to be more easily utilized if they are not in the esterified form. Both forms — the nonesterified and the esterified are on the market.

ican — and even at this level of supplementing, it may require up to two years to replenish the storage. Therapeutic doses may reach 1000 mgs. daily or more. (1 mg. = 1 unit.)

Inositol

There are those who will challenge the incorporation of inositol in a supplement, on the grounds that it has not been proved to be essential, either in nutrition or in the body. However, there are unpublished findings concerning this vitamin, some of which I have been able to corroborate by personal observation. The amount of the factor in a balanced diet may be as high as 1000–1500 mgs. Giving 100 mgs. as a supplementary amount may seem to be, therefore, rather hesitant — but the fact is that it is difficult to find supplements that supply more. I have employed as high as 500–1000 mgs. a day in supplementary form.

Choline

While I have employed choline in therapeutic nutrition in quantities as high as 3000 mgs. a day, and 2500 mgs. is supplied by a well-balanced diet, we have the same problem here that we do with inositol — there are few supplements readily available that supply more than 100 mgs. of choline. This explains my adopting that level as a recommended amount. If you are able to locate the few commercial products that contain more of this factor, there is no reason why you should not raise your supplementary intake to 500 mgs. or even 1000 mgs.

Folic Acid

The quantity of folic acid available to the public in multiple-vitamin supplements has been severely restricted by the Food and Drug Administration, on the grounds that this vitamin may serve to conceal the progress of an anemia in the blood caused by Vitamin B_{12} deficiency. It should be pointed out that there are two fallacies in this policy. First, it is based on the belief that the blood is the first target for a deficiency of Vitamin B_{12}. It is not — in fact, it is possible to develop paranoid disturbances in behavior from Vitamin-B_{12} deficiency with no evidence of a pernicious anemia in the blood. Second, it supposes that the intake of folic acid from a supplement constitutes the only folic acid source in the diet — and that is obviously not true, even when the diet is virtually atrocious. In other words, a government agency that limits the amount of folic acid in a supplement should also limit the intake of spinach, milk, liver, and green vegetables, any one of which can supply enough folic acid to obscure the progress in the blood of the impact of a Vitamin-B$_{12}$ deficiency. In addition, the supposition that folic acid is important only to the blood is also fallacious. For one thing, folic acid interacts with female hormone — a characteristic that makes it most useful to the nutritionist or medical man who is attempting to compensate for inadequate estrogen activity in a female patient.

At any rate, the amount of folic acid available in supplements that are sold without a prescription is microscopic. There is no particular point, therefore, in setting up an optimal intake when it is not available.

Rutin, Hesperidin, and Bioflavonoids

These are factors that help protect Vitamin C from destruction in the body, intensify the action of Vitamin C as an antihistaminic and antiallergic factor, and protect blood vessels smaller than those that are strengthened by Vitamin C. There has been a consistent effort on the part of the Food and Drug Administration to denigrate the value of these factors on the grounds that all the papers that have found value in the bioflavonoids are "garbage," in research terms. Factually, some of these papers have been found quite satisfactory by qualified scientists, who regard the Food and Drug Administration attitude toward the bioflavonoids as part of its general campaign to dampen the public's enthusiasm for the use of vitamin and vitamin-like factors. If the bioflavonoids are to be truly useful, however, the quantities taken must be larger than those that have been provided in the Vitamin-C-plus-bioflavonoid supplements and in the multiple supplements currently available. I should like to see a supplemental intake of at least 900 mgs. of the bioflavonoids daily — really not too extravagant a goal when one considers that a large orange should yield approximately this amount. With the bioflavonoids, an inadequate dose does no harm. With rutin, another form of this factor, harm may result from an inadequate intake. I prefer a rutin dosage to begin at a level of 200 mgs. a day and not lower, unless it is accompanied by at least 200 mgs. of bioflavonoids.

Protein Factors

Aspartic acid is an amino acid that may increase resistance to fatigue. Lysine, an amino acid that is administered in gram quantities, is the factor not well supplied by cereal and vegetable protein.

Therefore, taking it would make the inferior protein of the diet much more valuable.

Glutamic acid or glutamine, which is the substance the body manufactures from glutamic acid, may also be a useful supplement to some people. I have already commented on the benefits that may be experienced by some schizophrenics from supplements of ornithine, which is an obscure protein compound. Glycine, the simplest of the amino acids, is also a fascinating substance, yielding to some individuals a great improvement in blood circulation and a distinct lift in the basal metabolism. I originally recommended it as a supplement in the diet of hypoglycemia. As soon as the public began to demand it, the Food and Drug Administration, faithfully pursuing its policy of dampening interest in the use of supplements, relabeled this simple food substance a "drug" and made it unavailable except upon prescription. However, whole gelatin contains at least 27 percent glycine.

Lecithin

Lecithin is a phosphatide, a factor that helps us in the utilization of fats and fatty substances in the body. It may improve the utilization of the fat-soluble vitamins, A, D, E, and K. It has been used in the treatment of certain skin disorders, particularly psoriasis. It also has had a remarkable quieting effect upon the nervous systems of some people. To be effective, lecithin must be used in fairly large quantities — one to two tablespoonsful daily. It is rather pointless, therefore, to incorporate it in a multiple-vitamin supplement unless one is willing to use a formula that requires taking fifteen or twenty capsules daily, which seems improbable. Lecithin is available in capsules or granule form. Since the quantity required is fairly large, the granule form would appear to be the most convenient, mixed with tomato juice, or added to cereal.

PABA

PABA is the chemical shorthand for para-aminobenzoic acid, a vitamin factor that is part of the Vitamin B Complex. PABA has remarkable actions in its metabolism in adrenal hormones, pituitary hormones, and estrogens. For those of age thirty-five on, it has long been my practice to supplement the diet with 100 mgs. of PABA daily, sometimes increasing the amount in the later years. But, the Food and Drug Administration has limited to 20 mgs. the amount of PABA that may be incorporated in a multiple-vitamin or a B-Complex vitamin supplement. Of course, the vitamin is available separately and additional amounts can be taken — which makes the limitation on multiple and B-Complex supplements an arbitrary inconvenience. If you can find no higher potency, the 20 mgs. will still be useful.

I am certain that if the following remarks are not made, I shall receive exasperated letters from many readers informing me — as if I didn't know it — that supplements exactly meeting these specifications are nonexistent. Of this, I am well aware — but are you well aware that reasonably increasing the amounts of vitamins suggested presents no hazards? In other words, I should be concerned with your taking materially less, but not at all concerned with your taking more.

These potencies are a starting point. For instance, you may find that you feel and function better with 500 mgs. of choline in your daily supplement rather than 100 mgs. You may be one of the minority who do better on 6 mgs. or 8 mgs. or 10 mgs. of thiamin daily, rather than 2 mgs. So far as it is possible to generalize, the intake of water-soluble vitamins presents no risk of toxicity, for water-soluble factors are not stored in the body. This fact explains the use of Vitamin C in gram quantities, and of B_{12} in amounts 1,000 times the postulated minimum daily requirement. With the fat-soluble vitamins, one cannot so freely increase intake. The quantity recommended in this chapter is safe, but somewhat larger amounts may be required by some individuals. If large amounts of the fat-soluble vitamins are used, the entire Vitamin B Complex — with emphasis on the factors that help in the utilization of fat, such as choline, inositol, and lecithin — must be employed to allow the liver maximum efficiency in coping with them. For short periods of time astronomical doses of the fat-soluble and water-soluble vitamins have been given, but in this chapter we are dealing with a supplement intended to be used for a lifetime. As the years go on, utilization may become less efficient, and a rise in the potencies may become necessary. More emphasis must be placed on the factors that help utilization: The use of the fat-soluble vitamins (A,D,E, and K) in the water-dispersible, emulsified, or dried form; lecithin, to improve fat utilization; dried stomach tissue, to help the absorption of Vitamin B_{12} — and your physician may wish to add hydrochloric acid for that purpose; and the daily use of yogurt to change favorably the nature of the bacterial flora in your intestine.

For those who prefer to use vitamin-mineral supplements entirely of natural origin, and who wonder whether potencies anywhere near these standards are available in concentrates that do not contain synthetic vitamins, a brief trip to your health-food store is in order. You will find available natural supplements of vitamins and minerals in potencies for the major part favorably comparing with those outlined in this chápter. A typical formula yields:

VITAMIN A: 25,000 units
VITAMIN D: 1,000 units
VITAMIN B$_1$: 7 mgs.
VITAMIN B$_2$: 14 mgs.
VITAMIN C: 200 mgs.
NIACIN: 4.5 mgs.
VITAMIN B$_{12}$: 25 micrograms
VITAMIN E: 100 mgs.

BIOFLAVONOIDS: (water-soluble) plus Hesperidin and Rutin: 40 mgs.
CALCIUM: 550 mgs.
PHOSPHORUS: 200 mgs.
IRON: 40 mgs.
IODINE: .1 mg.
MAGNESIUM: 40 mgs.

Some of these products also supply, as previously noted, pancreatic and other digestive enzymes. Several add glutamic and nucleic acids to the natural ingredients from which the vitamin concentrates are derived. However, there is a limit on the amount of concentration that can be applied to natural sources, and supplements so formulated and achieving these potencies necessarily are taken more than once daily. Also available in supplements of natural origin are formulas specifically directed to children. From brewer's yeast, rose hips, kelp, fish liver oil, and natural tocopherols, children's formulas are available, approximating:

VITAMIN A: 6,000 units
VITAMIN D: 400 units
VITAMIN C: 120 mgs.
VITAMIN B$_1$: 1.5 mgs.
VITAMIN B$_2$: 3 mgs.
NIACIN: .5 mgs.
VITAMIN B$_{12}$: 10 micrograms

VITAMIN E: 5 mgs.
BIOFLAVONOIDS: 40 mgs.
RUTIN: 10 mgs.
l-LYSINE: 50 mgs.
CALCIUM: 150 mgs.
IODINE: .1 mg.
PEPTONIZED IRON: 15 mgs.

These potencies represent a starting point, but if larger amounts of individual vitamins are desired, they should be added to the intake of the basic supplement.

RANGE OF SUPPLEMENTARY VITAMIN INTAKES FOR TEENAGERS AND ADULTS

VITAMIN A — 10,000 to 25,000 units daily
VITAMIN D — 500 to 1,500 units daily

VITAMIN C — 250 to 5,000 mgs. daily
VITAMIN B1 — 2 to 10 mgs. daily
RIBOFLAVIN — 4 to 8 mgs. daily
VITAMIN B6 — 4 to 20 mgs. daily
NIACINAMIDE — 50 to 5,000 mgs. daily
PANTOTHENIC ACID — 20 to 100 mgs. daily
VITAMIN B12 — 10 to 50 mgs. daily
VITAMIN E — 50 to 300 mgs. daily
INOSITOL — 100 to 500 mgs. daily
CHOLINE — 100 to 1,000 mgs. daily
BIOFLAVONOIDS — 900 to 3,000 mgs. daily
RUTIN — 200 to 500 mgs. daily
PABA — 10 to 100 mgs. daily

What about vitamin toxicity? Here would be a good place to label the entire story of toxicity of vitamins as another device used to discourage the public from taking supplements. Vitamin A has been used as a supplement to the diet for hundreds of years. If that statement astonishes you, you have forgotten about the time-honored use of cod liver oil. There have not been hundreds of cases of toxicity among millions of users. Actually, there have been far fewer than one hundred — and in most of these cases, the individual took self-prescribed or medically recommended daily doses of many hundreds of thousands of units of Vitamin A and continued to do so over a long period of time. There is nothing that will not become toxic at some dosage level. To derive from these isolated incidents a principle that warns the public that vitamins are toxic seems capricious. As for the stories of Vitamin-D toxicity, some mothers administered teaspoonsful of concentrates that were supposed to be given in doses of fifteen drops daily to their young babies. As a matter of historical interest, you might wish to know that Vitamin D in doses of 50,000 units to 200,000 units daily was prescribed for the treatment of arthritis for many years, and to this day, dosages almost as high are used in the treatment of myopia.

When an individual — child or adult — achieves toxicity with dosages of vitamins far exceeding recommendations on the label or prescription of the physician, would you not say that a newspaper headline "vitamins found toxic" is at least another version of the man-bites-dog variety of sensationalism?

It may also be of interest to note that vitamin toxicity is more likely to occur when vitamins are used individually, which is not the way nature provides them. That is to say, the Vitamin B Complex is called a complex because the vitamins tend to come together, and the diet ordinarily will supply or be deficient in more than one factor at a time. Actually, animal experiments have shown that the administration of very large doses of Vitamin A does not produce toxicity if the Vitamin B Complex has been given simultaneously. Since Vitamin A is a fat-soluble factor and Vitamin B Complex contains several factors that help the liver in the management of fats, this result would be predictable.

The previous observation provides the answer to a question that may occur to you after reading the recommendations for supplementing the diet. Let us suppose that you are using brewer's yeast, liver, and a multiple-vitamin-mineral supplement — but you have an exaggerated need for one of the vitamins. What do you do? The answer is obvious: Add a dosage of that vitamin to your basic supplementing procedure. In this way, you not only avoid multiplying doses of other factors to arrive at a higher dosage of one, but you take advantage of the inter-relationships among vitamins and minerals, which are profound.

MINERALS

In formulating recommendations for a mineral supplement, we are faced with even graver technical problems than those presented by the vitamins. The range of requirement for some of the minerals is as great as that for the vitamins; the supply, particularly with regard to the trace minerals that are needed in very small quantities, is even more conjectural than it is for the vitamins. In addition, exactly as there are unknown factors among vitamins that may one day prove to be extremely important, so are there minerals we do not now consider to be vital in human chemistry but one day may very well prove to be so. A good example is trivalent chromium — intake of which has been shown to help the metabolism of sugars and starches. Some authoritative medical men indicate that doses of this mineral may prove important to diabetics. (Brewer's yeast, which contains trivalent chromium, has been used as a supplement to the diabetic diet for many decades.) This same statement might be made for vanadium, intake of which is known to lower blood cholesterol. Among the trace minerals, there are factors that lower the incidence of tooth decay — not calcium, not phosphorous, and apparently not any of the minerals one would be inclined to label as being important to tooth enamel. So here is an area in which we have a great deal to learn. This was demonstrated most vividly in the list of minerals suggested for use as supplements by a nationally known bio-chemist, who allowed 10 mgs. of iron — a sensible amount, but suggested 5 mgs. of zinc — a metal that is needed by the body in larger quantities than iron.

The processes that remove vitamins from foods also remove minerals. The cooking techniques that cause a loss of vitamins engender a smaller loss of minerals. In the processing of canned and frozen foods, there are stages in which there are significant losses of potassium and smaller but significant losses of trace minerals. The filters and distillation units many Americans use in an effort to make dubious drinking water safer and more palatable likewise deprive them of minerals.

A lowering of mineral intake is not the only direct concern. There are also networks of interrelationships between vitamins and minerals: There is probably interaction between Vitamin E and manganese, between Vitamin B_6 and potassium, between Vitamin C and calcium, between magnesium and Vitamin B_{12}, and between zinc and Vitamin B_1.

It is true that the requirements for minerals other than calcium, phosphorus, potassium, iron, and zinc are so small that, theoretically, an auxiliary supply would seem unnecessary. But it is this faulty reasoning that has persuaded many professional men to prescribe vitamins without minerals. There are two possible errors in this course of action. Neither the supply nor the utilization of trace minerals need necessarily be adequate. More importantly, there are a number of instances when the simultaneous presence of the vitamin and trace minerals in the digestive tract will be advantageous. For example, Vitamin C will aid in the utilization of iron only if they are ingested simultaneously. Magnesium helps the absorption of Vitamin B_{12} only if both are present in the colon at the same time. The action of Vitamin D in facilitation and absorption of calcium obviously cannot be exerted if the mineral is not simultaneously available.

We must also consider defects in enzyme manufacture such as those that are responsible for exaggerated needs for certain vitamins. Since minerals, more frequently than not, are components of such enzymes, we have as much reason for mineral supplementing as we do for vitamin supplementing.

The use of bone meal, kelp, sea salt, and blackstrap molasses, will, of course, provide variable quantities of trace minerals, as will calcium, phosphorus, iron, and zinc. However, I have a bias in favor of knowing the actual supplementary intake. I have therefore, for many years, suggested the use of mineral supplements with formulas approximating:

Calcium: From 250 to 1,000 mgs. in the total daily dose. The quantity used will in part be determined by the amount of milk and cheese in the diet. Setting the objective at 1,000 mgs., each glass of milk or each ounce of hard cheese should be considered as deducting 250 mgs. of calcium from the amount needed in the supplement.

The utilization of calcium will be aided by the Vitamin D in the vitamin supplement and may be further improved by one or two tablespoonsful of lactose with each dose of calcium. The lactose will also probably offset the constipating effect calcium has on some individuals.

Phosphorus: 180 to 750 mgs. daily.

Iron: 15 mgs. to 18 mgs.

Zinc: From 20 to 100 mgs. While in this formulation we are not considering the possible use of zinc as an aid to healing, which would call for therapeutic doses that would necessarily be higher, the range of zinc intake is suggested to meet the varying and rising requirements of older people and diabetics. Thus 20 mgs. will be generally adequate for the teenager and younger adult, with the recommended intake thereafter increasing.

Magnesium: 150 to 270 mgs.

Manganese: 1 mg.

Iodine: 0.15 mg.

While all minerals are ultimately of natural origin, there are concentrates of minerals from natural sources available. These are derived from bone meal, kelp, and other mineral-rich natural substances.

In the 1890s a clerk resigned from the U.S. Patent Office, saying that everything had been invented and there was obviously no future in his calling. I am reminded of this story when nutritionists conclude that we are now in possession of all the individual factors that comprise food, because we can keep animals alive on purified starch, purified fat, amino acids, and a handful of the known vitamins and the needed minerals. However, these people will criticize the formulas for the supplements in this chapter on two grounds: Many of these factors have not been proven essential in human nutrition; and recommended quantities of essential factors are above the standards suggested by the government and the medical societies. As a person who has had an opportunity to watch the response of thousands of people to doses of vitamins at varying levels, I have concluded that our principal sin is inadequate dosage rather than overdosage. With respect to emphasis on factors not proved to be essential to human nutrition, let me observe that there have been experiments in vitamin-mineral therapy for neurotics and psychotics in which dosages of vitamins and minerals confined to those factors generally accepted as being necessary in human nutrition produced no response, but formulas with many factors not demonstrably needed by the human organism did in fact act therapeutically. Under the circumstances, as a nutritionist who has been guiding the public in the use of the supplements as well as foods for more than thirty years, I should rather err by providing factors that are not useful, than commit the sin of failure through omission.

There are several questions that will have occurred to you by now. Surely you will wonder why so many vitamin supplements — including those manufactured by major pharmaceutical houses — do not comply with the specifications given here. In many cases some of the vitamins and minerals will not be provided; some vitamin supplements provide no minerals at all; and potencies in many cases will be below those I have suggested. Unfortunately, many commercial supplements are formulated by the bookkeeper rather than the chemist, which results in generous quantities of vitamins that are cheap to manufacture and fewer vitamins that are expensive to manufacture. Many supplements from major manufacturers will also lack all the nutrients labeled as "need in human nutrition not established." This omission simply represents the path of least resistance. It is easier to go along with the dictates of the orthodoxy rather than violate their taboos and create a need for expensive educational advertising.

You must not conclude that the supplements described in this chapter are going to be costly. Careful search of the shelves in the health-food store or drugstore will reveal numerous brands that will approximate these values at prices within reason.

Several questions remain to be answered before we leave the topic of nutritional supplements. Is the list, so far as we know, of factors complete? It is not — not even within the limitations of present knowledge. There is, for instance, Vitamin B_{15} (pangamic acid) which is in use in Europe, but not often employed in America except when it appears naturally as part of the Vitamin B Complex. There is Vitamin B_{17}, known as Laetrille, which has been reported to be useful in the treatment of cancer, and may be useful in its prevention. As usual, with all products not originating with the Establishment, the Food and Drug Administration promptly moved to suppress it, using a technique so blatantly unfair that several government officers have protested the entire procedure. At the present time, Vitamin B_{17}, like Vitamin B_{15}, cannot be obtained in this country except as it may occur in a natural source. There are also minerals like vanadium, which has demonstrated a real potential in reducing blood cholesterol, and there may be others with actions useful to the body, the existence of which we know, but the actions of which we do not yet understand. Consider the fact that vegetables grown on soil reclaimed from the sea have helped reduce tooth decay, yet we cannot ascribe this action to any particular mineral, including fluorides.

It is for these reasons, of course, that I have reiterated the statement that a supplement *is* a supplement, not a substitute to intelligent selection of foods.

I am frequently asked when supplements should be taken. They should be taken either before or after a meal, since certain vitamins appear to be better utilized when they are taken with food, and this is their normal "environment."

It will be perfectly reasonable, as you contemplate the plunge into good diet and into the use of supplements, to ask about the dividends. Frequently, they are not spectacular. After all, in your present hostile environment, you are faced with a large number of threats ranging from radioactivity to pesticide residue to water pollution to food additives, which may or may not cause disease. Good nutrition is one of your means of "detoxifying" some of the inimical chemicals in your environment. What does *not* happen may be a very rewarding dividend. Some of the other benefits are almost as subtle, and, indeed, you may not appreciate them until you decide to revert to your previous dietary habits and drop the use of the supplements. After a few months, you gain a very useful perspective on the well-being that you were enjoying without consciously realizing it. Perhaps the best way to appraise the benefits of good nutrition is to ask what has kept me dedicated to the cause of education in nutrition over so long a period of years, when it has involved me in crusades I did not ask for and battles with the Establishment, which took valuable time that might have been devoted to more constructive purposes. I can tell you about hundreds of families whose infertility was succeeded by high reproductive efficiency. I have watched the paranoid lose his delusions, the arthritic restored to social and vocational usefulness, the "senile" become functional again, the nervous become serene. There have also been the less dramatic, but equally meaningful changes: Healthier hair, better nails, skin with better tone, better elimination, more resistance to fatigue, improved sleep, all the "little" things that are so important in determining one's feeling of well-being.

If you select your food with reasonable intelligence, supplement your diet in the way suggested in this chapter, and make an effort to give yourself the degree of preventive maintenance conferred upon any good car — meaning reasonable medical checkups, and dental care — there is no doubt that you will be starting on the pathway to better health. I recall one doctor who examined me, when I was in my late fifties, for a very large insurance policy. In the course of the examination, I was subjected to rigorous testing and at the end the doctor said: "Not a darned thing wrong!" He added: "There must be something to this nutrition business!" To this I responded with a question. "What percentage of men in their late fifties have 'not a darned thing wrong'?" The doctor replied, "No percentage — every man over fifty has something wrong." There you have some of the dividends I have personally enjoyed. I wish them to you.

11.

HOW TO SHOP IN A
HEALTH-FOOD STORE
— AND WHY

The Commissioner of the Food and Drug Administration, in "supporting" his unbelievable decision to continue to allow the beef industry to fatten cattle with diethylstilbestrol, remarked that the use of the hormone saves the consumer about 1 cent per pound for beef. One might suggest that the Commissioner weigh the penny per pound versus the cost of a single case of terminal cancer, then reevaluate his decision. The trouble with the reasoning of the people who head such agencies is that they are dealing with statistics rather than people.

You may be considering the possible hazards of food additives from the same academic point of view. Let us make this matter of chemicals in food a little more real. About 700,000,000 pounds of peanut butter is manufactured in this country yearly, and most of it is consumed by children. One child probably consumes more than four pounds of peanut butter per year. The standard for peanut butter allows the use of food additives and cheap sweeteners. Consequently, a child, eating four pounds of peanut butter a year, is swallowing over sixty teaspoonsful of additives from this one source alone! Not only do these additives have no food value, but you are paying for them at the price of a food. Furthermore, the best that can be said for such food additives is that we hope they are harmless. No one has yet portrayed them as a boon to a child's body and yours.

Returning to the diethylstilbestrol, the most favorable thing that has been said for this hormone is that it boosts the weight gain of the animal. No one can describe that weight gain as a consumer benefit. It is mostly fat and water, rather than beef, and you pay for it at beef prices. The grower gleans the profit, and you and your family take the risk of ingesting diethylstilbestrol. This hormone, administered to pregnant women in the early 1950s, exerted its baleful effect on the babies, who, however, did not succumb to vaginal cancer until twenty years later. The time period involved is of critical importance. It is the best possible answer to those who say that no food additive has ever been demonstrated to have caused any harm. This is a frequent plaint from the Food and Drug Administration and industry spokesmen. Factually, when twenty or even thirty years can elapse between insult and effect, how can anyone know exactly what has caused the disaster? When a physician diagnoses cancer, with the exception of the diethylstilbestrol tragedy just cited, he is hardly ever able to tell you how it originated. In fact, he usually doesn't even speculate upon the cause.

This information should explain the increasing patronage of health-food stores. There are now millions rather than a handful of Americans who have decided that only the additives you do not swallow are totally without harm — and that is the only way in which one can make positive statements about the risks of the vast array of chemicals that season, color, change the texture of, or in other ways modify our food supply. It is therefore reassuring to me to be told that an increasing percentage of the patronage of the health-food store is made of young people who just a few years ago derided such shopping practices. At the same time, the newcomer to a health-food store may arrive there with certain prejudices still entrenched. Do you have a picture, for instance, of the health-food-store patron as an individual who eats alfalfa doused in blackstrap molasses, swallows dolomite tablets, and looks — appropriately — generally unhappy? You should now realize that the use of supplements does not mark the eccentric, and that the use of special-purpose foods — liver, brewer's yeast — does not mean eating a tasteless diet. You who enjoy our commercial bubble-gum white bread have a degenerated palate, which you will realize only when you become habituated to good whole-grain breads, cookies, cakes, and cereals. That is not an idle statement. In New York City, two major bakers recently introduced completely natural loaves of whole-wheat bread, with all the "garnishings" to which health-food store patrons are accustomed — polyunsaturated fat for shortening and sea salt* and the like — and report with apparent astonishment that the demand seems insatiable. It is obviously a demand from the average housewife and not from the seasoned health-food-store customer.

This chapter is primarily a shopping guide for the newcomer to a health-food store. But you who are old-timers may profit by reading it, too, for there are some products in health-food stores that should not be there, some which are overpriced, and some which are less preferable than others.

Do not begin with the assumption that all foods sold in health-food stores are nutritionally superior, or entirely free of undesirable additives. This is simply not so. I have found candy in health-food stores laden with additives, artificially colored and flavored; and in most stores you will find gum and candy labeled "sugar-free" that actually contain manitol or sorbitol, which are carbohydrates that yield calories that must be considered both by diabetics and by reducers. The only virtue of such carbohydrates is that they do not attack teeth as sugar does. I have always regarded the label "sugar-free" on such products as being somewhat deceptive.

The cornflakes in a health-food store — unless they are made from whole corn, which I have not yet found — are no better than the cornflakes in the supermarket. On the other hand, there are many cereals — some of European origin — in the health-food store that do represent excellent nutrition. One must be a label reader both in the supermarket and in the health-food store.

Most health-food stores now have refrigeration and freezer space. In this department, you are likely to find cheeses made from certified raw milk. While the price premium is high, there are good reasons for introducing sources of uncooked protein into the diet. Whether you are aware of it or not, practically all of the protein we eat is heat treated — and this represents a departure from man's customs during his eons of evolution.** Therefore, if you can afford to pay the extra cost of cheeses

*The Food and Drug Administration attempted to dampen the enthusiasm for the use of sea salt by announcing that it causes high blood pressure in rats. Americans who naively believe that this agency protects the consumer would not know that the poorer nations of the world have used sea salt for centuries, because their people can not afford the luxury of salt processed to remove its mineral values. Only the initiate in nutrition would also know that sea salt, according to the *Journal of the American Medical Association,* is less toxic than ordinary salt (meaning in overdosage), and for reasons not understood it reduces the requirement for the Vitamin B Complex.

**The pituitaries of animals and human beings who are the products of pregnancies in which all the protein was cooked may suffer functional limitations. In women, this can cause symptoms ranging from premenstrual tension to feelings of inadequacy. The external physical symptom of the process is a narrow palate. In men, according to studies by Dr. Weston Price, the same condition may be responsible for asocial behavior such as crimes of senseless violence.

made from certified raw milk, or for certified raw milk itself, by all means do so. (I do not mean the use of ordinary raw milk, which, however clean the barn and the farmer and the cow, may convey disease.) Also available in many of the stores will be "organic" eggs. In contrast to those you buy elsewhere, you will find that these eggs have shells so strong that breaking them becomes a real chore. They are quite unlike the paper-thin shells, so frequently cracked in the carton, which you have bought elsewhere. This thickness is of course a testimonial to a better diet provided to the hen. We definitely know that better diet for the hen shows up as increased nutritional values in the eggs. Whether that increase is commensurate with the higher price charged for the eggs, you must decide. I myself pay the premium. I do think that a dollar and ten cents a dozen for such eggs, as compared with perhaps sixty or seventy cents a dozen for large eggs sold in the ordinary commercial outlet is a sizable premium. However, it is my educated guess that this is probably a good investment.

I have no patience with bread described as being flourless, for carbohydrate is carbohydrate and I cannot find any excuse for bread that is sold at a dollar a loaf. But you *will* find in the freezer or refrigerator section of most health-food stores good, wholesome whole-grain loaves, with a texture that requires the kind of chewing that may spare you the need for water massaging your gums in a frantic effort to save loosening teeth. In addition, there usually are available whole-corn, whole-rye, and whole-wheat breads, and occasionally, "Cornell formula" bread, which describes a loaf made from unbleached flour with such nutritious additives as wheat germ, soy flour, and nonfat milk. This loaf of white bread will satisfy the palate of families conditioned to the commercial variety while freely feeding them infinitely better nutrition. Some stores sell a mix that is of the "Cornell-formula" type for baking at home.* This is an excellent way to initiate your family into eating better bread, for the bread appears to be white and actually has values beyond some of those provided by whole-wheat bread.

In many stores there will be "organic" produce in the refrigerator section. It is priced higher than ordinary fruits and vegetables for several good reasons. The yield is reduced as a proportion of the crop will be sacrificed to birds and insects, and labor charges are greater when insects must be plucked off by hand. In many instances there are considerable charges for transportation — a good deal of produce

---

*See appendix for "Cornell Formula." In your library you should also find *The Natural Foods Cookbook,* and *The Natural Foods Primer,* by Beatrice Trum Hunter. Both are kitchen guides for the beginner, and the latter teaches you how to make your own "Cornell" mix and the bread based on it.

originates in California and is then flown to New York. Ultimately, competition and increased production will bring these charges down, but again the premium seems to be well worth paying when one can feed a family on fruits and vegetables that do not carry residues of insecticides known to be poisonous.

So far as the nutritional value of "organically fertilized" fruits and vegetables goes, there is the usual debate in progress. The Establishment behaves as if all the evidence were on its side, and chemical fertilization showed all plusses, no debits, with nothing to the credit of the organic method of cultivation. Actually, there is evidence to indicate that the excessive use of nitrates as a chemical fertilizer is beginning to become a very distinct pollution problem — the excesses run off into our streams. There is also some evidence that in the body these nitrates may be converted into other compounds, which may include at least one that is among the most active cancer-producing chemicals yet discovered. In behalf of the organic method of fertilization, one experiment has shown that babies fed on organically fertilized carrots grew better than those receiving carrots from the same seed fertilized in the ordinary way.

When you first try organic fruits and vegetables, you will notice that there are many varieties that are distinctly more succulent than those you are accustomed to buying. You will certainly come to the realization that your salad greens have been flavorless, and your fruits woody. This difference derives not only from the method of fertilization used on the organically raised produce, but also from the use of varieties of seeds that have not been employed commercially. The criteria used in selection of varieties in large-scale commercial production ordinarily is how well does this keep, how well does it can, how well does it ship? You will note that there is no consideration of flavor and less of nutritional value.

At this point you may wonder how the health-food industry knows that the produce has in fact been organically raised — meaning properly fertilized and free of sprays. The industry, I am happy to report, is taking important steps toward policing its suppliers. There is also under way a modest program, which will be expanded as time goes on, to subsidize testing of organically raised produce, grains, and other foods at major universities in order to fix superior nutritional values, which present evidence indicates are a by-product of the old-fashioned way of cultivation.

Whether in the refrigerator section or elsewhere in the health-food store, you will find a substantial assortment of bottled fruit juices. Once again the prices will be higher than those you are accustomed to paying.

You might measure those prices against an arbitrary standard. Here, for instance, is the text of the label on apple juice that we drink in my home:

"Made from organically grown, whole, carefully washed and inspected apples, processed unclarified to preserve solids and pectin."

Beyond the intrinsic interest of the statements on the label, which imply a more nutritious product, you should consider what is not on the label: Preservatives, and a long list of pesticide residues permissible on apples and thereby permissible in apple juice. You pays your money and you takes your choice!

Not all health-food stores carry fresh produce, and there are still a few that do not have refrigerator facilities. Virtually all the stores, however, sell whole grains. You can buy brown rice, which is much better for you than white and is superior to converted; whole-grain barley instead of the pearled barley, which has lost nutritional value; whole buckwheat, which you can use as a cereal or as a substitute for rice; and whole-buckwheat flour, which lends a delightful accent to other flours for baking and pancakes. There are also such interesting and nutritious products as buckwheat groats, known to the orthodox Jew as "kasha" but more generally known as buckwheat grits. There is bulgar, which is a whole-wheat product with the seed cracked, used from time immemorial in the Near East. It is useful in casserole dishes, stews, and soups. Many people use bulgar as a cereal.

Cornmeal (not degerminated) is available in most health-food stores, and you will find that the undegerminated variety makes cornsticks, muffins, and cornbread that will stay fresh and moist much longer than the processed variety, which you invariably get in the supermarket. (Except in the state of Georgia, where bitter experience with pellagra and other dietary deficiency diseases led to the passing of a law that makes degerminated cornmeal illegal. Would that it were, elsewhere.) You will also find millet, old-fashioned oatmeal, peanut and barley flours, brown-rice flour, whole-rye meal, wheat germ (which should be vacuum packed), and other whole grains and flours with which you can start some of the most rewarding kitchen ventures: Baking good bread, cakes, and cookies and making good cereals for the family. The health-food store also has *some* pancake mixes that are superior to the ordinary commercial variety; bread mixes that will save you time; and occasionally cake mixes. These products need to be examined carefully to make sure that you are not sacrificing nutritional value for convenience. If you want to do that, you can do it at less cost in the supermarket.

Before you approach the section of the health-food store where cooking and salad oils are displayed, you will need a little background to interpret labels properly. On the labels of these oils will appear the words "cold pressed." To understand the term, one must know something about the method by which our oils are prepared. Generally, the cooking and salad oils of commerce are derived from seeds of one type or another, which are preheated (perhaps with steam) and pressed; the oil is expressed and then subjected to a long series of treatments, which include bleaching, chilling, heating, and saponifying (treatment with an active alkaline agent to produce soap, which is discarded, and then the residue processed further). At the end of the line, the oil may be filtered through activated charcoal and subjected to forty or fifty filtrations by other methods. It is obvious that the original composition of the oil must change drastically in this series of treatments. One evidence of undesirable alteration in the composition of oils is the long list of preservatives you will find on the label. The natural antioxidant for oils is Vitamin E in its various forms.* When processing has so reduced Vitamin E that the oil no longer has any natural protection against the attack of oxygen, the manufacturer must turn to the use of butylhydroxytoluene, butylhydroxyanisole, or perhaps propylgallate — and sometimes to a combination of all three. These additives, two of which are known to be hazardous, represent tombstones to departed natural vitamin antioxidants. Their presence therefore is a double affront to the knowledgeable consumer.

The term "cold pressed" put on health-food-store oils is supposed to represent the end product of processing techniques that eliminate the drastic methods used with commercial oils. Actually, this is not true. In fact, the term "cold pressed" is meaningless, and would, were it accurate, represent a suspension of the laws of physics. It is not possible to apply great pressure to a grain or seed without causing heat, nor is it possible to produce a clear oil of the kind you will find labeled as "cold pressed" without using many of the techniques employed on the supermarket oils. So far as I am concerned, the only virtue — an important one — of the health-food-store product is its freedom from the undesirable antioxidants that mark virtually all oils sold through other channels.

Always buy vegetable oils in small quantities and preferably in brown bottles or in metal cans. Use them promptly. If you fry with them, discard the fat after the first frying. If I could discard hundreds of

---

*Ironically, when oils are without protection against oxygen, the resulting chemical reaction turns the oil into a substance that actually causes Vitamin-E deficiency. You will recall that the chapter on aging suggests that a Vitamin-E inadequacy is a good way to accelerate the entire aging process.

gallons of fat at a summer camp to protect the children, you can do it for your family.

We are now left, however, with the problem of restoring to our diets the values that are lost when oils are processed. An important factor removed from the clarified oils of commerce is lecithin. This is an agent that helps emulsify fats. It is therefore used to help keep blood cholesterol from depositing on and in the walls of the arteries. It is also used to help fat utilization and to improve the utilization of the fat-soluble vitamins. It has an important role in the nervous system and the brain. Lecithin, however, can be purchased in the health-food store in granule or liquid form and be used as a food supplement. I use the granules in tomato juice; some people sprinkle them on cereal. They are sometimes labeled "soy phosphatides," a term deriving from the fact that lecithin is a by-product of the soy industry. The liquid form of lecithin can be mixed with vegetable oils or butter, which is poetic justice because these phosphatides are removed from commercial oils. When mixed in this way, you are restoring some of the unsaturated fat and helping the utilization of all the fats in the diet. To assure one's self of the Vitamin E lost in processing, simply consult the guidelines for Vitamin E in the vitamin-supplementing formula listed in Chapter Ten. To bring back to the diet arachidonic acid, an important factor in the treatment of the brain injured and in many neuromuscular diseases, it would be desirable to use wheat-germ oil to mix with the pressed oil, solely for use on salads. Subjecting such a product to heat would defeat one's purpose. Usually, I add about 25 percent wheat-germ oil to the salad oil, but if your family's taste buds are sensitive, it is better to begin with a smaller percentage and gradually increase it.

While we are discussing fats, let me note that although the margarines I have encountered in the health-food stores are sometimes free of the long list of chemicals found in commercial margarines, their flavors, at least to my family and me, are hardly pleasing. Taste is as individual a reaction as tolerance for and needs in food — you might try a few of the brands to arrive at an improvement on this basic food.

In most of the health-food stores you will find yeast for baking. This has the virtue of being free of butylhydroxyanisole, which thus far I have not been able to avoid in the yeast from other sources. My only complaint is that its leavening action seems to be somewhat less than that of the commercial yeast of yesteryear. I find that I have to use a rounded tablespoon rather than the level tablespoon the package calls for to obtain the action of a cake of yeast. This is not to be used as a supplement to the diet, but as a way of avoiding baking powder. Baking powder brings considerable sodium into the diet that we don't need, contributes no nutritional values, and creates an environment that may actually destroy some nutritional values in baked recipes. Yeast lends delightful flavor and added nutritional value without debits.

In the previous chapter I have described some of the forms of brewer's yeast that can be used as supplements to the diet. Let us expand upon that information slightly. Dried brewer's yeast is not a living organism and therefore is never used for leavening. Its sole purpose is for supplementing the diet. Primary brewer's yeast has been grown specifically for use as a supplement; secondary brewer's yeast has been grown for use in brewing and is then recovered and sold as a supplement. Since the brewer does not care about the vitamin value, check to see if the yeast is primary or secondary; whether it conveys the generous values in vitamins, minerals, and protein that can be achieved by careful selection of yeast and by use of appropriate media in which to grow. Some companies grow brewer's yeast in buttermilk whey or beef bouillon, thus incorporating into the yeast much larger quantities of the sulphur-containing amino acids than yeast would ordinarily supply. Other companies grow Vitamin B_{12} into yeast and manage to raise the Vitamin B_6 and the total protein value of yeast to significantly high levels. (Vitamin B_{12} is ordinarily associated only with animal protein.) Other yeasts are grown for high vitamin value and for palatability. It is therefore necessary to experiment with yeast, try a number of brands both in the flake and the powder form, and learn to use it for the invaluable supplement it can be. In most baked recipes — particularly in bread — small amounts of brewer's yeast can be incorporated without changing the characteristics, other than nutritionally, of the finished product. Torula yeast has been described as being nutritionally less desirable than brewer's yeast, but there is one variety of torula that has been smoked over hickory to achieve a bacon flavor. This smoking becomes a useful way of bringing additional nutritional values into the diet. The smoked yeast can be employed whenever a bacon flavor is acceptable — in lentil soup, on eggs, in salads. The addition of brewer's yeast or smoked torula yeast to such foods as stew in the last fifteen or twenty minutes of cooking does a great deal to restore vitamin values that ordinarily are seriously depleted during long cooking. This technique was used in the commissaries of shipyards in World War II.

There is one product in the health-food store that really ought to escape the confines of limited distribution, but has not yet been discovered by the public. This is carob. Carob comes from a tree in the locust family, the pods of which are ground and roasted. The finished product is almost indistinguishable from chocolate. Carob, however, is free of stimulants, low in fat, and has virtually no allergenic properties. (I have never understood parents who deny coffee and tea to a young child but allow him chocolate, cola drinks, and cocoa.) I have experimented successfully with carob to make "chocolate" icing, milk flavoring, cookies, candy, and cakes, and find — when you select the right brands of carob — that it is perfectly possible to deceive children into accepting this superior food in place of chocolate. (For those who are cynics, I did my recipe testing in a summer camp at which I was nutrition director. We violated all the traditions of the camping industry by serving nothing but top-notch nutrition.)

The mention of carob candy reminds me that health-food stores carry numerous products made with raw sugar, turbinado sugar, and brown sugar. There is no form of sugar that does not cause tooth decay. There is no form of sugar that does not increase the need for B-Complex vitamins without materially augmenting the supply. In fact, I know of only one brand of raw sugar that retains any significant amount of nutritional value. This is difficult to achieve, for the methods used in concentrating sugar are inimical to retention of these values. So do not go overboard on the use of raw sugar any more than you do with ordinary white sugar. It is true that in the less processed varieties of sugar trivalent chromium is retained, which helps us to utilize sugars, but this does not warrant a raw-sugar binge.

In some health-food stores, you will find royal-jelly products. These are looked upon with disfavor by the Establishment, which for me is almost automatically an endorsement of possible helpfulness. Royal jelly should be purchased in the fresh form in capsules, not in the "dried" or "desiccated" form in which it appears in some royal-jelly supplements. On the market there is also honey fortified with royal jelly, which is worth buying. Royal jelly is the special food the bees create to feed to queen bees. It is richer than honey in certain values.

Many varieties of honey are sold in the health-food store. Most brands will claim superiority because the honey was not heat treated nor clarified by filtration through charcoal. Such filtration would drop the small vitamin-mineral value in honey by about 35 percent and therefore serves no constructive purpose. Honey is a misunderstood food, even by the knowledgeable in nutrition. It contains a sizable amount of sucrose, which is identical with the sugar in the sugar bowl — intake of which is already too large. In honey there is fructose, also known as fruit sugar or levulose. It is regarded as a potential benefit to diabetics and hypoglycemics, because it is believed not to elicit insulin production, although converted into glucose in the body. However, if this is true, the relief is purchased at the price of consumption of excessive amounts of sucrose, so don't abuse honey. My personal preference is for honey in the comb, which we consume in its entirety. Don't make a face! There is value in the comb, and the taste of honey in the comb is pleasant.

Another sweetening agent popular with the nutrition minded is blackstrap molasses. This form of molasses is richest in nutritional value, since it contains nutrients that should have been retained in sugar. Its taste, however, is rather bitter. I use it as I use wheat-germ oil — I combine it with a lighter form of molasses and increase the percentage until the family detects what I am doing, and then I decrease it a little. There is about fifteen times as much iron in blackstrap molasses as in ordinary molasses, and some of the B vitamins are retained — amazing when one considers how much processing has preceded the making of this concentrate. The brand of blackstrap molasses chosen should be one that indicates that the product has been properly prepared for human consumption. This food is also used for cattle feed, which tells us automatically that it must be good nutrition, for in this country we feed animals better than we do children. If you have heard that blackstrap molasses contains the rust from the sugar-processing machinery, you might ask yourself when that machinery has a chance to grow rusty in a country where people eat an average of 104 pounds of sugar a year. If you have heard that blackstrap molasses is contaminated with lead, remember that it *is* used as cattle food, and cattle are at least as sensitive to lead as we are.

Yogurt in the health-food store is open to the same praise and subject to the same criticisms that may be directed against comparable products in the grocery store. You may have read statements by the Food and Drug Administration and the American Medical Association to the effect that yogurt is simply a very costly method of buying the benefits of milk — no more, no less. I do not know whether the Food and Drug Administration believes what it says, but I do know that a few years ago, the *Journal of the American Medical Association* carried an editorial commenting on the work of DuBos, at Rockefeller University, who had found that administration of the friendly bacteria (of yogurt), to animals had increased their resistance to infection and prolonged their life spans. (The medical journal was well aware of the implications of the report and tried to hide embarrassment with a facetious title on the editorial. The title was: "A Funny Thing Happened On The Way To Buy Some Yogurt. . . .") So much for the basic benefits of yogurt — which you will achieve only if you use it daily. However, those yogurts that are made with added fruit are simply a good food messed up with a great deal of jam or preserves. As much as an ounce of sugar (120 calories!) may be added to a container of some of these brands —

including those labeled "plain vanilla." If you want to buy yogurt, buy it unflavored and add your own fruit and a bit of honey. Honey, incidentally, has a special virtue in a situation like this: It is sweeter than sugar and you therefore need to use less of it.

While writing about jams in the preceding discussion, I am reminded that in the health-food store you will find a large variety of organic jams and jellies. These are free of corn syrup, but do represent a high concentration of sugar, and therefore should be used with discretion. As the man said when he married for the ninth time, there is a point at which one begins to exercise some caution!

One of the spreads for bread that I believe unique to the health-food industry is tahini, which is made from sesame seeds. This is virtually the only food richer in calcium than milk. It is also an excellent source of unsaturated fats, and it is a fine aid in keeping blood platelets at a normal level. In addition, tahini is a most enjoyable spread. If you have ever eaten halvah, which is the same product messed up with a great deal of sugar, you will be familiar with the basic flavor. I have used tahini not only as a spread for bread, but also as a flavoring for milk. Using a flavoring to induce children to drink milk, so far as I'm concerned, sets up an undesirable practice, for milk is palatable enough without additions. However, if you have already established the habit, tahini or carob would represent better choices than chocolate.

A popular misconception is that maple sugar is superior to ordinary sugar. Neither maple syrup nor maple sugar is necessarily the pure food we have always considered it to be. For many years the industry used a chlorine disinfectant to prevent bacteria from clogging up the tap holes of trees. The chlorine evaporated and therefore had to be replaced at intervals. For the same reason, it did not contaminate the maple syrup. To lower its overhead, the industry obtained from the Food and Drug Administration — that stalwart defender of the consumer — permission to substitute formaldehyde for chlorine, with the result that there is no way of knowing whether maple syrup is pure or is legally contaminated with five parts per million formaldehyde. You can ask the health-food store proprietor to query his source of supply, which he'll be glad to do. Maple syrup has a small mineral content, but presently no other known nutritional advantage.

There are many types of nut butters — peanut and others — sold in the health-food stores. Some of the stores have mills in which they will grind nut butters for you, fresh. Since all types of nuts are good nutrition, and since what you buy in the health-food store will be free of additives and cheap sweeteners, this service presents only one problem. Your family may find that nut butters minus synthetic soaps, detergents, and emulsifiers, are "tacky," which means that they tend to stick to the roof of the mouth. Do not surrender to this objection. You can add orange juice to peanut butter, for example, to reduce the tackiness and lend a very pleasant flavor. Experiments with other types of nut butters and additions are well worthwhile.

Besides yogurt, the health-food store carries other types of fermented milks, including kumiss and kefir. These actually represent a pre-digested type of milk, since the acid fermentation anticipates the acid digestion that is ordinarily the first stage in the utilization of milk products in the body. This fermentation reduces the curd tension, thus creating a very fine curd, which is digested more quickly than that of ordinary milk. In addition, the acidity of buttermilk, kumiss, kefir, and yogurt is an important factor in the utilization of calcium. The calcium of milk is better utilized because milk sugar in the body yields lactic acid, and an acid medium is more favorable to the solubility and thereby to the utilization of calcium. In these fermented milks, there is a head start in the fermentation process, providing an acid medium.

The health-food store carries many varieties of dried fruit, which have been prepared by exposure to the heat of sunlight. Ordinarily, vacuum drying would be preferable, because it is quicker — prolonged mild "cooking" actually is inimical to vitamin values. But this dis-advantage is offset by the fact that the sun-dried fruits of the health-food store are free of preservatives. The sulphur dioxide commonly used in the ordinary, commercial products not only destroys Vitamin B_1 but also has been indicted as a possible contributor to cancer.

The whole gelatin sold in the health-food store is the only such product worthy of the name. What you have been calling "gelatin dessert" is 85 percent sugar, 15 percent gelatin, artificial flavoring, artificial color, and sometimes several additives. Use the whole gelatin, add your own fruit and your own flavoring. You will find natural flavoring agents sold in many health-food stores. They are worth the premium.

Many health-food stores sell appliances related to nutrition or to health. Some of these are valuable contributions to the well-being of the family. The yogurt maker sold in many stores allows you to prepare yogurt at home, with results frequently as good as those achieved commercially and at much less cost. In addition, when you make yogurt at home, you can reinforce it with nonfat milk powder and build extra good nutrition into the recipe. Also, you will find in the stores devices for sprouting seeds. The increase in vitamin value of a seed when it sprouts is almost unbelievable. The sprouts are valuable and succulent additions both to salads and to cooked vegetables. The vegetable juicer is another worthwhile purchase. You may be tempted to save by buying the lighter-weight unit, which is largely plastic, and has a short or uncertain life span. It pays to buy the better machine, which carries a long-term guarantee on the cutter blade and other essential parts. Some machines automatically expel pulp and thus are more easily cleaned. Don't shrug at the thought of introducing vegetable juices to your family. If you are an average American family, you have been consuming them canned and cooked, without feeling very "different." It is better to obtain additional potassium this way than to take it in tablet form. Fresh vegetable juices may help offset the sodium-potassium imbalance that complicates many cases of heart disease.

When you consider the ticking time bomb that many food additives have already been recognized to be — which is why many now have been banned, after we swallowed them for years — and you keep in mind the dividends that accrue from good nutrition, you may very well reevaluate the price structure of these better foods. (The term "health foods" is largely invalid. Either a food preserves health, or it should be considered inedible. I have always thought the industry should call its stores "better-nutrition stores.") Least tenable of all objections to a return to a more natural way of eating is the added cost. Is this not ungraceful and inconsistent of a public that has paid up to $2.00 per pound for the added sugar in presweetened cereals, and up to $.70 for a pack of cigarettes, and some 13,000,000,000 dollars yearly for liquor and smokeables? The only food that is expensive is food that does not support optimal well-being.

In closing our journey through a health-food store, I would suggest that you learn simple ways to use special-purpose foods so that you can immediately begin to improve your family's diet without their knowledge. (It is important that you not let them know that you have changed recipes to raise your family's intake of important nutrients, for the average American husband will feel compelled to assert his masculinity by rejecting the entire proposition — after all, taking care of yourself is feminine!)

WHEAT GERM

An easy way to use wheat germ is by adding one teaspoonful to each cup of flour used for baking and other purposes. This amount ordinarily is not detectable. Because wheat germ contains fat (wheat-germ oil), in baked recipes where you use more than this percentage, it will be necessary to reduce slightly the amount of shortening and raise slightly the amount of liquid in the recipe. Once a housewife has seen the dividends her family enjoys from the addition of a little wheat germ to her recipes, she has a tendency to go overboard in the quantity she uses. The net result is likely to be cakes, cookies, and bread that cannot be lifted by a strong man. Wheat germ is so rich in protein that you cannot use an unlimited amount in baked recipes.

Wheat germ is one of the most nutritious cereals on the market. It can be served alone or added to other breakfast cereals.

The more experienced cook will find wheat germ a delightful and nutritious addition to meatloaf, and a "stretcher" for hamburgers that does not dilute but generously adds to the protein and vitamin value of the dish. Proportions are about the same, at least to start: A teaspoonful of wheat germ to eight ounces of meat. You can later experiment with raising the quantity, stopping short of the point where your husband and children begin to suspect that you are inflicting good nutrition on them. Wheat germ sprinkled on ice cream tastes like chopped nuts, and it's surprisingly good when sprinkled on liver sautéed with onions. Experience will show many other enjoyable uses of this superior food.

For some individuals the roughage of wheat germ may be difficult to tolerate. Occasionally this reaction can be overcome by thoroughly rolling the wheat germ with a rolling pin, or by chopping it finer in a high speed blender.

Remember to buy wheat germ vacuum packed, for like all good foods it is perishable. It should be resealed with each use to shield it from air. If it stays in the house too long, the wheat-germ oil may become rancid. On the other hand, if *that* happens you're not using enough to do you any good, anyway!

SOY FLOUR

Contrary to the beliefs of many of my friends in the health-food industry, soy flour is not a perfect food. When it comprises a major part of the diet, as in the case of a baby fed soy milk, it may — if the baby comes from a family predisposed to goiter — adversely affect the thyroid gland.

Soy flour is also deficient in Vitamin B_{12}, a factor important to the utilization of the protein in which soy flour is rich.

However, despite these debits, soy flour is a valuable source of protein and minerals, with special emphasis on potassium. As much as 6 percent soy flour may profitably be added to bread, cake, and cookie recipes. It is also a desirable addition to pancakes and waffles. Since soy flour is available at both low and high fat content, it is difficult to generalize about quantities, but most recipes calling for flour can be improved by the use of one or two teaspoonsful of soy flour per cup.

NONFAT MILK

Nonfat milk powder represents what is probably your best buy in the grocery or health-food store. Now that it is enriched with vitamins A and D, it contains all the nonfat nutrients of milk at a price far below that of whole milk. The missing cream and fat values can be restored to the diet by the use of butter or, if you want to, substitute unsaturated fat, margarine, or vegetable oil. Then you can feed your family the equivalent of whole milk at about fifteen or sixteen cents per quart. Let me make it clear that there will be no nutritional difference between whole milk and nonfat milk if for each quart of the skim milk you consume approximately one and one-half ounces of fat. You may choose unsaturated fat if your physician is attempting to hold down your blood cholesterol.

Like soy flour, nonfat milk can be used to improve texture, flavor, and — very significantly — nutritional values in protein, vitamin, and minerals. (This would mean six teaspoonsful of nonfat milk powder for each cupful of dry ingredients in a bread recipe. For cakes, cookies, pancakes, and waffles, start with less and experiment until you strike the level that produces the most pleasing flavor and texture.)

Some special uses of nonfat milk: If you use a blender, liquid nonfat milk can be prepared with double the nutritional value. In other words, the amount of powder normally used to make a quart is used to make a pint. Taken as a supplement, between meals, four glassfuls a day of the double strength nonfat milk may help in weight gain. For hypoglycemics who can tolerate this amount of milk sugar, such a beverage is useful in the small hours of the night or just before retiring, since it is a long-lasting fuel that may help avoid or mitigate the drop in blood sugar responsible for nightmares and awakening in the late night or early morning hours. It is helpful also for patients with peptic ulcer (for whom the nocturnal drop in blood sugar is likely to initiate attacks) if they train themselves to awaken at about two in the morning and drink a glassful of the double strength nonfat milk. Ultimately, this can become so much of a reflex that they will awaken, consume the drink, and return to sleep without actually being conscious of the episode.

If a little vanilla is added to this beverage, it resembles a malted and will be accepted by children whose nutrition needs a boost.

There are numerous other ways in which to employ nonfat milk usefully, such as adding protein value to homemade ice cream.

MINERAL WATER

A large percentage of health-food stores stock mineral water. It may be strange to list water as a "special-purpose food," but a good mineral water can be used in many ways other than as a direct beverage.

The expense is justified if you realize that our water purification systems were built before drugs like cortisone and birth-control pills were entering our sewerage. These systems will not cope with such chemicals. One evidence of that failure is a verified report that the drinking water in Boston, finished and ready for consumption, yielded a precipitate that was mutagenic — an action that increases the possibility of causing cancer.

Conversely, where water is hard (highly mineralized), the incidence of heart attacks is reported to be reduced. Considering these facts, the investment in a good, pure, mineral water seems prudent. Use it not only for drinking purposes, but also to dilute fruit juice concentrates and to make tea and other beverages.

Before writing this chapter, I consulted the Funk and Wagnall's Encyclopedia for a definition of *health*. It read: "A state of optimal function of an organism, never achieved." Wouldn't it be wonderful to make them rewrite that?

12.
THE WELL-FED BABY

Let me begin this chapter with a confession: I write it reluctantly, by popular demand — mainly my editor's wife. The reluctance is natural — nothing is more individual than a baby, and generalizing about baby food is a trap into which an author of a book dedicated to individual differences does not fall without a struggle. From the moment of birth (and, indeed before) your baby is as individual as any little animal can be.

Question: In view of the DDT content of breast milk, should you nurse your baby? The advantages of breast feeding,* which include contact with the warmth and the obvious loving care of the mother, so far outweigh any consideration of insecticide residues — since they are present in cow's milk, anyway — that the answer is automatic: If possible, nurse your baby. To minimize the amount of DDT that will reach the infant in mother's milk, do not permit the baby to completely strip the breast. It is in the last ounce or two that the pesticide is concentrated.

*Those who need guidance in breast feeding should consult the LaLeche League, Franklin Park, Illinois 60131.

No bottle propped up on a diaper is a substitute for the warmth of the breast, and so if you must resort to a formula, hold your baby while he is feeding. The benefits of breast feeding include a food that is the only edible we know was intended to be a food* — all else is guesswork. The nutritional differences between breast and cow's milk are profound. Not only is breast milk a source of uncooked protein, but its protein, fat, and carbohydrate content as well as its vitamin values differ, too. There are other plusses for breast milk. The most important effect is that of helping the baby's pituitary and adrenal glands to develop properly. Another and almost equally significant benefit is the comparative freedom of the breast-fed baby from the diarrheas that often represent a serious threat to infants in hospital nurseries. Now there is serious thought being given to a return to the practice of home delivery, with a midwife in charge. Intestinal infections are much less frequent in the breast-fed child. So is allergy. In fact, our national problem with allergy, and we do not believe that this is coincidence, began to rise appreciably when breast feeding yielded to bottle feeding.**

---

*Although different in proportions of carbohydrate, protein, and fat, there *is* one form of cows' milk that is an excellent food for babies who cannot be breast fed. This is certified raw milk. It is a perfectly safe milk, but there is always the possibility that you may contaminate it in handling. Therefore, I prefer that certified raw milk be "pasteurized" by you before it is fed to the baby. This process involves raising the temperature of the milk to 140 degrees for thirty minutes, or bringing it to a quick boil and then withdrawing it from the heat. If you are inclined to object to this suggestion on the grounds that it seems foolish to pay a premium price for certified raw milk that you must cook, let me remind you that in the ordinary formula, the milk is cooked (pasteurized) before you buy it and then you recook it. Accordingly, the baby on home-pasteurized certified raw milk is eating food that has been cooked only once, rather than twice — and the less heat we apply to protein, the better the food. There are physicians who prefer to dilute certified raw milk with water, without added carbohydrate, but I believe this ignores the specific importance of lactose (milk sugar) to babies. The fact that a baby thrives on a given method of feeding does not necessarily mean that this is an ideal type of nutrition. It was only a century ago that mothers were instructed to form a doughy mass with flour and water, roll it into a ball, bake it in the oven until the outer part was burned almost black, and then break pieces of the dough into beer before feeding it to small babies. So far as I know, the babies survived — which is no endorsement of this type of nutrition.

**Undoubtedly, you are wondering about babies who are raised on soy milk or goats' milk. For many babies who cannot be breast fed and are allergic to cows' milk, soy milk offers a chance for survival. However, if there is a hereditary tendency to underactivity of the thyroid gland, babies deriving a substantial part of their nourishment from soy milk must be carefully watched for signs of interference with the thyroid function. Goats' milk has a tendency to interfere with the utilization of Vitamin B_{12}. This action can obviously be compensated for by raising the potency of Vitamin B_{12} in the baby's supplement. Goats' milk does have an advantage in that it is naturally "homogenized," making its fat easier to utilize. On the other hand, allergy to goats' milk may also occur. In any event, should a baby who cannot breast feed prove allergic to or intolerant of all the other forms of milk, don't despair. Babies have been raised on strained meat as a substitute for milk, reminding us once again that they are remarkably hardy creatures — not that meat is a bad food, but it is so different from the nutrition offered by milk.

Next question: At what age does a baby begin to eat solid foods? The question presupposes uniform babies — and you must confess that you will never admit that your baby is average or a carbon copy of any other infant. Don't engage in a horsepower race with your neighbor, by deploring the fact that *your* pediatrician waits four weeks longer to introduce the solid foods that her baby is *already* being fed. No two babies are alike; that's why no two grown-ups are alike, and that is the theme of this book. Among the five children we have raised, no two had the same starting date for solid foods. (One of our boys was so hungry that we had him on meat at the sixth week.) An infantile digestive tract has not yet learned to be selective in what it absorbs and what it rejects. If that delicate mechanism is compelled to make choices too early, one of the consequences can be the start of allergies that will vastly complicate your child's life and your own. Let your pediatrician decide when solid food should be introduced, but don't listen to him if he tries to talk you out of breast feeding, unless there is a sound medical reason for the advice — painful breasts or a great psychological aversion on your part.

It is easy to be as pessimistic as a "consumer protectionist" who harangues the New York television and radio audiences with dire warnings of one kind or another, and who announces that DDT is inescapable and that pesticide residues on food are a fact of life. However, instead of looking at the hole, let us examine the donut. The lower you keep your baby's intake of such chemicals, the better off your baby will be. This is one good reason for preparing your own baby foods, providing that you have access to organic fruits, vegetables, and meats not subjected to pesticides, diethylstilbestrol, and other residues and additives. In preparing your own baby foods, you will be achieving other worthwhile goals. The addition of salt to baby foods is aimed strictly at the mother's palate. The baby will not miss added salt and will probably be better off without it. The natural sodium value of milk and other foods is great enough to supply the baby's needs, and extra salt may be, in susceptible families, a pathway to hypertension. Preparing pureed vegetables for babies (and for that matter invalids) is really easy to do if you have a food mill or a blender. Even if you don't, you can grate, shred, or grind the vegetables and fruits by techniques I shall describe. The baby will derive another benefit if you prepare his fruits and puddings at home because you will be omitting the substantial content of sugar and processed carbohydrate that unfortunately marks the commercial product.

There are two methods of pureeing vegetables. You can peel the vegetables, then wash, chill, grind, and promptly steam them. They are very palatable prepared in this way, and virtually no nutritional values are sacrificed. The other technique is to chop the peeled vegetable after it has been cooked. My preference is for the latter. In either case, a food mill or a blender can be used. On many blenders you will find a puree-ing speed marked on the dial. When the time comes to introduce vege-tables to the baby, remember that there is a special technique for introducing new foods to babies. The most successful method is to present the new food combined with a familiar one. Cook it in milk at a simmering temperature of approximately 200 degrees. The milk should subsequently be used for cream sauces and soups.

Cereal is usually the first solid food offered to a baby. (Remember — use no cereal containing BHT, BHA or any other additive other than vitamins and minerals.) However, some babies will reject it in favor of fruit or vegetable. Usually this revolution in the menu occurs at the second or the third month — and I cannot offer you anything more firm than that range. During the same period hard-cooked egg yolk can be mixed with cereal or with formula to make a paste and can be given to the baby a tiny bit at a time. Gradually increase the amount until the baby accepts an entire yolk.

Cereal and egg yolk are important because they are good sources of the B Vitamins. Milk — including breast milk — isn't. The cereals should be whole grain, and they should be completely free of all ad-ditives, including salt. We usually start with whole-wheat cereal, adding a bit of honey if the baby refuses it. If refusal still continues, then try oatmeal. Most of the other prepared cereals are not whole grain, and merely supply two or three "enrichment" vitamins. I take a dim view of these. If the cereal you first offered is refused, it may be due to a mechanical difficulty. Start the feeding with a single teaspoonful of the cereal to let the baby experience a new taste. Use a small spoon to put the cereal at the middle of the tongue; if you place it near the lips, the baby may — in the very act of trying to swallow it — push it out. You will emerge from this experience, shaken, sure that your child has a dislike for whole-wheat cereal.

When you have established the cereal pattern, increase the amount until the baby is taking two or three tablespoonful. Ordinarily, the cereal is fed before nursing or formula feeding because subsequent to the milk, he is less likely to eat the solid food. To anticipate a question: Wheat germ can be added to the enriched cereals to bring in the other B Complex vitamins. If this seems a "high roughage" food to offer to a baby, disabuse yourself: Wheat germ was used in the very first pro-prietary cereal ever to be marketed in this country — Pablum. It might be wise to roll the wheat germ with a rolling pin to reduce the mechanical roughage before you add it to cereal. A quarter of a teaspoonful to a portion of cereal will be adequate. Excessive laxative action will be a sign of intolerance, indicating that the amount should be reduced.

According to Dr. I. Newton Kugelmass,* who has, I think, a unique monopoly on chemistry in pediatric medicine and pediatric nutrition, you should introduce cooked or strained fruit during the third or fourth month — unless you are compelled to do it earlier because the baby has refused cereal. Begin with teaspoonful amounts and gradually increase to two or three tablespoonsful, according to tolerance, at each feeding. When the baby is two weeks of age, you can offer orange, tangerine, tomato, grapefruit, apricot, pineapple, prune, lemon, or lime juice. Prune juice is ordinarily used only when there is constipation. At three months: dried apricots (and be sure they are free of sulphur dioxide), ripe raw banana, and apples. At four months: fresh apple, apricot, pear, and plums. At five months: scraped apple or pear, sieved apricot or peach. At six months and thereafter any cooked fruit. Needless to say, you should be buying organic fruits and vegetables, and if you can't, be sure to peel them where possible and wash them thoroughly.

Vegetables, which are a source of iron and other minerals as well as the B vitamins, are introduced in the form of a puree during the fourth month, usually at the afternoon feeding. Initial quantities are about a teaspoonful, and gradually are increased to three tablespoonsful at the 2 P.M. and the 6 P.M. feedings. Babies who don't seem too happy about eating vegetables should not be coerced. In fact, children should never be coerced at the table, for you will ultimately pay a price. If the baby's stools contain undigested vegetable particles, the amount fed should be limited, or other vegetables tried in the search for one that will be better digested. Kugelmass reminds us that spinach may redden the buttocks and beets may color the urine and stools. If a vegetable produces allergic symptoms, it should be eliminated for at least two months and then offered again. If the symptoms recur, it should be eliminated from the baby's diet indefinitely. At four months, Kugelmass feeds carrots, spinach, broccoli, chard, and turnips. At five months: green peas, string beans, asparagus, kale, kohlrabi, squash, pumpkin, and rutabaga. At six months: potato, cauliflower, beets, and artichokes. At eight months: brussels sprouts, soybean, onion, and cabbage. For the very young baby, the vegetables are pureed to the finest possible softness. For the older infant, they may be pureed or chopped.

I have mentioned egg yolk, and you will be asking about egg white. This should not be introduced until about the eighth month. Begin

*I. Newton Kugelmass, *Complete Child Care in Body and Mind* (New York, Twayne Publishers, 1959).

with a mere pinhead and increase the amount slowly. It is served soft cooked or coddled.

Many babies will accept meat earlier then the fifth month, but many pediatricians do not introduce it until that time. If it is well cooked and finely divided, meat is easily digested. At home, you can cook beef, chicken, or liver, scrape it, and sieve or grind it, long before the baby has teeth with which to chew. You may mix your meats with baked or boiled potato in increasing amounts, always watching for such allergic reactions as vomiting, colic, skin rash, or diarrhea. If one of these occurs, discontinue the particular meat. On the same basis, postpone the feeding of fish until the baby is at least a year old. Fish is a highly allergenic food.

At four months of age, Kugelmass feeds beef juice, liver-and-beef soup (home-prepared — the commercial variety has as little as 5 percent liver), and powdered chicken liver. The latter is prepared by broiling livers until they are quite hard, then scraping them into a powder.* At five months, he recommends scraped beef, scraped liver, scraped lamb, and stewed chicken. At seven months: minced chicken and minced steak. At eleven months: minced roast beef, minced roast lamb, and minced roast veal. At fifteen months: any prepared meat or fresh fish such as flounder, haddock, and halibut. It is correct to broil, braise, or stew freshly cooked or prepared meat after twenty-four hours of refrigeration.

Kugelmass shares with many of us a distaste for ordinary soups in the diet of children. They take up a lot of space and yield very little food value. The vitamin content is depleted by the long cooking to which many soups are subjected. However, broths do stimulate the appetite. Canned meat soups containing meat, strained vegetables, and coarse cereal are offered during the third month. Beef juice — long eulogized — has very little nutritional value. For your baby make liver-and-beef soup, liver-and-vegetable soup, beef, chicken and lamb broth, and vegetable, potato, or tomato soup. All these foods are just as well tolerated in their original (solid) form.

Bread is usually introduced when the baby is about six months of age and his teeth are beginning to appear. It is usually offered in the form of zwieback or graham crackers. The former is overcooked and overprocessed bread; nutritionally the graham crackers offer more. Both foods encourage the baby to chew. Babies who are allergic to wheat can be given brown-rice crackers, rye crisp, or, if available,

---

*This denatures the protein so much that it may not cause allergic reactions in babies ordinarily allergic to liver. There is still valuable nutrition left in the food. It may be added to applesauce or other strained fruit for convenient feeding.

whole-rye bread as soon as they have mastered chewing. By the time the baby is two years old, he is ready for whole-wheat, whole-rye, and Boston brown bread (without spices, raisins, and seeds), which are more preferable laxative agents than medication. Hot breads are not usually fed to babies, and neither are ordinary muffins, pancakes, and waffles. There *are* mixes available that make good foods of muffins and pancakes. In our family we have allowed our babies to have these at the age of 6 months. The old-fashioned baked potato is certainly more nutritionally virtuous than ordinary rice, which is usually over-processed. If you are going to serve rice or spaghetti, choose the less-processed brands. Converted rice is better than white rice, but not as desirable as brown rice; spaghetti with 20 percent protein, made with wheat germ, is commercially available. In comparing potatoes with rice or spaghetti, remember that potatoes do supply a considerable amount of Vitamin C, and that the addition of butter — which in reasonable amounts is desirable — introduces Vitamin A into the dish. Both of course are important to your baby.

Desserts represent an opportunity to avoid starting dietary habits that may exact a toll in later life. Do not place a premium on sweet desserts and the mark of undesirability on other dishes by using the familiar statement: "You cannot have your ice cream until you eat your spinach!" This makes spinach undesirable and ice cream desirable, just the reverse of what you want. Desserts are introduced around the fourth month at the afternoon and 6 P.M. feeding, in the form of stewed fruit, whole gelatin, junket, custard, or pudding. If junket powder is used instead of the tablets, large amounts of added sugar can be avoided. If whole gelatin is used, add your own fruit or flavoring. Prepared gelatin desserts are actually 85 percent sugar and only 15 percent gelatin. Custards need not be oversweetened — you will find, for instance, that genuine vanilla acts like a sweetening and permits you to reduce sugar content. If you add honey, which is sweeter than sugar, you will use less. Commercial puddings are a triumph of technology over the needs of the body and should be avoided. Excellent recipes for nutritious puddings are available.*

Not only should desserts be undersweetened, but they should also be offered sparingly because they tend to lessen the desire for more essential foods.

When the ice cream age is reached — which is about one year — protect your child against artificial flavoring, artificial color, and ordinary ice cream, which is 16 percent sugar. Buy a hand-crank ice

*Adelle Davis, *Let's Cook It Right* (New York, Harcourt Brace Jovanovich, Inc., 1962); paperback edition (New York, The New American Library, Inc., 1970).

cream freezer (quite inexpensive — even the electric model) and experiment with your own recipes, using nonfat milk powder to raise the protein content. The milk powder will also provide some sweetening from milk sugar, which can be heightened with some natural vanilla flavoring. Fruits allowed in the diet may be added.

As your baby begins to eat bread, he will learn to accept the pattern you start. If you begin with bubble-gum bread, that will be his demand. If you begin with good whole-grain breads and cereals, he will be accustomed to those. You are shaping not only a baby's taste, but a baby's future in terms of well-being.

In changing from formulas to meals, add solid foods during the third month, one at a time. If a baby persists in refusing a food, do not force it — he may know more than you do. If you increase the strength of the formula by reducing the amount of water, babies will proportionately reduce their intake if they are not ready for the increase. If your baby takes much more of a food at one time than another, do not be astonished. Aren't you variable in your tastes?

If your baby shows extreme likes and dislikes for food — whether solid or liquid — he may be telling you that he is allergic to some. A baby's food aversions up to the age of two are probably meaningful. After that time, he has all of the protective instincts of an adult — meaning, none!

Remember that milk is not a perfect food. The baby who is overfed milk winds up pale, constipated, sleeping poorly, and subject to colds. If you have fallen into the vicious circle of saying, "At least he takes his milk!" when dealing with a baby who is on a hunger strike, there is only one way to educate him to accepting foods again: Stop the milk! I have reference, of course, to a two-year-old; it is an age when an infant tends to experiment with hunger strikes because he is too lazy to chew. This refusal is a wonderful way for a little human being to take complete control of the household. Stopping the milk may fill you with gloomy forebodings about beriberi, scurvy, pellagra, rickets, and sprue, but the fact is that no baby has yet voluntarily starved to death, and he will come to you for solid food long before you have given way to outright hysteria.

Add new foods at the 10 A.M., 2 P.M., and 6 P.M. feedings, because this ultimately is the pathway to breakfast, dinner, and supper, which will be the meal pattern at about one year of age. Omit the 10 P.M. feeding after the third month if the baby has not done so for himself. Usually, it becomes necessary for you to awaken him to take some of the 10 P.M. feeding, which he accepts with reluctance, falling asleep before finishing the formula. However, it is possible that he will awaken before midnight and expect to be fed. To remedy this, continue to feed him at 10 P.M. or 11 P.M. until he refuses the bottle, sleeps through the night, and allows you to obtain some rest. It may take several weeks during the third or fourth month to make the necessary adjustment. Once the 10 P.M. bottle is eliminated, divide the twenty-four hour formula into four bottles — or breast feedings at those intervals. If your baby indicates a need for more frequent feeding, honor it — he will ultimately find the pattern that will suit his unique physiological needs. Generally, he will tend to take more milk at the daytime feedings.

When a baby is on whole milk, meticulous sterilizing of bottles and nipples has outlived its usefulness. Simply prepare six 8-ounce bottles of boiled milk and keep them refrigerated and capped until feeding time, then replace the caps with clean nipples.

Encourage self-feeding by the tenth month. The baby can usually hold the bottle at six months, hold crackers at seven months, hold a cup at eight months, and hold a spoon at nine months. The latter will be messy, but it will be an opportunity to observe which hand he prefers. If there is left-handedness in the family, then let the baby use the left hand, if he so chooses. Since he is bent on exploring the world, you must allow him to enjoy touching, handling, smelling, tasting, biting, chewing, and when he is inclined — splattering food into your patient face.

Before one year of age, the baby should be on three meals a day, although babies may reach this precise point at different times. When a baby does not awaken at 6 A.M. and when he does not show signs of appetite between feedings, he is ready for the five-hour feeding interval. If he prefers the four-hour, but dawdles at the feedings, putting him on three meals a day will help make him hungry for a meal.* If the morning or afternoon interval seems too long for the baby, some milk or fruit juice can be offered between meals.

The basis of the baby's diet is milk, meat, fruit, and vegetables. If the baby refuses milk, serve gelatin milk, thicken soup or cereal with milk, and feed him custards and puddings made with generous amounts of milk. If he refuses meat, serve thick meat soup or calves' foot jelly. If he rejects fruit or vegetables, add gelatin or a harmless vegetable coloring. Your baby may be ravenously fond of a given food for a time and then suddenly refuse it for weeks. Allow him individuality.

Remember that your baby's appetite will tend to slow down at the end of the first year and after the second year. Don't coerce him!

A typical diet during the second year might be:

*Some babies prefer more frequent, smaller feedings, which provide a sounder pattern for them.

8 A.M. Stewed fruit, 3 oz.; cooked cereal, 3 oz. with butter; egg or bacon; milk, 8 oz.; toast or graham crackers with butter

10 A.M. Orange or tomato juice, 4 oz.; cod-liver oil, 1 tsp.

1 P.M. Meat, liver, or chicken, 3 tbs.; potato mashed or baked, 3 tbs. and butter; vegetable puree, 4 tbs.; toast or dry bread with butter.

3 P.M. Prune juice, 4 oz., if constipated

6 P.M. Vegetable puree with milk and butter; cottage cheese, 3 tbs.; stewed fruit, 4 tbs.; milk, 8 oz.; bread and butter

Baking for your baby is a contribution you alone can make; you can provide him with cookies, cakes, and bread that contribute to his well-being and that do not inflict on his immature systems of detoxification the burden of artificial color, artificial flavoring, and the more than a hundred food additives that you may innocently bring home in commercial baked products. The Cornell formula bread, a recipe that I have supplied in the appendix, is a good way to introduce white bread into the baby's diet. If he has been raised on good whole-wheat bread and on the Cornell formula, he will find distasteful the flavorless, air-filled, additive-laden bread of commerce. Your home-baked cookies will be infinitely better both for baby and the family than those you find on commercial shelves. The preceding paragraph indicates the answer to the question frequently asked by mothers of young babies. "Can the baby eat with the family after the age of two or so?" If he can't, your family is eating improperly. That is why the baking suggested should be aimed at the entire family.

With regard to vitamin supplements: American pediatricians have literally been brainwashed into the belief that babies only require supplements of Vitamins A and D. I do not propose to review the evidence that makes this philosophy an injustice to growing babies. Suffice it to say, the remarkable (if impossible) Fredericks children were given the benefit of all the known vitamins plus the unknown as supplied by a natural B-Complex source, plus calcium, phosphorus, iron, and the various trace minerals. There are a number of such products commercially available in liquid form for infants. They are usually not introduced in the stipulated dose, which is often a teaspoonful of the vitamin syrup and a teaspoonful of the mineral syrup, for this might prove to be a laxative for a very young baby. One starts with a very small quantity and gradually increases the amount. The syrup may be fed from the teaspoon or it may be mixed with formula or milk. Years ago, Hoobler, a pediatrician, began to feed brewer's yeast to babies. Although the infants were receiving formula, orange juice, and cod-liver oil — still considered to be top-notch nutrition for a very young infant — the response of the babies to the yeast was described by the pediatrician in these glowing words:

"Thin, weak, crying, cranky, fretful babies with indifferent appetites turned into happy, rosy-cheeked, smiling infants whose appetite was never satisfied and whose weight gain was nothing short of remarkable." The pediatricians who have been brainwashed by the medical hierarchy into believing that babies require no supplements beyond Vitamins A and D should reread Hoobler.

It is on this basis and with memories of the many thousands of happy, healthy babies who have been conceived on and raised on my diets, that I tell a new mother that brewer's yeast is as good for her infant as it is for her. Experiment. The yeast can be added to many recipes in reasonable quantities.

When your baby is walking, snacking begins. This may become a serious threat to the good nutrition habits you are trying to preserve. If you create a cookie-cake-cracker baby, you have only yourself to blame as the dental bills mount. (There are other bad effects, too.) In the Fredericks' household, we always kept available a platter with bits of cheese, small pieces of meat or chicken, and small amounts of fruits. Our children learned to snack on these nutritious goodies, so we created the protein habit rather than the cookie catastrophe.

This chapter is not intended to be encyclopedic in the range of its suggestions for infant feeding. At the very least, I hope it will give you cause for thought as you prepare or select foods for your baby. For what you are doing will affect not only his welfare, but also that of generations as yet unconceived.

13.

SUPERSTITION OR FACT?

No matter how sane people are, when you bring up the topic of health or anything related to it, a little area in the brain lights up as an invitation for pixies, elves, gnomes, witches, and leprechauns to take turns shaping what passes for thinking and knowledge.

Perhaps the best illustration of this process is the twentieth-century housewife, who in preparing eggplant salts the slices and then stacks them to let the liquid drain. Her custom dates directly from the twelfth century and has changed little since. It was believed then that the juice of the eggplant had the capacity to cause insanity — particularly in doctors and lawyers. So it is that this practice of the twelfth-century housewife, in protecting her family against the juice of insanity, is still employed today. All that we have done is to discard the original name for the eggplant, which directly reflected the superstition, the apple of insanity.

For many decades tomatoes were regarded as aphrodisiacs. The French called them apples of the Moors. The name simply indicated that the Moors were recognized as having first cultivated this delectable vegetable. However, when rendered phonetically it can be translated as "apples of love." And so tomatoes gained an undeserved reputation for stimulating the sex drive.

Consistency does not contaminate thinking about nutrition. There are those who will assure you that drinking milk after eating fish is virtually a guaranteed passport to the next world. Then they will promptly sit down and eat crabmeat mornay — seafood in a cream sauce containing cheese, which is thoroughly decomposed milk. Factually, there is no basis for the belief that foods that are good alone are bad together. This may be true of people, but food incompatibilities simply do not exist. In other words, the gastrointestinal explosion you anticipate when you eat pickles with ice cream either will not materialize, or, if it should, would have been achieved by eating one of the two foods alone.

There is a short, delightful joke about a little Jewish mother who has just been informed by a psychiatrist that her son is a paranoid schizophrenic, with overtones of the manic-depressive, the catatonic, the hebrephrenic, and a dash of the Oedipus complex. Her response is simple and direct, reflecting an ancient folklore solidly grounded on superstition. "Doctor" she asks, "instead of sending him to the hospital, could you let me take him home and give him a little chicken soup?" In such esteem is this sovereign remedy held among this ancient people that it has been known as Jewish penicillin. What healing virtues does it have? You tell me.

From the doctrine of food incompatibilities came a belief, staunchly held by many people, that there is a battle engendered when you take fruit juice, toast, and coffee at the same meal. While this represents an inadequate breakfast, there is no doubt that for some people it also creates an intestinal uproar. The explanation does not lie in any antagonism of those foods toward each other. If you attempted to awaken quickly by pouring ice-cold orange juice over your head, you would learn to appreciate that very frigid juice may be a similar shock to the fasting digestive tract. The uproar very often ceases to occur when the fruit juice is taken after rather than before breakfast.

There are other familiar superstitions that masquerade as fact in the field of nutrition, many of which you may have repeated as indisputable. Is fish a brain food? Before you answer, consider that the Japanese, replete with seafood, nonetheless declared war on the United States.

Are the meat eaters generally belligerent and the vegetarians always peace-loving folk? If this is your belief, you should have told Hitler and Mussolini — both were vegetarians. If as a vegetarian you believe that meat is filled with toxins, have you ever paused to ask how the toxins managed to concentrate in the meat of an animal that is a pure vegetarian? Perhaps you are one of those who believe that within you is an inner voice of wisdom guiding your cravings in food, so that what you keenly desire obviously reflects a need of the body. If inner wisdom guides our cravings, please explain the fat lady who craves candy, the diabetic who cheats on his diet by eating forbidden sweets that may threaten his very life, and the allergic who is fond of just those foods that careful testing indicates are causing his troubles. If you point to the food practices of primitives as reflecting instinctive selection of good nutrition, you will discover that what you are observing is the phenomenon that distinguishes man from animal — the ability to transmit information from generation to generation.

In short, you are observing inherited wisdom. The Chinese do not eat millet alone but with other cereals. Modern technology has taught us that the protein of cereals is very much more efficient when the cereals are mixed. The ancient Chinese knew nothing about protein (amino) acids, but they did have the opportunity to observe over the centuries that people who mix cereals did better than those who did not. While we are addressed to the Chinese, we might consider the belief that the Chinese eat rice, the Chinese have low blood pressure, and therefore — Q.E.D. — eating rice lowers blood pressure. To speak of a nation of 800 million people as sharing a single dietary preference is nonsense. It is analogous to a foreigner who flies directly from Europe to Birmingham, Alabama, and concludes that all Americans eat grits. Actually, the northern Chinese eat noodles, the southern Chinese eat rice, the Chinese do seem to run a lower blood pressure than we do — but at that lower blood pressure they have the same strokes that we blame on higher blood pressure. Nonetheless, the shaky foundation for this theory has not prevented at least one medical institution from capitalizing upon the rice diet as a sovereign remedy for hypertension.

You need sugar for energy. You will find this statement in textbooks, you will find posters announcing it to the children in the home economics classroom, and you will hear millions of Americans voice it as a truism. Even momentary reflection should remind you that no nation in the world consumes more of such "quick-energy" foods than Americans do — and probably no other nation is more troubled with fatigue. It is the first symptom millions of patients describe when they are voicing their complaints to physicians. If sugar is necessary for energy, let us remember that the caveman had no sugar bowl, but obviously had the energy to evade the saber-toothed tiger and survive long enough to sire our forbears.

The Harvard University Nutrition Department informs you that white bread is equivalent to whole-wheat bread. The comparison is usually in terms of thiamin, riboflavin, niacin, calcium, and iron. Don't ask for a comparison of Vitamin-E values, Vitamin-B$_6$ values, or a dozen other factors of the Vitamin B Complex. If you do, you will discover that in no way is white bread as nutritious as whole-wheat — and you have been guilty of a superstition created by indoctrination posing as education.

You have been informed by propaganda masquerading as the voice of science that there is no distinction between the natural vitamins and the synthetic, and that paying a premium for the natural vitamin is therefore a working example of gullible's travels. Theoretically, this is true — the chemist who is synthesizing a vitamin copies the natural atom, molecule for molecule. But how do we explain the fact that there are people who are allergic to synthetic vitamins but are not disturbed by the natural, and people who have the converse reaction? You have also been advised that organic farming is an exercise in cultism — the type of fertilizer used has no influence on the quality of the food, and that, in fact, the only difference made by fertilization is in the quantity of the crop. This is simply not so.

My friends in the health-food industry have heard me complain about books that eulogize the "mucus-free diet." It never seems to occur to the authors of such books or to the people who practice such diets that a body free of mucus would not survive, for mucus is one of our natural protections against infection. In such diets, milk is defined as a mucus-producing food. In the strict chemical sense, since milk is a source of Vitamin A and Vitamin A helps to keep mucous membranes moist, the statement is true — but that does not make milk undesirable. You have also been informed that man is the only creature who drinks milk after he has been weaned. He is also the only creature who drinks Scotch whisky and drops atom bombs, but I know not what those distinctions teach us. If you do not use milk, cheese, yogurt, or similar dairy products, it is virtually impossible for you to obtain an optimal intake of calcium from the diet. The vegetables and fruits that are recommended as alternate sources of calcium by careless dieticians or inexpert physicians would have to be eaten literally by the pound to give you the equivalent of what you obtain from two glasses of milk or a few ounces of cheese. Milk and cheese avoiders need calcium supplements.

Many superstitions hover around the influence of food on the sex drive. There is a proverbial reputation of oysters as an aphrodisiac. There is currently an identification of Vitamin E as sex's middle letter. Actually, the flame of love is slender, and anything inimical to the body's well-being — however slightly — may dim or extinguish it. But the only nutrient that has ever shown any aphrodisiac action is PABA, a B-Complex vitamin. That action is exerted in men only, and in only a small percentage of those who take it. Generally, when it stimulates the libido it also tends to recolor gray hair, indicating that the stimulation comes from an effect of the vitamin on the pituitary gland.

Those who with sangfroid ignore the tenets of good nutrition, believing that there is validity to the government statement that our supply of food is so varied and so plentiful that an inadequate diet becomes impossible, should reflect on this analogy: American banks have so much in them that obviously nobody in this country is poor. Another generalization of this nature derives from observing people who violate all the rules of good nutrition and virtually all the laws of hygiene and escape consequences, and, indeed, wind up at the age of ninety marrying for the fifth time, being careful to locate an apartment near a public school. There *are* such people. They reflect a good heredity. These are people who came from good eggs and who can laugh at the environmental factors which you and I, and all bad eggs, must carefully consider. They also set a very bad example for the rest of us. but their experience proves nothing except the wisdom of choosing ancestors carefully.

Pregnancy is surrounded with beliefs, many of which are pure fairy tales. Examples: One can, for instance, stop worrying about the diet in the first four months of pregnancy when morning sickness frequently interferes with food intake because the baby is so minute that his nutritional needs will necessarily be met, even at the expense of depletion of the mother's reserves. Actually, in the first four months the baby's "blueprints" are being laid down — the matrices on which all the organs are formed. One may remember that thalidomide caused no harm to babies when the drug was taken in the seventh month of pregnancy. It precipitated its tragic effects when taken in the first few months. However, a belief about pregnancy usually labeled as a superstition *has* turned out to be factual. Proverbially, the expectant mother's need for peace and quiet has been regarded as one of the pleasant myths, but there is now evidence that the unborn baby's heartbeat rises astronomically with loud noises, including, surprisingly, such sounds as may be made internally when the mother drinks carbonated beverages. There is also evidence that extreme emotional pressure on the mother may — perhaps because of the release of certain adrenal hormones — actually deform the child.

On the other hand, from these lines millions of husbands will now learn that the pregnant woman's cravings for raspberry sherbet at 3 A.M. of a midwinter night with the temperature 10° below zero do not reflect a physiological need, and failing to act upon her wish will not cause the baby to be born with a raspberry birthmark. It is our considered conclusion that such demands are simply devices by which the pregnant woman punishes her husband for the interesting condition in which she finds herself. Husbands have cooked up some beliefs of their own, with parallel-vested interest. Rebelling against the introduction of new recipes or more nutritious foods in the menu, some men have strongly voiced the opinion that what they do not enjoy will not physiologically or nutritionally be profitable for them. This is an interesting way to avoid eating liver when you hate it, but it has no foundation in fact. Those who have believed this superstition should obtain a list of the foods that our flyers were instructed to consume when shot down over the South Pacific in World War II. Then you will learn that some remarkably distasteful foods may indeed preserve life.

Watching your teen-agers, some of you have come to the conclusion that their legs are hollow and used for storage of cold drinks, pizzas, and anything else that doesn't bite back. Actually, the nutritional needs of a teen-ager are the highest in the life span — even higher than those of the expectant mother. This, however, is no license for consuming foods that, fed to animals will ultimately bring premature old age and susceptibility to degenerative disease. It is also a superstition to believe that you cannot guide a teen-ager to select a better diet. You can, if you wait for the teachable moment. You cannot discuss this subject with a twelve-year-old, but when he becomes thirteen, discovers girls and realizes that they are not boys, that they are interesting, and that he has his first pimple — this becomes a teachable moment and should be seized upon.

Superstitions about infant nutrition are numerous. A common one concerns the child who refuses to eat his ordinary foods, but compensates by drinking vast quantities of milk. "At least he drinks his milk," is mother's approving rationalization. But milk is not a perfect food — no food is — and the child who is overdosed with milk will wind up pale, lethargic, constipated, and perhaps troubled with colds and insomnia. The remedy, which would seem obvious but is sharply rejected by mothers positive that their offspring will come down with beriberi, scurvy, pellagra, rickets, and xerophthalmia, is to stop the milk. A hunger strike may follow, but no child yet has voluntarily starved to death.

Pediatricians likewise accept and dispense superstition. One that has been promulgated by the orthodox in medicine concerns the infant's need of vitamin supplements. Pediatricians have been persuaded that the only supplements required by the infant are vitamins A and D. The breast-fed baby enjoys an advantage in certain of the B vitamins as well as in a more optimal intake of the major fractions of food. But both breast- and formula-fed babies deserve Vitamin-B-Complex supplements just as much as they do supplements of the other vitamins.

Among the millions of letters I have received in some thirty years of broadcasting are some which provide a chuckle as well as a challenge to the nutrition educator. A boy in Elizabeth, New Jersey wrote: "I am seventeen, a firm believer in good foods, and I don't eat sweets, soda and the like. My mother thinks I overdo it. She claims I should strike a medium and eat some bad foods."

Answer: Let's be consistent — you should also go out with some bad girls.

On the other hand, apropos of nothing except the manner in which a radio listener can immobilize an educator, there is this note:

"I have done everything you have said. I've revised my menus, I take vitamin supplements, I use wheat-germ oil, I eat whole-grain bread, and I still find my shoes in the washing machine."

Question: "I have been troubled with halitosis. I have been using tablets and gum containing chlorophyll. Is it true that this neutralizes the offensive odors?" Answer: Have you ever smelled a goat?

Once in a while a superstition comes along that turns out to be solid fact. Consider the answer to this question:

"I have been told that Vitamin A may make warts disappear. I've also been told that this is a superstition. Which is correct?"

It has been established that any remedy in which you believe is likely to make warts disappear. It has been accomplished by hypnosis and by administration of colored water, which the patient believed was potent medication.

Canned foods also have their share of criticisms based on fiction rather than on fact. Take, for instance, the frequent statement that foods should not be stored in an open can, but should be transferred to a clean dish or other receptacle. Actually, in the course of the canning procedure, the bacteria content of the canned food has been deliberately and sharply reduced if not wiped out, while your "clean" dish is crawling with bacteria. Those foods that are high in acid — such as tomato juice or pineapple — should not be stored in the open can because they will pick up a metallic taste. All the others are safer in the open can than they would be in your own dish.

I am on friendly terms with all the publishers in the health-food field. That, however, does not dilute my interest in truth. A persistent belief among millions of Americans, originally planted by one of these publishers, revolves around the purported dangers of cooking in aluminum vessels, on which, among other horrible consequences, the publisher has blamed cancer. Factually, cancer predates by millions of years the use of aluminum cooking vessels in man's history. Equally factual, people with stomach ulcers are frequently dosed with vast amounts of aluminum salts over a period of many years, with no discernible ill effects. And finally, aluminum happens to be a human requirement and would be present in the body with or without the use of aluminum pots, because the metal is in virtually all soil, every vegetable, and every fruit.

Many beliefs are based on facts, which, however, have no real significance. A letter reads:

"I am fond of clams. I recently learned that there is something in raw clams that destroys Vitamin B. Is this true — and should I stop eating this good food?"

There is an enzyme in raw clams and in certain other seafood that does destroy Vitamin B. However, unless you are a mink, primarily eating such seafood, the action has no significance. Indeed, if it were a hazard, it would simply mean that your intake of Vitamin B is precariously low. If you intend to eat large amounts of clams, it might be well to raise your Vitamin-B intake.

A similar type of reasoning is applied to this question:

"My son, who hates spinach, has just learned that there is an acid in spinach — I believe that it is oxalic acid — which interferes with the utilization of calcium. Before he succeeds in barring spinach from the house, please tell me if this is based on fact."

Again, this is based on fact and again, it has no significance. A given amount of oxalic acid will render insoluble and thereby nonabsorbable a given amount of calcium. The amount of oxalic acid in spinach is small. If it were large enough to interfere significantly with utilization of calcium, then eating spinach would be a quick passport to the next world. Accordingly, all that you need to do if you happen to be a spinach lover, is to increase your intake of milk and dairy products so that you have enough calcium to protect you against this minor interference.

There are those who would like to return to the primitive ways and discard cooking entirely. Such philosophy sometimes invites shock:

"I understand that you have told the public that cooking causes loss of nutrients, but also confers some dividends. How can this be possible? Is not a raw carrot better for me than a cooked one?"

Answer: I'm glad you chose carrots as an example, for the cell wall of the carrot is so tough that the body may have difficulty extracting the nutrients, with the result that the cooked carrot is frequently better utilized than the raw. It is quite true that cooking may exact a toll and yet confer some benefits.

Occasionally a very brief answer clarifies a question of fact and makes the fiction look foolish:

"I am told that since I am an allergic person, I should not nurse my baby. True or false?"

Answer: As an allergic person, you are virtually obligated to nurse your baby. Bottle-fed babies are much more subject to allergic reactions, so much so that we believe it significant that the apparent rise in the incidence of allergy started when mothers were convinced that a concoction of cow's milk, water, and some type of overrefined carbohydrate, packaged in a bottle with a rubber nipple, is equivalent to the breast and the highly nutritious food it creates.

Sometimes the layman will challenge medical doctrine — as in this letter.

"I have arthritis of the spine. My doctor told me to omit milk because obviously I already have too many calcium deposits. One of my friends tells me that *his* doctor gave him the opposite advice; his explanation is that the calcium will continue to be deposited even when I don't drink milk, but it will be withdrawn from other bones and the result, will be that I will still wind up with calcification plus a weakened skeleton."

Answer: Patronize the second doctor. His thinking is contaminated with a knowledge of biochemistry.

Calcium is the start of another argument. A listener wrote:

"I quoted you as saying calcium is lost in pasteurization. A physician and a chemist present at my home pointed out that calcium, being a mineral, is inert, and cannot be lost or diminished to any perceptible degree in milk as the result of pasteurization."

Answer: Let the chemist and the physician read the trade journals of the dairy industry. They will find advertised numerous detergents intended to remove "milk stone" from the pasteurization tanks. This is calcium that has been precipitated out of the milk in the pasteurization process. The percentage lost is small — perhaps 6 percent — but because of the huge volume of milk consumed, it represents millions of pounds of calcium that do not reach the public.

There are numerous beliefs surrounding garlic, the most frequent of which deals with its alleged action on hypertension. A listener wrote:

"I am told that if you eat garlic regularly, you will never have high blood pressure. Is this true?"

Answer: Italian families have their share of hypertension. If garlic does prevent high blood pressure, it does so because it keeps other people away from you.

"I have read," writes one of my readers, "American Medical Association and Food and Drug Administration statements to the effect that yogurt is simply a very expensive way to buy milk, and that it conveys no benefits that are not obtained from ordinary milk. Superstition or fact?"

Answer: This distortion may come as something of a surprise to Dubos, at Rockefeller University, who found that animals fed yogurt showed higher resistance to certain infections, plus a prolonged life span. Interestingly, I gleaned this report from a journal published by the American Medical Association.

The topic of food incompatibilities frequently brings up a dietary practice in the Jewish household. "Those of us who keep a Kosher household as you are probably aware, do not serve meat with milk. Is this purely a religious custom, or is there any scientific basis for it?"

Answer: Milk is modified blood. Blood is an animal tissue. So is meat. End of comment.

"I appeal to you as a nutritionist," writes a trusting reader, "to give me unbiased advice. I have been taking three tablets of brewer's yeast daily, and one of my friends remarks that this may be an overdose."

Answer: Isn't it interesting that the American public yearly eats over 800 million pounds of foodless cereals, plentifully dosed with undesirable preservatives, and never asks a question about advisability or overdose? Likewise, you eat 104 pounds of sugar a year, per capita, and ask no questions. The minute we feed you something that is rich in protein, vitamins, and other body-building substances, you grow nervous about overdosage. Why are you uneasy when threatened with good nutrition? Afraid of becoming healthy? In medical nutrition, up to *four ounces* of brewer's yeast daily have been prescribed.

In every profession there are the incompetent or those who are sincerely misguided. After consultation with such a person, a reader sent me this letter:

"I have been told by a practitioner that none of the calcium in pasteurized milk is absorbed. Is this true?"

Millions of babies, deprived of the benefit of consultations with the particular practitioner cited by my reader, have managed to build their skeletons on pasteurized milk. Certified milk — raw or pasteurized — is a better food than ordinary pasteurized milk, but about 23 percent of the calcium in pasteurized milk will be utilized. The utilization of milk calcium, whether it derives from raw or pasteurized milk, will always be aided by the presence of milk sugar. In the body this provides the acid medium that is favorable to solubility of calcium and thereby to its absorption. In their vast land where dairy products are not plentiful, the Chinese show inherited wisdom when they give a pregnant woman pickled pigs' feet in vinegar. Here again you have calcium in an acid medium.

When physicians prescribe foul-tasting medicines they show little concern — after all, they didn't ask you to become sick. Sometimes the same cavalier attitude carries over to the diet they prescribe. Witness this note: "My doctor has me on a low-salt diet. The monotony of such food, it seems to me, is worse for me than my high blood pressure. He tells me that there is no substitute for a low-salt diet, and that I must simply learn to enjoy food that is not seasoned. Is this true?"

It has been long established that spices that are not high in sodium can be used by individuals on a low-salt diet. Thus, other than celery salt, garlic salt, onion salt, and monosodium glutamate, all spices and seasonings that those on a low-salt diet can tolerate may be used. It is not true that a low-salt diet is irreplaceable. When such a diet is being used to encourage the body to part with water that it has been retaining, a low-carbohydrate diet may prove more effective and certainly more enjoyable for the patient. In cases of hypertension, however, there are those who must have a restricted intake of sodium.

Mention of acidity, a few paragraphs ago, brings up a subject dear to the hearts of many concerned about their nutrition and their well-being. The nutritionist is constantly plied with questions concerning foods with an alkaline residue and foods with an acid residue. Since most of these questions reflect pure superstition, they receive an acid reply. If, by virtue of any food combination, you succeeded in changing the blood from its normal alkalinity toward acidity, all questions about nutrition would become academic — except, possibly, food for worms. Actually, the body has a magnificent system of checks and balances so that that which should be acid remains so, that which should be alkaline remains so, and nothing short of a major disorder is likely to change the circumstances. In fact, the body has at least one group of cells that manage to manufacture the most highly alkaline and the most highly acid organic substances simultaneously.

Some fictions in nutrition originate with propaganda from government or industry. A frequent target involves vitamin intake that is "beyond your requirement," and the question arises very often in this form: "I have read that intake of vitamins beyond one's needs is at best wasted and at worst toxic. What is truth and what is falsehood here?"

There are individuals whose enzyme chemistry is faulty. Many enzymes include a vitamin and frequently include a mineral. If one wishes to increase the body's manufacture of an enzyme that is being produced in inadequate quantities, one feasible way is to supply more of the building materials.

So it is that there are enzyme disorders that raise the vitamin requirements to as much as 100,000 times the "average." This subject is discussed at length elsewhere in this book. Not only is the statement about vitamin intake untrue on these grounds; it is also untrue in terms of individuals whose enzyme chemistries are normal. In chemistry there is the law of mass action. Simply stated, there is a more rapid transfer of a vitamin through a blood-vessel wall and into the tissues, or through a cell membrane, when the concentration of the vitamin is high. When government sources tell you that vitamin intake beyond the requirements set by the government are wasted, they are taking the liberty of repealing a law of chemistry. Nature's laws are not subject to bureaucratic manipulation. As far as toxicity goes, the subject is one on which a book could be written. Suffice it to say, reports of toxicity have originated when doses of nutrients have been employed so high that milk taken in the same overdose would have proved deadly. Most of the victims were small babies whose mothers disobeyed the pediatrician's instructions. The prescription called for ten or fifteen drops of a vitamin concentrate, and these mothers thought that a teaspoonful or two would be better. I guess if vitamin needs can be exaggerated, government propagandists may likewise exaggerate.

There are dozens of beliefs concerning honey — most of them fallacious. A common one is that honey is a better form of sweetening than sugar. This is vociferously denied, particularly by the sugar manufacturers and the university nutritionists to whose departments the former make large contributions. There is a small number of vitamins and minerals in honey, not significant to warrant claims of nutritional superiority. Honey also contains a sizable amount of fructose — fruit sugar — which is reported to place no burden on the pancreas and insulin mechanism of the body. On the other hand, there have been several reports that indicate that overdosage with fructose may carry some hazards. In honey there is a large amount of sucrose, which is the same sugar that Americans consume in entirely too great a quantity. One virtue of honey, courageously ignored by fluoridationists, is that like other natural sweets it is much less conducive to tooth decay than ordinary sugar. If a diabetic abuses honey, he may cause himself serious trouble. At one point, the health-food industry decided that tupelo honey had some special virtues for diabetics. If it does, they are known only to apiaries producing tupelo honey.

The subject of food additives has given rise to a new folklore. Innocent chemicals are blamed; suspect ones are swallowed without thought. The mound of fact mixed with fiction is topped with a garnish of propaganda, again originating with universities heavily subsidized by processed-food manufacturers whose excessive use of food additives makes their labels read like prescriptions. Witness the following letter: "I have just read a book by a man named Deutch, in which he demonstrates that food is nothing but a mixture of chemicals. He comes to the conclusion that nobody should object to food additives on the grounds that they are chemicals, because it is not logical to accept the first fact and reject the second one."

Having encountered this particular author in a debate and ascertained that he is a bosom friend of all processed foods and food additives, it was not surprising to find that many of his opinions reflect a sophistry analogous to that in the doctrine just expressed. If one is to accept all food additives because they are simply chemicals added to food that is composed of chemicals, one invites the use of strychnine as a seasoning. However, the chemicals in food are not new to the body; the body has had physiological experience with them for millions of years.

Food additives, on the other hand, represent a plunge into uncharted areas — areas that may be fraught with physiological dangers. And it is a matter of record that missing from the market today are food additives that for many years were labeled by equally complacent authors as perfectly safe. They were discovered to be toxic, teratogenic, cancer-producing, or in some other way undesirable.

Going to the other extreme, in reply to a letter asking about the safety of calcium propionate, is this note: Propionic acid is normal to the human body. Its action as an antimold ingredient for bread and certain other foods was employed because it was noticed that garments thoroughly wet with perspiration became resistant to mold and mildew. The active antifungus agent turned out to be propionic acid. One must therefore believe this to be safe. On the other hand, there are numerous writers who are concerned about BHT and BHA, butylhydroxytoluene and butylhydroxyanisol. A number of nations have banned these antioxidants completely and will not permit foods containing them. In this country we are swallowing them in practically all breakfast cereals, save a very few, in salad oils, and in chewing gum. Manufacturers will not defend the use of additives on the grounds that they, like food, are chemicals. They will tell you that these additives preserve nutritional values. A quick riposte would be the observation that Germany permits preservation of food values, but only with Vitamin C, Vitamin E, and other safe substances. In addition, such preservation here is often a euphemism for prolongation of shelf life — an action much more serviceable to the manufacturer than to the consumer. Once in a while the chicanery becomes painfully obvious. What nutritional value is being preserved in chewing gum by the use of such antioxidants as BHT? And why have we permitted the use of preservatives banned in Canada, Germany, Sweden, and Romania?

Some legends are built on what would appear to be logical premises. Many readers and listeners write in protest against exorbitant prices for organic foods, defined as foods that are free of undesirable additives, that have been properly fertilized, and that have not been excessively processed. There is no defense for whole-wheat bread selling at one dollar a loaf. There is a legitimate reason for a 10 percent premium on organic beef, for there is a sizable delay in weight gain when the breeder does not use the antibiotics and synthetic female hormone. There is good reason for a premium on organic vegetables and fruits: Insects must be removed by hand or measures must be employed that are more labor consuming and thereby much more costly than spraying with toxic insecticides. This is not to say that there is not some unconscionable overpricing, for it is inevitable that in every industry that has captured the public interest there will be the "fast-dollar" group. But progress is being made in making available supplies of more nutritious and purer foods for those who wish them. Attenuated gastronomic suicide, the only legal kind, will continue to be your option.

Sometimes logic breaks down when applied to something as complex as the human body and its reactions to diets. A physician wrote to me when I first published a low-carbohydrate diet and said: "It seems unreasonable that a diet high in fat would cause the body to burn fat — yet this is the implication in the low-carbohydrate diet. Please comment." The interesting part of the research is that it originated with the United States Navy, whose nutritionists established that starvation causes a loss of weight resulting from the breakdown of tissues — meaning protein — while a high-fat diet causes loss of weight due to the burning of fat. A helpful ingredient in the prescription, however, is that some percentage of the fat in the diet has to be unsaturated. Don't ask why — what we do not know about nutrition will fill a number of volumes in the centuries to come.

A chapter on this subject presents the difficulty that spelling the word "banana" does for some people — where do you stop? Unbelievable as it sounds, melba toast, weight for weight, actually has more caloric value than bread. Brown sugar is merely white sugar with a dab of molasses — but is it? It contains trivalent chromium, but still remains bad food. Cocoa and chocolate do contain a stimulant; why are they given to children who would be denied coffee? Why does dog food represent much better nutrition than foods packed for human consumption — frequently by the same companies? Why do we speak of three square meals daily when there are millions of people who would be much better off with six smaller meals? Why do nutritionists warn the public that the avidin in egg white destroys the biotin in egg yolk, when experiments have shown that it requires three-and-one-half pounds of egg white daily to create a biotin deficiency? Why does the Arthritis Foundation assure the public that diet has nothing to do with arthritis when common sense tells us that arthritics must include the badly nourished as well as the adequately fed? Common sense tells us that improvement of one's nutrition is certainly likely to better one's battle with a degenerative disease. Dr. Tom Spies was medically honored for the research in which he demonstrates that, "vitamins can be used for the smaller pains of arthritis — for the larger pains, we use hormones." And is it because of the modern chemical food preservatives that people have lost sight of the truth of the ancient axiom: "If a food spoils — eat it before it does. If it keeps, throw it out"?

In another book I intend to explore superstition or fact in nutrition in greater depth. In the interim, remember that it is not safe automatically to regard folklore as being baseless. The ancient Britons, treating a child for rickets, included a ritual in which the child was passed through a cleft in an ash tree, but only in the presence of full sunlight. When one studies superstitions in nutrition in depth and finds the same beliefs, modified according to tenets of the culture and availabilities of food, repeated from one people to another, from one land to another, and under circumstances where they must have arisen independently, one can only conclude that exposed to certain phenomena, man's mind tends to arrive — wherever he is — at the same conclusions; and a good part of the time, they are faulty.

We may end our journey through superstitions with a story that may answer the nagging question: How do these beliefs start? It is the tale of a man who is watching his wife prepare a ham for roasting. After applying the brown sugar and inserting the cloves, she cut off a chunk of ham from one end and proceeded to throw away a sizable amount of good meat. When she was asked why, she said the practice had started with her grandmother. They called her for a long-delayed explanation. "I started that a very long time ago," said grandma reflectively. Then she said: "I remember now — my pan was too short!"

14.
NUTRITION IN PREVENTION AND TREATMENT OF DISEASE

As one who has served as a consultant in nutrition to a medical group practice, a sanitarium, internists, psychiatrists, osteopaths, and dentists, I have watched a good many triumphs of nutritional therapy. I have regarded every one of them as a monument to a failure — for what nutrition cures, it ordinarily prevents. When a woman with a record of five miscarriages changes her diet, plies herself with vitamin concentrates, and manages in the succeeding pregnancies to bring three healthy children into the world, one must think that had the corrected nutrition been instituted earlier, the tragedies would not have occurred.

This does not mean that the success of nutritional therapy necessarily implies nutritional deficiency. There are many instances in which nutritional treatment is used for disorders *not* caused by dietary deficiencies. A classic example would be the use of large doses of Vitamin C to treat the dermatitis of ivy poisoning, or the use of a carbon-twenty unsaturated fat to stimulate the function of the brain in a brain-injured child. But generally, it has always seemed to me that triumphs in nutritional therapy are flawed. Either they represent the lost opportunity for prevention, or they are applied as a last resort: "I've tried neurology, psychiatry, gynecology, obstetrics, physiotherapy, chiropractic medicine, osteopathy, and periodontics — and they all failed.

Now give me a diet that will straighten everything out in two weeks." If we nutritionists have any batting average under those circumstances — and we *do* — we may well feel gratified.

There is often a long delay between new findings in science and their ultimate application in helping suffering mankind. Particularly exaggerated is the cultural lag in the field of nutrition, and if someone doesn't intervene, millions of people will wait for decades for information to trickle down from the research laboratories to the physician's practice. This chapter is not intended to encourage self-medication, but to bring you the benefit of nutritional therapies that should be applied under the supervision of a competent physician. It is comforting to know that while the side reactions of today's powerful medicines can and sometimes do fill cemeteries, the nutritionist's mistakes rarely result in anything more serious than bellyaches. Moreover, nutritional therapies almost invariably help the actions of needed medication and may often reduce or eliminate the side effects of drugs.

There will be no attempt here to cover all the diseases to which you are susceptible. They are numbered in the thousands, and this is only one chapter in a book. Also, contrary to the philosophy of those who believe that good nutrition solves all problems, there are numerous diseases for which there is no specific nutritional therapy. However, there is no disorder that does not ultimately involve the patient's nutrition, which means that a well-fed person is more responsive to treatment, for all disease must interfere with the nutrition of the cell, the organ, or the system.

A disorder may be psychosomatic, and yet proper diet may prove helpful. In other words, your spouse may have given you the ulcer, but your menus may ultimately be part of the healing process. The sickness may be an infection, but the antibodies that are needed for recovery are proteins, and several vitamins will be required in their synthesis. The insult may be a burn, but vitamins and proteins are involved in the healing. The trouble may be glaucoma, and its origin may be emotional but proper use of two vitamins may drop the intraocular pressure. The difficulty may be periodontal disease, starting with malocclusion (a bad bite), but after the dentist has adjusted your bite, good nutrition and exercise of the mouth and jaw may retard decalcification of the jawbone. Your diabetes may be an unwelcome gift from your genes, but your Vitamin-B-Complex intake will still be helpful in stabilizing your liver function and increasing your tolerance for both fats and carbohydrates.

In this chapter, I review some nutritional therapies with which the professions and the public are usually unacquainted. I have also included certain nutritional treatments that are based upon my un-published research and reports that have reached me from the many thousands of professional men who have heard my papers on various subjects in the field of nutrition, or who are readers of my books or newsletters.

Let us begin with a group of disorders for which medicine has neither satisfactory explanation nor truly satisfactory treatment, and at present, little hope of a cure. I refer to the myoneuropathies — the vast number of nerve-muscle disorders, some of which are relentlessly progressive, and a few of which are deadly. In this group would be included multiple sclerosis, muscular dystrophy, amyotrophic lateral sclerosis, myas-thenia gravis, amyotonia congenita, dermatomyositis, postencephalitic syndrome, petit mal and grand mal epilepsy, epileptiform equivalents including migraine headaches, and cerebral palsy with all its varia-tions — the spastic, the atonic, the rigidities, tremors, and ataxics.

Ordinarily, when a single treatment is applied to what appears to be a number of different diseases, medical men logically become wary. Panaceas do not exist. Actually, the common targets in all these dis-orders, even though symptoms and causes of the diseases are different, are the nervous system, the brain, and the muscles. It should also be remembered that in recent years medical research has identified factors that are common to many apparently unrelated disorders. Such, for instance, is the implication of Hans Selye's discovery of the stress adap-tation disorders. Such is the ultimate implication of the recent discovery of the prostaglandins, the quasi-hormone substances that appear to be involved in the functioning of virtually every cell and organ in the entire body, and which are synthesized from dietary unsaturated fats.

Some of the actions of these nutritional therapies can be explained only if another medical shibboleth is discarded. At this very minute fledgling neurologists are being taught that repair of brain cells is impossible; that damaged neurons elsewhere in the body may possibly be healed, but those in the brain cannot be healed or replaced. My experience indicates that this may not be entirely true. The responses I have seen to nutritional therapies in spastics, for instance, both in motor and in mental function can be interpreted in only three possible ways: Either damaged cerebral neurons are indeed restored to function by this treatment, or the therapy is stimulating the maturation of young nerve cells (neuroblasts) that then take over the function of the damaged cells. However, in some cases, the response is so quick that there is literally no time for the latter process to occur, leaving two possibilities: either the previously mentioned restoration of the function of the damaged nerve cells, or stimulation of the "totality of function" of the brain.

The overprocessing of wheat and other grains deprives us of a group of unsaturated fats found in the oil extracted from the germ of those grains. (This is one of the reasons why favorable comparisons of enriched white bread with whole-wheat are made only by the ignorant, the incompetent, the commercially biased, or those unaware of the nutritional importance of certain of the fats.)

The unsaturated fats with twenty carbon atoms or less act on us in ways unknown to most of our endocrinologists and neurologists. They may affect hypothalamic function. They stimulate the maturation of immature nerve cells and the function and repair of the mature. These fats also stimulate the pituitary gland and are somehow involved in the metabolism of the nervous system. They increase the cardiac reserve and add to the capacity of the muscles for work. (It has been established that middle-aged men can turn back the physical clock ten or even twenty years by following a program of exercises geared to their capabilities and needs, and accompanied by supplements of a concentrated wheat-germ oil.) How they do all this I leave to future investigators. There is every possibility that these fats are the precursors for prostaglandins synthesis. The pathway of action may also be via other effects on the anterior pituitary. But we are not concerned with the mode of the action, but rather the effect. This neuromuscular fraction in such fats as wheat-germ oil should now receive the medical attention that the researchers in physical education, who have established its favorable effect on muscle performance, have given it for twenty years.

Given with Vitamin E and a proper formulation of the Vitamin B Complex, the neuromuscular fraction of wheat-germ oil has improved both the motor and mental performance in the brain-injured, in the cerebral palsied, and in the epileptic. In approximately one-third of the cases of multiple sclerosis in which I have observed this treatment, significant benefits have accrued. These can be distinguished from spontaneous remissions quite easily, by comparing handwriting at intervals before, during, and after the treatment. In a spontaneous remission the legibility of handwriting does not ordinarily improve.

In amyotonia congenita it has already been established that wheat-germ oil itself is semitherapeutic. In myasthenia gravis, the therapy is augmented with therapeutic doses of pantothenic acid and choline in order to facilitate synthesis of acetylcholine. (The same treatment, incidentally, may be useful in glaucoma.)

In brain-injured children, coupling this type of therapy with needed medication, patterning, and other physiotherapeutic treatments should accelerate and augment the positive responses.

It was in the treatment of patients suffering from the aftermath of encephalitis, perhaps resulting from a virus infection such as measles, that I first observed the startling benefits these fats bring to the nervous system and to the muscles. You may have seen people so afflicted. There is the painfully slow speech, the slogging walk, and difficulty with any action calling for neuromuscular coordination — even the familiar task of buttoning a button becomes a gigantic challenge. When you watch a patient recapture the ability to button his own jacket after sixty days of treatment with wheat-germ oil plus Vitamin E and Vitamin B Complex, you develop a respect for the nutritional importance of these factors to the nervous system and the musculature.* This treatment, coupled with large doses of niacin is, in my observations, potentially helpful in treating brain damage following use of LSD, and in treating the retarded, the brain damaged, the autistic, and the epileptic. (A hypoglycemia-type diet is also necessary. Allergenic foods to which the patient is sensitive and caffeine should be excluded from the diet.)

Nutritional resources are also not employed adequately for some very common problems — for example, acne. Professional men have forgotten that more than twenty-five years ago, Norman Jolliffe established the usefulness of Vitamin B_6 in reducing facial oiliness that invites or aggravates the infection.

Likewise, the emphasis on Vitamin A's toxicity has obscured the fact that reasonable doses of the vitamin, particularly when given in the emulsified or in the water-dispersible form, have also been helpful in treating acne. Instead of debating, the dermatologist should try prescribing 100 mgs. of Vitamin B_6 and 15,000 to 25,000 units of Vitamin A daily. (Preferably in the water-dispersible form for better utilization).

Another application of nutritional therapy is in breaking the common cold. I have read all of Linus Pauling's writings on the subject — indeed I have shared the scientific platform with him, and I was among those who rose to the defense of his thesis when it was brought under attack. Yet I will be the first to tell you that Vitamin C is neither useless in warding off the common cold, as his critics would have you believe, nor an infallible preventive treatment, as Dr. Pauling appears to

---

*In disorders where there is no spasm of the muscles, the B-Complex supplement should supply larger amounts of choline and inositol than are usually present in commercial formulas and generous amounts of the other crystalline B vitamins. The formula should provide a daily intake of at least 1,000 mgs. of choline and 500 mgs. of inositol. Where spasm of the muscles is present, as in multiple sclerosis, the choline should be omitted.

believe. First, there is no such thing as the common cold; it is a group of disorders, with a group of causes. There are, for instance, colds that arise purely from the frustration that comes from rage that cannot be expressed; and I question that any vitamin will be fully effective in treating this type. Second, there are colds perhaps of viral origin, which nothing blocks or cures. Third, there are colds that will not respond to Vitamin C, but do respond to Vitamin A. People differ — there are Vitamin-C responders, and there are Vitamin-A responders.

In breaking a cold with vitamins, there are four requirements:

1. The cold must be of a type that responds.
2. We must be responders.
3. We must use the correct vitamin for us as individuals.
4. The vitamin must be given at the earliest sign of a cold.

The current emphasis on Vitamin C puzzles me for two reasons. Firstly, it isn't a new discovery — over thirty years ago the vitamin was recognized to be an antihistamine when taken in large doses. If that claim is fraudulent, so must be all the advertising for the antihistamines that are sold as cold remedies. The other reason is the failure to recognize that among reports contemporary with those that motivated Dr. Linus Pauling's research with Vitamin C, there is equally valid work to indicate that Vitamin A in large doses breaks colds.

This contradictory information sounds like a large tempest in a vitamin teapot. Actually it is more than academic. The Vitamin-A responder not only gains no benefit from Vitamin C in large doses for colds, but he also runs the risk of moving the cold from his head to his chest. On the other hand, if a Vitamin-C responder should use Vitamin A, he will suffer no penalty — and no benefits in breaking his cold. Accordingly, if you want to try vitamin therapy to break a cold, the first step is to identify your earliest symptom. This isn't as easy as it sounds — it varies from individual to individual. It can be a feeling of malaise, an unnatural elation, a tightening of the scalp, which becomes painful, the blurring of eyesight, indigestion, or abnormal fatigue. The second step, if you do not know to which vitamin you may respond, is to try Vitamin A. If you are wrong in your choice, the only penalty will be failure to break the cold. The vitamin is used in quantities of 200,000 units daily, taken in one dose for each of five successive days. If this suppresses the cold, you must be careful not to become overtired or you will invite a return of the symptoms.

If Vitamin A is not effective, with the next cold Vitamin C may be tried. Quantities used are from 1,000 mgs. per dose, with frequencies ranging from two to as many as three or four doses per day for five days. It is advantageous to accompany each dose with a tablespoon of honey.

With regard to preventing colds: I have had more success with the routine use of Vitamin A than with Vitamin C. Contrary to the statement of the "medical authorities," supplements of Vitamin A or even cod-liver oil have significantly reduced the incidence of colds in industrial groups, as reported in papers dating back to the 1930s. I have less experience with Vitamin C used for that purpose, although it is logical that continued intake of quantities of that vitamin large enough to act as an antihistamine should be beneficial, for Vitamin C under this circumstance both inhibits the growth of bacteria and acts as an antiallergy factor. And we must not forget that allergy is a frequent component of colds. Therefore, a daily supplement supplying 15,000 units of Vitamin A or a gram or two of Vitamin C daily may very well bring your cold score down.

At this point there will be enthusiasts who will want to use large doses of both vitamins to break colds. Don't — what will happen will be a prolongation of the cold with the intensity of the symptoms somewhat reduced.

We positively know so many things that just aren't so — which is a very good way to begin a discussion of three disorders for which we have pat explanations that do not explain, and treatments that do not treat. I refer to hardening of the arteries, heart disease, and senile dementia, which is often associated with, and therefore mistakenly blamed on, hardening of the arteries.

John Dewey remarked that Americans would rather know than think, because thinking is precarious and leads to an unsafe world with too many "ifs" and "maybes." Knowing eliminates all of these uncertainties. Unfortunately, that craving for certainties frequently overcomes our medical men, too. As a result, the unbelievably complicated disorder — heart disease associated with hardening of the arteries — was "explained" as the product of too much fat and cholesterol and "prevented" by a simple reduction in the intake of eggs to three a week.

It might be instructive to review briefly the profile of the man who is coronary-thrombosis-prone. The factors could include the hardness of his drinking water; his smoking habits; the aggressiveness of his personality; the activity of his thyroid gland; the number of deadlines encountered in his work or profession; his handling of psychological and physiological stresses; the levels in his blood of beta-lipoprotein, triglycerides, and cholesterol; the ratio in his diet of saturated to unsaturated fat; the amounts he consumes of lipotropic factors, of Vitamin

C, of Vitamin E, and, possibly, of lecithin. As you look back over that list, you can understand why the public prefers four eggs a week as *the* factor that does you in with a heart attack.

Had any one stopped to think about it, surely the thought would have occurred that the diet cannot be the *dominant* variable. After all, there isn't that much difference in the diets of men and women — and yet men are much more susceptible than women to coronary thrombosis.

I have no doubt that Vitamin-E deficiency plays a part in inducing some heart attacks. One cannot experiment with induced vitamin deficiency in men — not when heart disease is the result — but it *is* significant that every mammal — from the monkey to the horse — subjected to Vitamin-E deficiency develops heart disturbances ranging from electrocardiographic aberrations to death. Those who deny the role of Vitamin E in human cardiac disturbances are saying in effect that man is the only mammal immune to the cardiac impact of Vitamin-E deficiency. Actual assay of the Vitamin-E levels in the blood of human cardiac patients has revealed low levels in a sizable percentage. Recently, too, actual assay of foods commonly used in the American menus indicates that the Vitamin-E intake of the general public is far lower than had been thought — indeed, far below the level considered satisfactory. Unfortunately, the remarkable therapeutic response in certain types of heart disease to doses of Vitamin E does not necessarily mean that deficiencies in the vitamin were the cause of the pathology. The large quantities of Vitamin E required would argue for its pharmacodynamic (druglike) effect. In nutrition, it is not uncommon for large doses of a nutrient to have a drug effect completely unrelated to the normal nutritional function of the factor. (As examples, consider the effect of very large doses of Vitamin C in breaking a cold, or the healing effect of very large doses of Vitamin B_{12} in the treatment of "shingles." Here you have disorders caused by bacteria or viruses, and yet amenable to treatment with large doses of a vitamin.)

I do not intend to review here (for I have done it in another book) the hundreds of responses of those who have suffered coronary thrombosis or angina to Vitamin-E therapy. Suffice it to say, the vitamin is neither the panacea which the overenthusiastic consider it to be, nor the complete failure which the American Medical Association and American cardiologists have labeled it. I have seen it yield dramatic responses in the first ten days of a massive coronary in an aged physician. I have seen it totally relieve mild angina and significantly help sufferers with severe angina, to the extent that some of them were able to go back to work. I have also seen it fail.

Wilfred Shute, who pioneered in research with Vitamin-E therapy in heart disease, has devoted his entire clinical effort to Vitamin E. To the careless observer, the cardiac application of vitamin therapy has therefore been dominated by Vitamin E. Actually, many other nutrients affect the heart. Vitamin B_{12}, for instance, has almost as much influence on the electrical activity of the heart as Vitamin E, and Vitamin B_6 is not far behind. Sodium-potassium and magnesium-calcium ratios are critically important to the healthy and to the diseased heart. Not only is Vitamin E important as an antioxidant, reducing oxygen needs, but the vitamin is also essential to the integrity of endothelial tissue. Furthermore, there is evidence that this nutrient is requisite in supporting the basic transport of electrons in the energy metabolism of the cell.

Although Vitamin E and wheat-germ oil are mistakenly considered to be equivalents, twenty years of exhaustive research have shown that there is a factor in wheat-germ oil that is not Vitamin E and that helps improve muscle function — including the heart.

There is as much individuality in responses to nutritional therapy for cardiac disease as in any other disorder, and the services of a competent medical nutritionist are essential. The important point is that the public, with heart disease one of our great killers, must no longer be deprived of the benefits of competent prophylaxis and therapy with Vitamins E, B_{12}, B_6, and B_1, folic acid, B Complex, correct proportions between calcium and magnesium, potassium and sodium. Likewise, the public must take full advantage of the arachidonic acid content of wheat germ and other germ oils.

Make no mistake: I repeat that I have seen coronary insufficiency helped by such treatments. I have watched patients with congestive heart failure, who were going downhill with orthodox treatment, successfully treated with vitamin and mineral therapy. I have seen severe angina mitigated and mild angina eliminated. All this information should lead you to a conclusion and a question. It is obvious that a medical nutritionist ought to be part of the team in any intensive care unit dealing with cardiac disease, and a useful partner of the cardiologist in routine practice. We also ought to ask whether our daily diet does what it should in supplying us with these nutritional factors for the preventive effect they exert. It usually *doesn't*.

When you examine that proposition, you will find that we have been making mistakes since the cradle. For instance, we may be predisposing our babies toward high blood pressure and consequent heart disease by the large amounts of salt that are added to baby foods. This is a gratuitous insult, for babies couldn't care less about flavoring and condiments, and the salt is added to please the mother, who will invariably taste the baby food before feeding it to her child. The net effect of this intake of salt and the substantial amounts of sodium in cow's milk (greater by far than the content of breast milk) is that we are inverting the ratio between sodium and potassium. The potassium intake should be higher than the sodium, and the opposite is usually true. Moreover, the American community has virtually tried to excommunicate those "health-food nuts" who have consumed substantial quantities of vegetable juices, nuts, raisins, and other foods that represent good or excellent sources of potassium. Indeed, our customs tend to deprive us of this mineral important to the heart.

Let us consider the foods carried to the moon by our spacemen. Contrary to the opinion you may have formed from the advertising of Tang, the moon shots were not really arranged to furnish a backdrop for the advertising of synthetic orange drinks, which are portrayed as "better sources of Vitamin C" than the natural product. They may be better sources of Vitamin C, but the other nutrients of orange juice — including potassium — are not provided. Now the space administration is busy revising the menus of the astronauts, so that more potassium will be supplied. The current belief is that lack of this vital mineral has been responsible for their irregularities of the heart. But we who are earthbound have likewise arbitrarily deprived ourselves of potassium. It is not only that the housewife ignorantly buys the synthetic orange juice drinks in the belief that she is saving money without sacrificing nutritional value, she also buys canned and frozen foods, which in blanching and in other stages of processing are subjected to techniques that cause a loss of trace minerals and of sizable amounts of potassium.

We not only tolerate but we also encourage by our patronage the marketing of carbohydrate foods — grains, cereals, flour, and sugar — marked by the removal of most of the Vitamin-B-Complex factors and about 97 percent of the Vitamin E they should normally yield.

NIACIN IN PREVENTION OF HEART AND ARTERY DISEASE

The vitamin action of niacin and niacinamide is identical. In the brain, in the treatment of perceptual disorders like schizophrenia the two have identical effects. (Niacin in large doses doesn't usually cause nausea. Niacinamide may.) However, there are drug actions of niacin that the other form of the vitamin does not yield. These include beneficial effect on microscopic circulation, on the flow of red blood cells through the capillaries, and influences on carbohydrate, fat, and cholesterol metabolism, on tissue oxidation, and on the chemistry of biogenic amines in the brain.

The beneficial effects of niacin, oddly enough, are not yielded by the vitamin itself. For many years we have known that virtually everyone who takes niacin experiences a flush not yielded by niacinamide. That is the reason why the form of the vitamin used in ordinary vitamin supplements has been niacinamide. People who are merely supplementing their diet had not wished to experience heat waves. Only recently was it realized that the niacin flush originates with a release of histamine caused by the vitamin. This is the chemical that creates much of the misery of allergic reactions.

The histamine release was traced to an action of niacin on the mast cells, which are found around the blood vessels. These cells also produce heparin — a chemical that is to blood fat what insulin is to blood sugar.

Because heparin helps reduce blood fats, it aids in preventing the blood from clotting abnormally. Therefore, the action of niacin in releasing heparin might very well help prevent the blood clots that are so often the prelude to coronary thrombosis attacks.

When we are too generously supplied with the antihemorrhagic blood chemicals such as the platelets or fibrinogen, a delicately balanced mechanism goes awry, and the tightrope we walk between bleeding to death and clotting to death may suddenly snap.

Where we do not manufacture enough heparin or do not properly release it, the action of niacin in raising the heparin levels of the blood may very well be life saving. But this is not the only helpful effect of heparin. It also induces the manufacture of lipoprotein lipase, an enzyme that clears both milky fat and triglycerides (fats manufactured from sugar). In addition, heparin stimulates the manufacture of fibrinolysin, which is the enzyme that dissolves clots and may help dissolve the plaques which, forming in a blood vessel, may initiate a heart attack or hardening of the arteries, or both.

And these are not all the dividends from the niacin action that persuades the mast cells to release histamine and heparin. The depletion of histamine makes it virtually impossible for an allergic person to experience a dangerous allergic reaction. The heparin also manages to act like a policeman in preventing the red blood cells from creating traffic jams. These cells should go through the small vessels in single file; they will do so if they carry sufficient negative electric charge to repel each other. But if the charge is insufficient, the cells tend to clump like a cluster of grapes. These aggregates cause the blood to "sludge," and in the lungs, since only the outer red cells of the cluster are properly exposed to oxygen, insufficient oxygen is picked up and conveyed to the tissues. By the simple action of reinforcing the negative electrical charge on the red blood cells, heparin reduces the tendency of the blood to sludge and helps to maintain tissue oxygen at a normal level. Every heparin effect may be life saving or at least life prolonging, and niacin is the key to release of this factor.

Niacin, which is used in quantities of 500 mgs., three times a day after meals, while a safe vitamin-drug for the majority of its users, must be employed with caution by people with special problems. For instance, the medicine used for high blood pressure prevents blood vessels from constricting in response to the release of adrenalin. The niacin flush brings a compensatory release of adrenalin, which is ordinarily nature's way to constrict the blood vessels and thus prevent fainting. So when the physician is giving niacin to hypertensive patients, the initial doses should be small, and the patient should lie down to avoid fainting. A small dose is defined by the authorities as 25 mgs. niacin every one or two hours for several days, until the histamine reserves are exhausted and the flush has stopped.

Since niacin raises the threshold for fasting blood sugar, it can be a useful vitamin for hypoglycemics. However, this effect for a diabetic might increase the need for diet restriction, exercise, weight loss, or all three. Some diabetics might react with an alteration in their insulin requirement. Such an alteration must be watched for in diabetics who have had coronary thrombosis or strokes, in order to be sure insulin requirements have not been significantly changed.

Niacin is an acid, and as such may disturb people with active peptic ulcer or a tendency to hyperacidity. For such individuals, the physician can request the pharmacist to prepare a liquid solution of niacin — 250 mgs. to the ounce — buffered to make it neutral and nonirritating. This is not available commercially since it cannot be patented and offers no chance for substantial profit.

Niacin can also be neutralized with ordinary baking soda — one quarter of a teaspoonful to each niacin tablet, dissolved in two ounces of hot water. With the addition of ice, this becomes an odorless and tasteless solution, which will not trouble those who have hyperacidity or peptic ulcer.

What you have so far read represents a preliminary review of a huge and yet unpublished study of coronary survivors who have been dosed with one of three proprietary drugs or with niacin, in an effort to reduce blood fats and cholesterol, and thereby lower the death rate from cardiovascular disease. Niacin has outperformed the proprietary drugs, and use of the vitamin for the foregoing purposes has quietly been approved by numerous government and private health agencies.

The patient who is given niacin, they report, will experience better oxygenation of the tissue and microscopic circulation, while enjoying lower blood fat and cholesterol, and a reduced tendency to blood clotting, embellished with a heightened sense of well-being. In addition, the niacin will reduce platelet stickiness, which helps avoid phlebitis, and, also via the release of heparin, will help restore the normal fat-clearing enzymes.

Individuals who are taking antiblood-clotting drugs cannot be given niacin without rechecking of the prothrombin time. Ultimately, on diets high in unsaturated fat and supplemented with niacin, the anti-clotting drugs can often be discontinued.

For those who have suffered a heart attack, niacin will help protect against a new one if the body weight is kept normal, if one exercises, and also takes polyunsaturated fat and Vitamin E. Niacin also helps Meniere's syndrome, one type of which develops because of poor circulation and fluid retention in the semicircular canals of the ears, abetted by the sludging of blood. Vascular headaches are also helped. Three grams of niacin daily will prevent — not cure — a headache and also the type of migraine caused by histamine. The authorities believe it is easier to exhaust the reserves of histamine than to desensitize the patient against the chemical. Some allergies temporarily worsen with niacin, and it is known that people who are prone to chronic hives (urticaria) often cannot stand the vitamin; but seasonal asthma and other allergies are ultimately relieved by the vitamin. In some cases, the individuals who react badly to niacin are really troubled by the filler in the tablet, rather than the niacin itself.

Niacin has also been used in the treatment of high blood pressure that is based on aldosteronism. Here niacin, Vitamin E, and Vitamin C are given in small amounts, with the niacin dosage gradually raised. The Vitamin E is used to protect endothelial integrity, and the Vitamin C helps protect the blood vessels. Sodium must be restricted, and — in the latest research — so must sugar. The dose of niacin, beginning with 25 mgs. with each meal is gradually raised to the standard dose of 500 mgs. with each meal. In moderate cases of hypertension where kidney damage is present, niacin is effective in lowering the pressure toward normal, but requires about ninety days to exert its action.

Finally, the repetition of strokes may be blocked with niacin. The use of niacin will also mean that the red blood cells will convey oxygen more efficiently, so that even with the reduced brain function caused by a stroke, the tissue will function more effectively. This is particularly true of the immature or "sleeping" cells that are adjacent to the areas where destruction has occurred. They may then take over the function of the damaged area, often leading to a noticeable improvement.

Following, you will find brief descriptions of some of the medicinal uses of the vitamins and other nutrients. These represent condensations of reports by qualified investigators, usually physicians, as I encountered them in medical journals over the past twenty years or more. In certain instances, where the nutrients or the quantities employed do not represent the ideal approach as indicated by information I have garnered from physicians with whom I have performed research, I have entered those observations separately.

MAGNESIUM

To reduce cholesterol: 500 mgs. daily.

To increase citric acid in urine: 20 to 400 mgs. per 100 grams of food.

Epilepsy: 450 mgs. daily, by mouth. (There are other nutrients, as indicated in discussion of nerve-muscle disorders, useful to the epileptic. Exclude from the diet: white sugar, caffeine, sodium, allergens, and excessive fluid intake. The hypoglycemia diet is used.)

ROYAL JELLY

Royal jelly is the special food that bees feed to queen bees. This remarkable substance is also responsible for converting ordinary larva into queen bees. It is probably the richest natural source of pantothenic acid yet discovered, and in the jelly is a factor that apparently makes the vitamin more effective. Some years ago British physicians discovered that the pantothenic acid levels in the blood of rheumatoid arthritics tend to be low. Since this vitamin is known to be important to the adrenal gland, the physicians tested its effects on rheumatoid arthritics. They found it to be significantly helpful, but its effectiveness was limited. No matter how much they raised the dose of pantothenic acid, the blood levels struck a plateau. In the effort to break through that ceiling, they administered royal jelly and discovered, to their satisfaction, that a factor in it does help the utilization of pantothenic acid. The rheumatoid arthritics responded with a rise in the vitamin blood-levels beyond the plateau and enjoyed proportionately greater benefits. It is interesting to note that the Arthritis Foundation has told the public that dietary factors bear no relationship to the cause of any type of arthritis and have no usefulness in its treatment. (High-potency Vitamin C, niacinamide, bioflavonoids, and Vitamin E, plus a low-carbohydrate diet are also used in rheumatoid arthritis.)

Royal jelly has also been used successfully in the treatment of leukemia in mice. And there *are* physicians who are treating leukemic human patients with royal jelly. I have heard occasional reports of helpfulness. All this information should encourage the Food and Drug Administration to reappraise its ill-considered contention that royal jelly is of interest only to bees. (See Chapter 10 for a discussion of the forms in which royal jelly is available.) Royal jelly is used in quantities of from 200 to 400 mgs. daily.

PANTOTHENIC ACID

Stress: Up to 10 grams of pantothenic acid in divided doses daily has been used.

Rheumatoid arthritis: Up to 750 mgs. daily, accompanied by supplements of 200 to 400 mgs. of royal jelly daily have been helpful, particularly when it is used as a supplement to the hypoglycemia type of diet — low in processed carbohydrate and high in protein and unsaturated fat.

Lupus erythematosus: 10,000 to 15,000 mgs. daily. (My own observation in research with Herman Goodman, M.D., indicated that this treatment is more effective for chronic discoid lupus erythematosus than for the more acute type. It is also more effective when accompanied by 600 mgs. to 2,000 mgs. of Vitamin E, and 300 mgs. of para aminobenzoic acid daily plus the entire Vitamin B complex.)

Scleroderma: See lupus erythematosus.

Dermatomyositis: See lupus erythematosus.

Hyperuricemia (elevated blood uric acid): It was reported years ago that generous supplements of pantothenic acid will reduce uric acid levels. I know of no later papers to confirm the report, which would be of great importance to sufferers with gout. Since the quantities of pantothenic acid used obviously extend over a wide range in various disorders, more research is needed in this area.

VITAMIN B_6

To reduce urea nitrogen: 200 mgs. daily.

Chorea: 10 to 60 mgs. daily.

Parkinson's disease: 10 to 100 mgs. daily.*

*Vitamin B_6 has an action antagonistic to L-Dopa, the medication that has been found helpful in some cases of Parkinson's disease. Therefore, ordinarily, the person who is being treated with the vitamin cannot be treated with the drug and vice versa. However, there is some evidence that L-Dopa can cause a Vitamin-B_6 deficiency, particularly if the diet is low in the vitamin. Therefore the physician administering the medication may wish to give small amounts of Vitamin B_6 in order to offset this possibility.

To reduce face oiliness in cases of acne: 100 mgs. daily.

To help the retention of nitrogen in the aged: up to 100 mgs. daily. The same amount, medical nutritionists have reported to me, may be helpful to the child who is not growing properly.

Sensitivity to sunshine: 1,000 mgs., in divided doses. (100 mgs. each hour for ten hours, the day before exposure.)

VITAMIN B_{12}

Canker sores: Vitamin B_{12} solution on a pledget of cotton, applied to the sore every three or four hours very often promotes very rapid healing. The injectible solution used has a potency of 1,000 micrograms per cc.

Bell's palsy: Vitamin B_{12} in high-potency injections, accompanied by the Vitamin B Complex (also injected), plus oral doses of the same vitamins accompanied by therapeutic amounts of Vitamin E (300 mgs. per day and up) have been useful adjuncts to physiotherapeutic measures in the treatment of Bell's palsy and trigeminal neuralgia.

VITAMIN A

To break a cold: 200,000 units daily for five days.

To compensate for the diabetic's inability to convert carotene into Vitamin A: 16,000 units daily.

Nephritis: 50,000 to 75,000 units daily.

Note: For those past fifty and for those whose utilization of fats is impaired, Vitamin A is more efficiently absorbed when it is taken in the emulsified or water-dispersible form. This is also true for all the fat-soluble vitamins — including Vitamins A, D, E, and K.

Postviral sinusitis, postnasal drip, clogging of eustachian tubes: See dosage for breaking colds.

BONE MEAL

Among dentists, there is almost complete agreement that decalcification of the jawbone cannot be reversed, and any competent dentist can trace the anatomical as well as biochemical reasons why repair of the process is impossible. Still, from time to time, I have received reports from dentists concerning individuals threatened with complete or partial loss of teeth as a result of weakening of the structures holding them, in whom decalcification of the jawbone has been reversed, with an increment of calcium deposition of as much as two millimeters in a period of a few months. This reversal was accompanied by parallel improvement in the condition of the gums. I do not propose to take a position in this debate, except to suggest that even improvement in the gum condition is a consummation devoutly to be wished. Use a gram of calcium from bone meal daily, divided into two or three daily doses. Accompany each dosage with two teaspoonful of lactose (milk sugar) dissolved in water. Also take high-potency Vitamin B Complex, multiple vitamins, Vitamin E, liver tablets, multiple minerals as supplements to the hypoglycemia diet. The diet is an important adjunct to the treatment.

VITAMIN B_2

Seborrheic dermatitis: 15 mgs. daily, plus 100 mgs. B_6.
Trichomoniasis: 6 mgs. daily.

VITAMIN C

To increase adrenal capacity for dealing with stress: 500 mgs. daily. Note: There are medical practitioners who have employed far larger amounts than this — up to the level of 4 or even 5 grams of the vitamin daily. (See pantothenic acid.)

To help increase the effectiveness of drugs: 300 to 800 mgs. daily. Note: This report deals primarily with the effectiveness of Vitamin C in increasing the action of diuretics (drugs that induce the body to part with water.) However, any attempt to take advantage of this action should be supervised by a physician competent in biochemistry, for there are instances when a reducing agent (this is one of the effects of Vitamin C) might alter the nature or the effectiveness of a drug.

Insect bites: When dangerous, patients have been protected at least partially by 4 grams of Vitamin C given every few hours.

Asthma: 1500 mgs. daily. (In personal research, I have learned that this must be balanced with sizable amounts of Vitamin A, particularly if the patient is a latent TB sufferer. Otherwise large doses of Vitamin C may activate latent tuberculosis. I have proposed large doses as a provocative test when the physician wishes to ascertain if the patient is in fact carrying a "sleeping" TB infection.)

Hay fever: 250 mgs. every four hours. (Dr. Wolfgang Seligman reported that his experience did not indicate that this amount was adequate for some hay fever sufferers, who needed three or four times as much.)

Hepatitis: 1000 to 2000 mgs. every three or four hours. (Please note that Vitamin B_{12} and other nutrients may be of equal importance.)*

Diuretic effect: 300 to 500 mgs. daily. Medical colleagues who have used Vitamin C for this purpose have advised me that the dosage may be inadequate — and should be given every three to four hours.

Ivy and poison oak dermatitis: Large doses of Vitamin C — 500 mgs. to 1 gram every four to six hours have been reported both to prevent or alleviate the poisonings and to diminish the severity of the itching and the dermatitis.

CHOLINE

To help reduce cholesterol: 2,000 mgs., plus 750 mgs. of inositol daily.

To help reduce intraocular pressure in glaucoma: 750 mgs. of pantothenic acid and 1,000 mgs. of choline, daily. (This is unreported research that I have personally observed. The action is that of increasing the synthesis of acetylcholine.)

Myasthenia gravis: See preceding note on glaucoma. High-potency Vitamin B complex containing a natural source, Vitamin E — 300 to 1,000 mgs. — plus concentrated wheat-germ oil have also been found helpful. (Personal observation.)

Gall-bladder syndrome: 1 gram of choline daily, accompanied by ½ gram of inositol, the entire natural Vitamin B complex, and a diet emphasizing vegetable fats rather than saturated fats, plus 2 or 3 tablespoons of lecithin daily have been observed by medical nutritionists to be a more rewarding approach to gall-bladder syndrome and fat intolerance then the usual regime.

---

*For years in various types of liver disorders including hepatitis, physicians have believed that a low fat, high carbohydrate, moderate protein intake is proper. There is now a great deal of evidence that this pattern of diet will retard recovery. High protein, a reasonable amount of fat — with 20 per cent of it in the unsaturated form — and lower carbohydrate intake will actually promote recovery faster. Nonfat milk is particularly useful in hepatitis, since it is a source not only of high quality protein, but of Vitamin B_{12}.

DRIED STOMACH AND COLON TISSUES

Colon and stomach tissues, dried under vacuum at very low temperatures, are both a source of protein and of unknown factors that may be helpful to individuals with peptic ulcer, colitis, or ulcerative colitis. There is really no stipulated quantity to be used, for the tissues are not medication as such, and usually the amounts employed are listed in tablespoonsful — perhaps two or three after each meal. Nonetheless, these simple supplements have brought about a remission in such serious disorders as ulcerative colitis in periods of as little as ten days.

VITAMIN E

Keloids: 1,200 mgs. of Vitamin E daily.

Dupuytren's contracture: 200 or 300 mgs. daily. (In my research with medical nutritionists, no dose under 300 mgs. was ever regarded as being therapeutic.)

Peyronie's disease: 200 or 300 mgs. daily.

To relieve symptoms of lack of oxygen: 600 mgs. daily.

Diabetes: 300 to 600 mgs. daily. (Note: This is not the only nutrient reported helpful to diabetics. Medical nutritionists have observed helpfulness from methionine, $\frac{1}{2}$ gram daily, and Vitamin B complex — with generous amounts of lipotropic factors, choline, and inositol, plus significant amounts of Vitamin B_6 and B_{12}.

Varicose ulcers: 400 mgs. daily. (It would seem reasonable that this dose would apply also to diabetic and stasis ulcers. In fact such reports have been rendered by some Canadian physicians.)*

Bright's disease: 300 to 600 mgs. daily.

Mongoloidism: 3000 mgs. daily. (Note: German medical research indicates that glutamic acid and B vitamins are also important to the mongoloid. My personal research indicates the usefulness of potent concentrates of wheat-germ oil.)

Menopause: 50 to 500 mgs. daily.

To reduce the likelihood of postoperative clots and phlebitis: 200 mgs. daily, after the operation. (Dr. Albert Ochsner's report indicates

---

*Vitamin A, riboflavin, Vitamin C, and the bioflavonoids are also important in healing. The amount of protein in the diet is critical — generous amounts result in faster healing, too. Likewise, there are reports that zinc — 200 mgs. daily — will promote faster healing even in young and healthy individuals. All these factors would be considered by the medical nutritionist who is treating ulcerations that ordinarily are slow in healing.

that calcium should be given with Vitamin E, and that the treatment should precede as well as follow surgery.)

Phlebitis: 300 mgs. daily.

Cystic fibrosis: 300 to 1500 mgs. daily. (Personal observation: The vitamin is certainly more useful to the child with cystic fibrosis if given in the water-dispersible form.)

FOLIC ACID

Sprue: 25 mgs. daily by injection.

LECITHIN

To reduce cholesterol: 4 to 6 tablespoons daily.

Diabetes: 3 tablespoons daily given with Vitamin E.

In psoriasis: 4 to 8 tablespoons daily.

In multiple sclerosis: 3 tablespoons or more daily. (As you have discovered elsewhere in this text, there are other nutrients useful in multiple sclerosis.)

NIACIN

Arthritis: it was reported many decades ago that megavitamin dosage of niacinamide has been helpful in a number of types of arthritis. Doses ranged as high as 5 grams daily or more.

Vincent's disease (trench mouth): 100 mgs. three times daily.

"Senile" pigmentation: 100 mgs. three times daily.

Schizophrenia: up to 20 grams or more daily; with Vitamin B_6, up to 1 gram daily; Vitamin C, up to 40 grams daily. Vitamin E has also been used — from 300 mgs. daily. Glutamic acid is sometimes employed — from 3 grams daily. Personal observation: The carbon-twenty fat of concentrated wheat-germ oil may be therapeutic when the schizophrenia has been released by brain damage caused by LSD.*

---

*It should be noted that tranquilizers, dilantin, other medications, and a hypoglycemia diet accompany the vitamin therapies when necessary. The authorities in this type of treatment emphasize that severely disturbed patients may require five years of such vitamin treatment, and there are those who will need it for a lifetime.

Hyperactive children (not in infancy): up to 3 grams daily; Vitamin C, up to 3 grams daily; Vitamin B₆, 100 mgs. daily; Vitamin E (personal observation), 300 mgs.; calcium, from 250 to 500 mgs.; and lecithin, 1 to 2 tablespoons daily have been helpful. The hypoglycemia diet is mandatory.

PABA

To increase tolerance to sunburn: 1,000 mgs. daily. (See Vitamin B₆.)
Vitiligo: 1,000 mgs. and up daily.*
To prevent graying of the hair: 300 mgs. daily, plus 100 mgs. of pantothenic acid, and a source of natural Vitamin B complex.
To promote fertility: 100 to 300 mgs. daily, with a natural B-complex source.

ZINC

To promote healing: 200 mgs. of zinc daily.
To help restore the senses of taste and smell: 100 mgs. daily.

It may puzzle you that the nutritional treatments just described as essentially free of toxicity and side reactions should nonetheless be administered by a medical man. However, you might expect such an admonition in a book devoted to individual differences in nutritional needs, for this thesis must recognize the possibility that your tolerance for high dosages of nutrients may likewise be unique. By way of example, though large amounts of Vitamin C have an antihistamine action, which is an antiallergy effect, there are people who manage to be allergic to Vitamin C, just as some people succeed in being allergic to antihistamine drugs. Such considerations make medical supervision of any therapy a sensible investment.

---

*When quantities of a gram a day or more of PABA are used, the physician will wish to check the bone marrow at intervals. The use of added supplements of the entire Vitamin B complex, Vitamin C, Vitamin E, and vacuum-dried liver will therefore be desirable, since these nutrients help protect the bone marrow. Other nutrients theoretically may help the recoloring of the skin or the hair.

APPENDIX 1

DIET PLAN: HYPOGLYCEMICS

BEFORE BREAKFAST: Use your blender or beater to mix 1 tsp. each of dry skim milk powder, mildly sweetened protein powder, primary food brewer's yeast powder, 4 tsp. of whole gelatin, 2 tsp. of glycerine in water, unsweetened fruit juice, or fluid skim milk. Add any flavoring (vanilla, for example) that pleases your palate. Never miss this supplement; it is a critical part of the dietetic procedure. If for any reason you must skip a meal or a snack as recommended by the diet, take a couple of ounces of this drink. It is only for emergencies; skipping scheduled food is not recommended.

BREAKFAST

Fruit or juice
1 egg
1 oz. meat or meat substitute, such as cheese or fish
½ slice whole-wheat bread with one teaspoon soft margarine
1 cup weak tea, sweetened artificially if desired

1 cup skim milk, flavored, if desired, with vanilla or other sugar-free natural flavor
1 oz. meat or meat substitute (see recipes)

LUNCH

3 oz. meat (cooked weight) or meat substitute
1 serving vegetables
1 slice bread with 1 tsp. margarine
Green salad with cottonseed oil or mayonnaise (1 tsp.)
Dessert from approved selection (see following recipes)
Weak tea or artificially sweetened soft drink
Note: A second vegetable may be selected from the list proposed as bread substitutes

AFTERNOON SNACK

2 oz. meat or meat substitute (see snack recipes)
½ cup skim milk, flavored if desired
½ slice bread with small amount margarine

DINNER

3 oz. meat or substitute
Vegetable
Green salad, cottonseed oil or mayonnaise dressing
1 serving approved fruit
Approved dessert
Tea (weak) or other approved beverage

EVENING SNACK

½ cup skim milk, flavored if desired
1 oz. meat or meat substitute (see recipes)

SUGGESTIONS FOR BETWEEN-MEAL SNACKS

These snacks are all high in protein, though it is possible, of course, to use up some of the allotted bread intake at these little meals. To keep low the amount of carbohydrates from bread, one can use brown-rice cakes, which are available in health-food stores. These weigh half as much as slices of bread, and, when prewarmed, are quite palatable, satiate the craving for carbohydrates (which will lessen as the low-sugar diet is followed) at the snacks, and provide a vehicle for the protein foods.

Note that snack portions are 1 ounce — for reducers.

COTTAGE CHEESE, a frequent choice of those on the hypoglycemia diet, can be made more palatable by adding chopped dill, chopped chives, chopped onion or scallion, shredded spinach, poppy seeds, caraway seeds, or horseradish.

HAM HORN: Press pot cheese through strainer. Add enough yogurt to make a soft paste and a little chopped dill pickle. Roll this in a paper-thin piece of ham, securing it with a toothpick to make a small horn.

TONGUE-CHEESE HORN: Fill paper-thin tongue slice, rolled into horn shape, with Neufchâtel cheese.

DOUGHLESS PIZZA:
½ lb. lean beef
¼ small can tomato paste
2 fresh tomatoes
1 medium onion
1 pinch pepper
⅛ tsp. each of sweet basil, oregano, paprika

Pepper meat and knead. Line small Pyrex dish with meat as substitute for pizza shell. Chop tomatoes with onions and mix with tomato paste and spices. Fill meat shell with mixture. Add a touch of oregano on top and bake to preferred doneness at 350°.

TUNA IN CUCUMBER: Hollow out ½ cucumber, stuff with 1 oz. tuna fish mixed with 1 tsp. mayonnaise.

CHEESE FOR SNACKS: These should not be restricted in variety. Use Brie, American, cheddar, pot, farmer, cottage, and be wary only of cheese *spreads*, for these may be diluted with cornstarch or other carbohydrates. Gouda, Swiss, and processed cheeses (Velveeta and others of this type) are all good choices. The cheese, for variety, may be combined with another protein: Ham as a blanket for a piece of Gouda is delightful, and good nutrition, too.

CELERY STICK AND POT CHEESE (1 oz.): Press cheese through strainer. Moisten it with a small amount of yogurt, buttermilk, or skim milk.

Flavor it with chopped green pepper, watercress, parsley, or pimiento, chopped fine. Fill celery stick with mixture.

SNACK BEVERAGE: Take ½ cup plain yogurt (fruit varieties contain an unbelievable amount of sugar) and fizz it in tall glass with carbonated water (club soda) or carbonated mineral water.

STUFFED EGG SNACK: Mash hard-cooked yolks of 3 eggs until fine and crumbly. Add 1 oz. melted margarine, ⅛ tsp. salt, dash pepper, ⅛ tsp. prepared mustard, ½ tsp. minced onion, 1/6 cup flaked tuna, cut-up shrimp, or crabmeat. Mix until smooth, and fill hollows in egg whites, garnishing with slices of olive, pimiento, or parsley. Yields 6 stuffed-egg halves. Reducers should eat only one.

SNACK DESSERT AND BEVERAGE: Pour a little low-calorie ginger ale over 2 tbs. of nonfat milk powder. Use rest of soda as beverage.

CHEESE-APPLE SNACK: Combine a wedge of Gruyère cheese with ½ small apple.

CHICKEN SNACK: Spread 1 oz. of commercial chicken-spread on thin whole-wheat cracker.

KOSHER SNACK: Broiled beef fry — 1 oz. of beef (smoked beef plate, used instead of bacon in orthodox Jewish diet). Beverage: V-8 vegetable juice cocktail or equivalent.

YOGURT SNACK: Plain yogurt (4 oz.), with vanilla or almond extract to taste.

COLESLAW SNACK: 1 oz. sliced meat, such as roast beef or tongue, rolled and filled with coleslaw.

SHRIMP SNACK: Commercial frozen shrimp cocktail (1 oz. portion for reducers) is a convenient snack food, very rich in protein. So are canned smoked oysters.

MUSHROOM SNACK: Stuffed mushrooms (2 oz.) filled (topped) with paste made from pot cheese, curry powder, and salt or salt substitute.

PEAR SNACK: Partially scoop out small pear and fill with 1 oz. soft Camembert cheese.

HAMBURGER: 1 oz. ground chuck, with a touch of garlic, 1 tsp. tomato juice, and a dash of tarragon. Broil.

Use as you please, within reasonable bounds:
    Salt substitute

Sugar substitutes (saccharin) — except during first five months of pregnancy

Clear broth (not bouillon cubes)

Unsweetened whole gelatin

Artificially sweetened gelatin

Lemon

Vinegar

All spices, save celery salt and garlic salt

All herbs

Sugar-free soft drinks (not cola types) — not more than 8 oz. daily

Coffee free of caffeine (Sanka, Decaf)

Desserts from approved ones mentioned later.

Avoid like the plague:

Butter

Sugar-sweetened soft drinks

Sugar-sweetened juices, canned, and frozen fruits

Vegetables packed in sugar-sweetened liquid or sauce (You must read labels carefully!)

Sugar (regardless of its color)

Molasses

Honey

Cookies, cakes, crackers, pretzels, popcorn, potato chips, and all starch-sugar snack foods

Recommended vegetables and fruits follow:

FRUITS	AMOUNT IN ONE SERVING
Apple	1 small (2-inch diameter)
Applesauce	½ cup (no added sugar)
Apricots, fresh	2 medium
Apricots, dried	4 halves
Banana	½ small
Blackberries	1 cup
Blueberries	2/3 cup
Cantaloupe	¼ (6-inch diameter)
Cherries	10 large
Cranberries	1 cup
Dates	2
Figs, fresh	2 large
Figs, dried	1 small
Grapefruit	½ small

LOW BLOOD SUGAR

Grapefruit juice	½ cup
Grapes	12 large
Grape juice	¼ cup
Honeydew Melon	⅛ medium
Mango	1 small
Nectarine	1 medium
Orange	1 small
Orange juice	½ cup
Papaya	⅓ medium
Peach	1 medium
Pear	1 small
Persimmon	½ small
Pineapple	½ cup
Pineapple juice	⅓ cup
Plums	2 medium
Prunes, dried	2 medium
Raspberries	1 cup
Rhubarb	1 cup
Strawberries	1 cup
Tangerine	1 cup
Watermelon	1 cup

Be warned that frozen fruits often yield more calories from sugar than from the fruit itself. Avoid canned fruits packed in syrup, whether light or heavy syrup. Choose the water-packed or artificially sweetened variety.

You *must* consume at least *two* cups of vegetables daily, and you can have as much as *four* cups of vegetables daily, chosen from the following list:

Asparagus	Beet Greens
Avocado	Chard
Broccoli	Collards
Brussels Sprouts	Dandelion
Cabbage	Endive
Celery	Kohlrabi
Chicory	Leeks
Cucumbers	Kale
Escarole	Mustard
Eggplant	Spinach
Green Pepper	Turnip Greens

Lettuce	Green or Wax Beans
Mushrooms	Tomatoes
Radishes	Tomato Juice
Sauerkraut	Summer Squash
String Beans	Watercress

Remember that the frequency of eating is as important as the composition of the meals. Do eat six times daily. If at work, protein tablets or foil-wrapped cheese wedges will bridge emergencies when recommended foods are not available.

If you are overweight, the margarine and salad oil recommended in this diet are absolutely essential for a low carbohydrate diet like this one to cause weight loss. In addition, such fats help better control the blood cholesterol.

Glycerine is recommended in the prebreakfast drink, because it is converted into sugar in the body. The conversion is so slow that it does not stimulate the excessive insulin production that is the principal cause of low blood sugar.

While no one vegetable should be overeaten, avocado may receive more emphasis in the diet. This vegetable contains a type of sugar that actually depresses insulin production. Avocado is also rich in unsaturated fat, helpful as noted above to those who are trying to control weight.

APPENDIX 2

DIET AND THE PERIOD

The diet that normalizes the premenstrual week and helps control menstrual discomfort is the same diet that protects your complexion, helps your muscle function, stimulates your energy — to put it briefly, the diet for normal and short menstruals is the diet to help avoid cystic mastitis and to promote good health.

We wish to raise your intake of protein, vitamins, minerals, and unsaturated fats; we wish to lower your intake of starches and sugars; and we must change the form in which you are now consuming these carbohydrates — from overprocessed to whole grain. The less sugar you take, the better, and this applies to sugar in any form. There is no variety that is good food, and no variety that does not cause abnormalities in the body's regulation of carbohydrate.

A quick way to give you a perspective on the proper kind of menu is to refer you to the diet plan for hypoglycemics — appendix pages 271–77. If you are not troubled by low blood sugar, such a menu outline will still prove profitable. You may not need the *severe* restriction on sugar and starch that the hypoglycemic must observe, but you'll benefit by eating frequent small meals, which generally make weight control easier, too.

The protein in your meals should always include just one from an animal source: meat, fish, fowl, milk and dairy products other than cream — including cheese, and eggs. Remember that cold cuts and frankfurters are lower in protein value, frequently inferior in protein quality, and often an unsuspected vehicle for corn syrup and other inexpensive sweets. And do not forget that the word "healthy" means "whole." Healthful nutrition is whole nutrition. In addition to steaks, chops, and roasts, buy organ meats. Not only is their protein of higher efficiency, but they are rich sources of the B vitamins that you need to help you keep the mischief of estrogenic hormones at a minimum.

Do not accept cheese spread as equivalent to cheese in protein value; it usually isn't. Do accept all animal proteins as approximately equivalent nutritionally. Fish is not inferior to meat, nor chicken to eggs in terms of a good diet.

When you shape your recipes to your budget, do not make the error of diluting protein with carbohydrate "to save money." It is false economy. Macaroni and cheese may be monetarily cheaper than meat, but actually it becomes more costly if the starch of noodles is being substituted for the needed protein of added cheese. The hamburger extenders based on bread crumbs give only an illusion of economy, for bread is no substitute for meat. If you must stretch ground meat, add wheat germ and soy. These extend without diluting; they are economical and rich in protein.

Concentrated nonfat milk diluted only ½ or ⅔ as much as the label suggests is a fine, inexpensive supplementary source of high-quality protein. Incidentally, if you wish to lower protein costs, serve nonfat milk instead of whole milk, and for each quart of the fat-free milk used, serve 1½ oz. of butter or margarine. This gives you the equivalent of whole milk at a fraction of the cost.

Don't overcook protein foods. This tendency has had an impact — particularly on women — that is so common, it is mistaken for normalcy. (It may result in the "constitutionally inadequate woman.")

There is no difference between brown eggs and white. There *is* a difference between firm and soft cheeses; the former are better sources of protein and, usually, calcium. Among the milk products, yogurt carries singular value because of its friendly bacteria. But do not buy yogurt messed up with added fruit, jam, preserves, vanilla or whatever — it may contain as much as six teaspoons of sugar per container. Buy plain yogurt, or make your own and add fresh fruit.

The carbohydrates should be bought in the form of whole grains. You will then be avoiding the frozen pies and the packaged cookies, much to your benefit. It also directs you toward home baking, with the same dividend. If you cannot tolerate whole grains, you may be able to tolerate wheat-germ enriched recipes made with unbleached flour. Wheat germ may also be added to breakfast cereals to improve their protein, Vitamin-B-Complex, Vitamin-E, and unsaturated fat values.

If you cannot bear even the wheat-germ-reinforced recipes, all is not lost. There remain the supplements — multiple vitamins, multiple minerals, and Vitamin B Complex. Sometimes, when the level of estrogen activity is very high or when we are coping with an aggravated problem such as cystic mastitis, it is necessary to use B-Complex supplements free of PABA and folic acid, for these, I have already noted, increase estrogen effectiveness. In such instances, we may also add supplements of lecithin and desiccated liver.

Let me make it clear that the use of these supplements is not solely as compensation for lack of whole grains and organ meats in the diet. To properly control the menstrual cycle and other aspects of the chemistry of estrogens, it is advisable to raise the intake of vitamins — in some cases, so high that no woman, however active, could satisfy these needs from food alone. In other words, trying to eat your way toward such a vitamin intake would only create obesity, which can and does distort hormone metabolism.

If you do not have the facilities or the time for between-meal high-protein snacks recommended in the hypoglycemia type of diet, protein supplements can be used. These are available in powder and tablet form. Choose one that supplies high-quality (animal) proteins of several types.

The disturbed menstrual cycle will not necessarily yield to either dietary persuasion or to supplements in a month or two; both are usually required. If you are patient for a few months, the dividends should begin to show. You will also run the risk of saying farewell to the collection of minor disorders that the average American woman credulously calls "good health." And you will be left with virtually nothing to discuss between speeches at your club meetings — but then, we always pay a price for gains.

APPENDIX 3

CORNELL BREAD FORMULA

For each cup of flour, place in the measuring cup 1 tbs. each of soy flour and nonfat dry milk powder, plus 1 tsp. of wheat germ. Fill the remainder of the cup with unbleached flour. The formula works well with any recipe that calls for white flour. Use about 6 cups of well-stirred and sifted mix in the recipe below.

Recipe for Cornell Mix

Measure 3 cups of warm water (85°F) into a large bowl. Add 2 tbs. of dry yeast granules (or 2 packets of yeast, or 2 squares of yeast) and 2 tbs. of honey. Stir and allow the mixture to stand for five minutes.

By now the yeast mixture should be frothy. Stir into it 1 tbs. of sea salt. Add half of the flour mixture. Beat it vigorously, using about seventy-five strokes by hand or beat for two minutes if you are using an electric mixer.

Add 2 tbs. of vegetable oil and the remainder of the flour mixture. Blend all of the ingredients thoroughly and turn the dough out onto a floured board. Have additional flour handy. Knead vigorously for about five minutes until the dough is smooth and elastic. Place it in an oiled bowl, oil the top of the dough lightly, and cover the bowl. Put it in a warm place (80°F–85°F) until it is nearly double in size. This will take about forty-five minutes.

Punch down the dough, fold over the edges, and turn it upside down in the bowl to rise another twenty minutes.

Turn the dough onto the board and divide it into three portions. Fold each one inward and form smooth, tight balls. Cover them with a clean cloth and allow them to rest ten minutes.

Shape into three loaves, or two loaves and a pan of rolls. Place in buttered tins (about 3½ × 7½ inches). Allow the dough to rise in the tins until it is doubled in bulk, about forty-five minutes. Bake in a preheated moderate oven (350°F) for about fifty minutes. If the loaves begin to turn brown in fifteen to twenty minutes, reduce the temperature to 325°F.

Remove the finished breads or rolls from the pans and cool them on racks. If desired, brush the tops with melted butter.

APPENDIX 4

TESTIMONY OF DR. FREDERICKS

A former commissioner of the Food and Drug Administration — once he was out of office — remarked that what bugged him most during his term of office was the popular belief that the Food and Drug Administration protects the public. What he was saying has been obvious to consumer groups and nutritionists for more than thirty years. The Food and Drug Administration, like the Better Business Bureau, protects business. Indeed, many Food and Drug Administration executives ultimately are employed by the industries they have policed.

Only if the Food and Drug Administration has appointed itself as the protector of cyclamates rather than the public and as a haven for toxic and carcinogenic dyes rather than the defender of your family's nutrition, do its policies seem logical. Those who buy health foods and vitamin supplements are obviously disenchanted with the merits of the American food establishment. On those grounds, the Food and Drug Administration has relentlessly persecuted not only those they label as crackpots, but physicians, dentists, reputable professors, biochemists, and anyone else whose nutritional advice to the public implies or states the heresy of criticism of cornflakes, white bread, or white sugar. Users of vitamin supplements are excommunicated as are those whose instruction in nutrition implies the need for use of such supplements. On the hapless head of such a rebel descends enormous pressure from a high-powered propaganda machine. Exactly how the machine operates, and what techniques are used to excommunicate anyone who does not believe that the American diet is perfect will be illustrated by my experience with it.

The treatment I received from the Food and Drug Administration was not extraordinary — yet Senator Edward Long, Head of the Senate Subcommittee on Government Invasions of Privacy, pointed to it as a striking example of profound misbehavior by a government bureau ostensibly charged with protecting the public.

My sworn testimony before that committee tells the story very succinctly. What follows is a transcript of my remarks, as they appeared in the records of that committee, under questioning by the committee and its counsel, Mr. Fensterwald.

TESTIMONY OF DR. CARLTON FREDERICKS, NUTRITIONIST, NEW YORK CITY

Mr. FENSTERWALD. Before you begin, Doctor, would you give us just a brief history of your background for the record?

Dr. FREDERICKS. Yes, sir.

I was educated in New York City through high school where I was a member of a class for gifted children — this is immodest, but I think it is relevant to some of the history that I am going to give you and I won an award from the Bossom Foundation for citizenship.

I attended the University of Alabama where I took a B.A. and had a fellowship in the Department of English and was a Phi Beta Kappa.

I took an M.A. in Public Health Education at New York University, 1948 to 1949. I completed a Ph.D. in Public Health Education in 1955.

Mr. FENSTERWALD. What universities?

Dr. FREDERICKS. At New York University in the same school of education.

I taught nutrition at New York University, at the adult extension divisions of CCNY and Brooklyn College, and as an associate professor at Fairleigh Dickinson University in New Jersey.

I have been a worker in the field of nutrition since approximately 1938. I was associated with the staff of the U.S. Vitamin Corp., the scientific staff of which was directed by Dr. Casimir Funk who was the originator of the term "vitamin." I was director of professional and lay education, charged with the responsibility for delivering lectures before nurses, physicians, osteopathic groups, dentists, and the like.

I was also charged with the responsibility for writing the technical booklets which went out to the physicians, that being a firm which advertises only to the medical profession and dental profession.

I became a broadcaster on the subject of nutrition as part of the broad field of public health education on station WMCA in New York. My broadcasts were extended to WJZ and the Blue Network from coast to coast which presented the program unsponsored as a public service in wartime. The program was used for official releases of the OPA and Government agencies which would reach the public.

I subsequently broadcast for 12 years on station WMGM in New York and since that time I have been on WOR New York and during this period my programs were carried on between 200 and 300 radio stations, not only in the United States but often the world at large by shortwave. I have also appeared in television.

I had a column on nutrition in the New York Mirror and other newspapers.

I am the author of a half dozen books, the gross sales of which run into some millions of copies. I am editor of a monthly publication, Health and Nutrition News which goes out by subscription.

This background should be, I think, prefaced with one or two details concerning the nature of radio broadcasts because this is an aspect of the testimony which I have come to give.

These radio programs on the air in 1941 were organized in the form of a radio nutrition class which was attended by many, and it was intended to be a program aiding the wartime effort by guiding the American housewife to good nutrition in the presence of wartime scarcities and rationing. The scripts of those radio classes in nutrition were gathered together as a textbook and that textbook was translated into braille by the Library of Congress. The book was used as a medium of instruction by the health education units of various elementary and high schools, particularly in the New York area. The program was the occasion for an award from the Eloy Alfaro Foundation for public service in radio education, this being an award that had gone to three Presidents; and to Senator Smathers of Florida, who was kind enough to record my receipt of it in the Congressional Record.

I received an honorary degree from the Canadian Institution for the same reason — a Canadian college.

With this background I should like to say that while I have no prepared statement I do wish the liberty of making a suggestion to the committee, which I should like to do at the termination of my testimony, concerning possible legislation, with the full understanding that I am not an attorney and that my suggestions arise merely from a very deep and thorough understanding of the manner in which the U.S. Food and Drug Administration has abused the tremendous powers which have been bestowed upon it by Congress. . . .

Within the history I have just given there are two omissions which are relevant.

When I was graduated from the University of Alabama with a B.A. degree I had 1 year of general chemistry in my background. Because of the exigencies of trying to find employment in the depression years, 1931, I found myself to my astonishment working as a chemist. Because of certain experiences which I had with the pharmaceutical companies by whom I was employed during some years of working as a chemist I became interested in nutrition and cast about for a means of obtaining an academic education in it. I discovered, however, that such education was available only under the aegis of the home economics departments of the university and I was not particularly amenable to taking up sewing and a few other things in order to learn nutrition. So I decided to associate myself with the pharmaceutical companies who were specializing in nutrition — nutritional research — because this was another way of becoming educated.

At the time I came to New York University to take a Ph.D. I wanted to take my Ph.D. in nutrition. The professor who interviewed me was Prof. Morey Fields, who said that he had heard my broadcasts on nutrition — I have been in broadcasting for over 7 years, and he had read my book on nutrition, this being the one that I had referred to previously which was translated into braille by the Library of Congress, and I am trying to quote him — the level at which I was working in the field of nutrition was above the level of any courses in nutrition which were available in his department.

He therefore suggested two things: that I should not take any courses in nutrition because he said that I would either fall asleep in the classroom or quarrel with the professors; and that neither was a judicious policy for a Ph.D. candidate, and second, he suggested that since I was working at a level above their courses, that I should teach a course in nutrition at N.Y.U., which I did.

In 1949 the question of the bread standards was being taken up by the U.S. Food and Drug Administration. These standards which have been a matter that has preoccupied me for many years, not only as a private citizen, but professionally, because it has been my observation that a standard which is, after all, nothing more than a definition, accomplishes several things which go beyond the ostensible purpose.

A standard is a definition that may become a ceiling rather than a floor under the value of the product. This is to say very simply that the ostensible purpose of the standard is to define a food so that transgressors may be identified. You cannot define a violation unless you have a norm, and the norm is the standard. But the tendency of the standard is often to inflict a level of mediocrity and the manufacturer says, "What is the use of making my food better, the Government has defined what is good?" Therefore, when the bread standards were being discussed somewhere around 1949 I called somebody — I don't remember the name of the man who spoke to me in Senator Paul Douglas' office, because I wished to get the Senator's reaction. I know he had voiced one to the bread standard, as it was proposed by the Food and Drug Administration.

I was informed that the Senator made a speech and that there was something in the Congressional Record on this, which I obtained. The Senator had said that the proposed bread standard represented as protecting the public was doing so with "reverse English." Instead it was protecting the inferior product from the competition of the superior one.

I repeated Senator Douglas' comment on the air in five States. The next day the New York Times carried a release by the U.S. Food and Drug Administration announcing that food faddists had a terrible hold on the American population and that this was a problem which must be cleaned up immediately. This was the beginning of a relentless, unmitigated, uninterrupted effort by the U.S. Food and Drug Administration to silence my radio broadcasts, by the use of every device, legal, or tangentially illegal that has occurred to the mind, the fertile mind behind the mimeograph machines in that department.

After the New York Times article appeared the Food and Drug Administration issued a letter to the public stating that I was, naming me, specifically — misinforming the public. What was the misinformation? Actually, it consisted of my repeating what Senator Paul Douglas had said.

Second, there were vague allegations of my having some commercial or financial interest in the outcome of this, which was untrue. I had no financial interest whatsoever.

The FDA represented to the public that the proposed bread standard would not limit the amount of nutrition in a loaf of white bread which I said it did. This technically was true, but if you made a loaf of bread more nutritious than the standard you couldn't call it white bread; and the public could not understand why this was a very severe deterrent to the sale of the product. So I went on the air and pointed out that when Mrs. John Public comes in a grocery store and she is a white bread eater and she wants white bread she is not going to accept something called health bread, she is not going to accept something called protein bread or vitamin bread or whatever. She is going to look for the name she is familiar with. So that this ruling was tantamount to blocking or impeding the sale of the nutritionally improved products, which is exactly what Senator Douglas and I had said.

Well, I couldn't bring it home to the public until the same move was made on the spaghetti standard. Then I was able to cite a case where the Administration had said, the Food and Drug Administration, to a spaghetti manufacturer, you can make spaghetti more nutritious than the standard, but you can't call it spaghetti.

So I went to the public and said, now, you tell me how do you sell spaghetti when you can't call it spaghetti? What do you call it? And at that point the analogy came home.

A couple of weeks after these things occurred two things happened. We are still around 1949–50. A Federal judge asked an attorney for the Food and Drug Administration in a case involving a standard on a food, why do you people inflict these standards on an industry? Why don't you just require that they list on the label their full ingredients and let the public make its own decision in the market place, which incidentally is what Senator Douglas had said and what I had said.

The response of the Food and Drug attorney broken down from the legal language was that the public is essentially too stupid to read a label. I went on the air and quoted the attorney and formed an organization called, "Idiots of the World, Unite."

Two days after a Food and Drug Administration agent appeared at New York University and told a professor in the school of education that the U.S. Food and Drug Administration took a very dim view of my fitness as a candidate for a Ph.D. degree.

Senator LONG. Do you know the name of this person?

Dr. FREDERICKS. Dr. J. B. Nash who was dean of the school of education.

Senator LONG. Do you know the inspector's name?

Dr. FREDERICKS. I don't know the inspector's name because I wasn't personally in contact with it.

Senator LONG. Is there any written record of it, Doctor?

Dr. FREDERICKS. There must be in the university files, because it became a cause celebre. It held up my degree 5 years. I had completed my work.

If I may explain, when you take a Ph.D. degree you are required to submit an outline of your proposed research. That outline goes to an outlines committee which then sends it back to you, usually torn to pieces, and you reassemble it in accordance with their recommendations.

Senator LONG. This is New York University?

Dr. FREDERICKS. Yes. My outline went in in 1949, but after the visit of the FDA men I couldn't get it back. It came back to me in 1954 with not a mark on it, not an amendment, not a change indicating that it had been perfectly satisfactory, had been held in a status quo, in effect, I think that it was returned to me only because the university attorneys warned the faculty that there was no legal ground for withholding my right to pursue the degree and that if I were to invoke the Civil Liberties Union or some similar agency or an attorney, that they thought the university would be in an indefensible position to justify what they had done. So at this moment I would say in addition to Dr. J. B. Nash, the entire graduate faculty of the university must have been very well aware of what was going on, and in fact I know this to be so because a number of them spoke to me.

Step No. 2——

Mr. FENSTERWALD. Did you get your degree?

Dr. FREDERICKS. Yes, sir. When the outline was returned I had already written my thesis which I had no right to do, but I just didn't want to waste time, so one year later I received a Ph.D. degree.

Now, I mentioned before — I must backtrack briefly one other event which is significant.

When I came to radio I was totally unaware of the possibility of this medium for evoking the hostility, not only in Government agencies, but in others. And since I am forthright I invoked hostility. One of the hostilities I encountered was one which I think Senator Javits would be familiar with in his previous role — I believe he was commissioner of the State department of education in New York in his previous history — and that that came under that department's aegis.

In 1945, two agents provocateur came to my radio office — I ordinarily saw no people privately in my office. Both of them presented me with a long history of serious symptoms, and both were asking for nutritional treatments. I responded that the symptoms they were describing could be those of a very serious disease and I gave both of them a written reference to a diagnostician.

They asked me whether they could take some vitamin supplement and I said anybody could take a vitamin supplement, but with the symptoms they presented I thought rather than vitamin supplements they should see a doctor and if not the doctor I recommended, to see somebody.

They left my office and I found myself 3 weeks later charged with the unlawful practice of medicine. Specifically, it was recommending vitamin supplements which can be purchased over the counter in any drugstore.

Senator LONG. Who brought that charge?

Dr. FREDERICKS. The State department of education in New York. There was evidence that the county medical society felt that the remarks in broadcasts were tangential to their field, and this they felt involved a trespassing.

Well, nonetheless, to come back, my Ph.D. degree was awarded after this event and since the Ph.D. is a certification of character it is somewhat relevant to this history that the FDA, in thousands of letters to the public and in releases to the public, has described me as a criminal.

Mr. FENSTERWALD. They are still trying your case in the newspapers?

Dr. FREDERICKS. There is never an end to the case. This is one feature that is pertinent. I have never been the target for any legal charge which would allow me to go into a courtroom and define myself.

Mr. FENSTERWALD. Under what authority did they issue these press releases about you?

Dr. FREDERICKS. They do this by tangential devices which I would like to describe because I think I was the person upon whom they perfected this.

In 1950 they were circulating, through the entire country, press releases which were picked up by major newspapers, by labor newspapers, union newspapers, journals published by county medical societies, dental journals, a description of me as a food faddist, cultist, crackpot, dispenser of nutritional nonsense.

Senator LONG. This is the FDA?

Dr. FREDERICKS. Yes, sir.

Senator LONG. Do you have copies of those releases?

Dr. FREDERICKS. I have some in my files. I only managed to get hold of those which were sent to me by indignant listeners. I should mention also that the tide has gone in the other direction.

Senator LONG. Do you have copies that our committee could have?

Dr. FREDERICKS. Yes, sir; I will bring you as many as I can.

(The information referred to follows:)

EXHIBIT A

U.S. DEPARTMENT OF HEALTH, EDUCATION, AND WELFARE,
FOOD AND DRUG ADMINSTRATION,
Washington, D.C., November 25, 1961.

A health food dealer's use of a diet book called "Eat, Live, and Be Merry," has brought about seizure of 43 copies of the volume on charges that the Federal law prohibiting false labeling of foods and drugs was being violated, the Food and Drug Administration said today.

Author of the book is Carlton Fredericks, according to documents filed in the Federal district court at Peoria, Ill. The action challenges use of the book along with other printed matter to make false claims of the medical value of vitamins and mineral food supplements.

FDA emphasized that books as such are not subject to the Federal Food, Drug, and Cosmetic Act unless they are used as labeling material for products covered by the law. FDA said that the Fredericks book recommends and suggests treatment of numerous serious ailments with vitamin and mineral supplements, which products are not effective in treating such conditions. The products seized contain the ingredients so recommended by the Fredericks book.

Fredericks has a daily radio program on nutrition and other subjects that is carried by many stations. He is listed on the front cover of his book as "America's foremost nutritionist." This is one of the statements the Government charged to be false and misleading. FDA said its investigations show that Fredericks has no formal training or educational qualifications as a nutritionist. He has a doctor of philosophy degree in the field of health education and recreation.

The products and literature, with a total value of approximately $1,000, were seized at the Century Food Co., Varna, Ill.

Products alleged to be misbranded by the Fredericks book, and seized with the books, were "Toddler's vitamin and mineral supplement for children," "Vita-Glo food supplement," "Nutra-Glo food supplement" and "Century Brewer's yeast tablets." Also seized as misbranded by the other labeling material were "Century natural pure dehydrated cabbage tablets."

The seizure proceedings charge that the Fredericks paperback book "contains statements which represent and suggest that the articles seized are adequate and effective for the treatment and prevention of diseases of the liver and gall bladder, peptic ulcer, diarrheal diseases, intestinal tuberculosis, mental disorders, heart failure, pulmonary disease, diabetes mellitus, chronic alcoholism, loss of protein in myelitis and nephrosis, rheumatoid arthritis, arthritis, rheumatic fever, rheumatic heart disease, cancer, leukemia, cystic mastitis, kidney disease, and for other purposes; which statements are false and misleading, since the articles are not adequate and effective for such diseases, conditions, and purposes * * *."

The Government also charged "that the labeling of said articles, namely, the paperback book entitled 'Eat, Live, and Be Merry,' by Carlton Fredericks, accompanying said articles contains statements which represent and suggest that Carlton Fredericks is 'America's foremost nutritionist'; and that the book furnishes scientifically proven nutritional and medical guidance for the supplemental use of vitamins and minerals by individuals generally in the treatment and prevention of serious diseases; which statements are false and misleading, since they are contrary to fact."

Dr. FREDERICKS. At the time when I suggested that this "stupid" public should unite, I understand that the Food and Drug Administration received many, many thousands of protesting letters from the public as a result of which the bread standard was relaxed and it became permissible for the bread industry to restore to bread a nutrient which is taken out in the processing of the bread or flour ordinarily, without going to jail for it or without being cited for misbranding, which I thought was something of an advance. But also they never forgave me for it.

Senator LONG. I am glad you educated them to that extent.

Dr. FREDERICKS. From 1950 to 1955 this was the sequence. There were thousands of letters to the public. There were many releases in the newspapers pursuing this vein, denouncing me as a crackpot, cultist, food faddist and dispenser of nutritional nonsense in which I joined a distinguished list of scientists in this country.

There are many scientists long known for their contributions to science and nutrition who have been so listed by the Food and Drug Administration which is an act which I question the propriety of to begin with.

The second thing that happened was, that station WMGM in New York on which I was then broadcasting received a letter from the Federal Communications Commission which must be in the station's files. It wasn't sent to me. It was addressed to Mr. Bertram Lebhar, Jr., who was then the manager of the station, saying, we understand from another Government agency that you have on the air a broadcaster of dubious reputation. We should like to have you remember that the matters like these are taken into consideration when the time comes for a renewal of your broadcasting license.

The letter then referred to me specifically. The station wrote to the FCC, pointing out that the scripts of my broadcast had been translated into braille by the Library of Congress, and they felt sure that the FCC had received some misinformation from another Government agency, and we heard no more about the matter at that time.

(The following letter was subsequently received:)

THE LIBRARY OF CONGRESS,
DIVISION OF BOOKS FOR THE ADULT BLIND,
Washington, D.C., July 26, 1946.

INSTITUTE OF NUTRITION RESEARCH, INC.,
New York, N.Y.

GENTLEMEN: Under our program in the Braille Transcribing Section of this Division, it is planned to have single copies of the book, "Living Should Be Fun," by Carlton Fredericks, hand transcribed for the use of blind readers. Your permission as copyright holder is requested before this work is undertaken.

All of this work is done by specially trained volunteer braillists, and when these books are completed they are generally placed in one of our various distributing libraries for the blind. Any books so produced will, of course, carry the proper copyright notice.

Trusting this request will meet with your favorable consideration and looking forward to an early reply in the matter, I am

Sincerely yours,

XENOPHON P. SMITH,
Director, Division of Books for the Adult Blind.

(NOTE. — This is text described by FDA as incompetent; as offering a diet for clubfoot and cancer. C.F.)

Dr. FREDERICKS. We then received visits from inspectors from the Federal Trade Commission, one of whom came into my office, barraged me with a long list of questions which I was perfectly willing to answer, although I didn't understand how the activities of a broadcaster fell within the province of a Federal Trade Commission representative since I wasn't engaged in manufacturing products nor in business for myself. I went down to Washington and I saw Senator James Mead who is Chairman of that agency and in effect, since I had known Senator Mead a long time, I suggested that he call his boys off, and they were called off.

The campaign then flagged for a while until 1957 when I began to add to the list of stations which were carrying my broadcasts. At this point I was discussing on the air a number of causes which I described as being unpopular in one sense or another, and I was delivering aspects or perspectives on these causes which brought to the public, let us say, the nay side of a yea which they might not have otherwise received.

Quite suddenly, the U.S. Food and Drug Administration seized the merchandise of a small vitamin company in Illinois, a vitamin company whose existence I never knew of and alleged that they found on the premises 12 copies of one of my books and alleged further, which the company denied, that these books were being used to persuade customers to buy the products of the company and thereby that the books were part of the labeling.

Press releases went out immediately describing this seizure — press releases from the FDA, but it is noteworthy that there was one paragraph on the company and two to three pages on Dr. Fredericks, with my full history and a description of me as a character with a criminal record and some other allegations, including incompetency with which I will deal later.

These releases were picked up by newspapers from coast to coast and seriously affected my broadcasting career since I was a national broadcaster.

This doctrine of seizing books is one which I have spoken about on the air. I have pointed out that this thesis, which was sustained by the courts in earlier decisions, which later were reversed very fortunately for the book-reading public, this doctrine had been set up on the premise that when a health food store or drugstore or department store sales clerk holds up a book to a customer, reads a paragraph in it which applies to a product, if not by brand name, then by type, that the book becomes part of the labeling of the product and I should say if the two are used simultaneously in that way the doctrine must have seemed to the courts to have been reasonably fair and they sustained it.

However, a fair doctrine in the hands of an unfair agency is quite another matter. Because it puts in the hands of the agency a weapon by which they can attack any critic who happens to have committed the sin of writing a book. As a matter of fact, in the decision in the appellate court in which this doctrine was reversed recently, the court pointed out that the U.S. Food and Drug Administration has the power to seize the Bible, because the Bible recommends honey and moreover recommends it therapeutically. So if the Bible were displayed in a store window along with a jar of honey, the Bible could be seized without the protest from the author, which I put up in the *Varna* case.

Senator LONG. You do not want to underestimate the ability of this particular Department. You may not have been here this morning, they just got through raiding one church. They might try all of them.

Dr. FREDERICKS. After my experience with the Food and Drug Administration, I can only echo what the previous witness said. You sometimes pinch yourself to remind yourself you are in America.

When they seized this book in Varna they decided to send out this press release. They expect to get a quick victory over the small companies because the small companies don't have the money to fight the U.S. Food and Drug Administration with the taxpayers' bottomless dollar behind them.

Senator LONG. Did you notice a tendency on the part of the Food and Drug Administration to spend a great deal of their time after the little manufacturer rather than after some of the large ones?

Dr. FREDERICKS. I have definitely noticed that. I noticed something else; when the small company is subsequently purchased by a large company, the needling attacks on niggling violations stop.

Senator LONG. The merchandise becomes all right then?

Dr. FREDERICKS. Becomes sacrosanct.

I decided to enter the case in Varna, I construed it this — I construed this not only as a character assassination in such a tangential way that a man is not given an opportunity to defend himself, because I had no legal standing in that court — I wasn't a defendant, but my book was being publicized from coast to coast and moreover my book was being described in language which could have been nothing but a deliberate series of lies, as presenting misinformation to the public of which no man in his right mind ever would have been guilty. I will give an example.

It was described as offering a diet for cancer. Now, the fact of the matter is that the book — and I am virtually quoting — I wrote it many years ago, but nevertheless, the book said there are those who are heartless enough to prey upon the desperate public where cancer is present by offering hope through diet. And that is the prefatory phrase to that discussion.

Nevertheless, I also mentioned — this is an interesting distortion — there was a report in either the Southern Medical Journal or the Georgia Medical Journal that a vitamin B complex deficiency in the first 3 months of pregnancy could be responsible for clubfoot involving the unborn baby. In other words, you have this maldevelopment in the baby's feet. This was presented to the public by

Food and Drug Administration as a claim for therapeutic action of diet on clubfeet.

This was in a libel which was used in a trial. The U.S. Food and Drug Administration however was somewhat disconcerted, I understood, when I decided to enter the Varna case ——

Senator LONG. You mentioned about the effect of drugs on unborn children and so on. The Food and Drug Department is developing quite an authority on Thalidomide after someone pointed out to them there was some danger to that particular drug.

Dr. FREDERICKS. Indeed, and perhaps the conversation becomes even more related when you remind the chairman that the diet of the woman, if it is rich enough in the vitamin B complex may protect her unborn baby against the harmful effects of Thalidomide, and that the U.S. Food and Drug Administration, not only kept Thalidomide off the market, but has done its best to drive vitamins off the market. If you disagree with this you are also a charlatan, crackpot, and cultist.

I retained the firm of Arnold, Fortas & Porter here in Washington. Mr. Paul Porter was the former Chairman of the Federal Communications Commission and oddly enough my professor at New York University, Charles Liepmann was the man who wrote the Blue Book for the FCC at the time that Mr. Porter was the Chairman of the FCC. I retained Mr. Porter and he sent one of his attorneys to Varna and we made a petition to the court asking for permission to enter the case, which the court not only granted, but became overenthusiastic about. I was not willing — not interested in a full entrance into this because I couldn't defend the company. I was merely trying to arrive at a point where an author can defend his book when an attack is slanted in a way which denominates him as incompetent.

The judge rendered a decision, and I bore you with this detail, Mr. Chairman, because what the Food and Drug Administration did with this decision is a point of this history. He rendered a decision that my competence and the competence of my book were not issues in that action which is what I was looking for, and therefore I instructed Mr. Porter to retire from the trial which he agreed was the proper thing to do.

The FDA then sent out a release which read approximately as follows, and I am not distorting it: "Dr. Carlton Fredericks entered the action at Varna, Ill., and withdrew with the result that the Government won a victory by default.

The fact of the matter was that the company defaulted it. . . .

Senator LONG. Seems how the Food and Drug Administration has an active public relations bureau.

Dr. FREDERICKS. Perhaps more active again than the chairman realizes, because at the time that this came along — that at the time this campaign of slander was in operation my broadcasts were being heard here in Washington on station WMAL, and what I am about to tell you is hearsay which I cannot verify, because I was told it orally. It wasn't in writing, but station WMAL called me one night and said they had a telephone call from Mr. Wallace Jansen who is the Public Information Officer of the Food and Drug Administration suggesting that the FDA took a dim view of any radio station which carried my broadcasts and urging that they be canceled.

Senator LONG. That was the Public Information Officer of the Food and Drug?

Dr. FREDERICKS. From the Food and Drug. He so identified himself.

Now, because the chain of stations was growing, my program was being heard in 70 some odd cities at the time — certain remarks which I made on the air about standards for food, certain remarks I made about Food and Drug policy which I felt were inimical to the protection of the consumer, had irked the agency to the point where they had decided to silence me. This attempt took shape in the following maneuvers: There was first the seizure at Varna, Ill.

There was then an action started by the Federal Communications Commission admittedly at the suggestion of the U.S. Food and Drug Administration, in which certain allegations were made concerning hidden sponsorship of my broadcasts, high technical violations of certain SEC regulations, all of it carefully couched in language which obscured one essential point; that is, that there were no charges against me and it took me 4 years to get a letter from the FCC admitting that there were no charges against me. . . .

The FCC, however, sent out this notice to radio stations that they were "investigating" the Carlton Fredericks program at the request of another Government agency, as a result of which in a period of 4 weeks 52 stations canceled the program.

Now, Mr. Chairman, I want to make one thing plain——

Senator LONG. How many stations did you have altogether?

Dr. FREDERICKS. Approximately 72.

Senator LONG. That strikes the chairman, it is not an American activity. This is something that — that type of persecution that I hate to see go on and we are definitely interested in it. If you are guilty you had a right to certainly be tried in some competent court rather than some bureaucratic agency giving that type of action.

Dr. FREDERICKS. Trial by newspaper has been characteristic — not by newspaper alone, the slick paper magazines, national magazines which were happy to take such stories, not only for sensationalism, because as a nutrition educator I have criticized certain foods which are made by manufacturers who have certain potency in terms of agricultural consumption and volume of advertising and a neat little coalition formed. This coalition consisted of the American Bakers Association, American Medical Association, the American Dental Association, and I was "under investigation" which never materialized in charges by the Food and Drug Administration, by the Federal Communications Commission, the Federal Trade Commission.

I remember awakening one morning and when I walked into the bank the Internal Revenue Department was there to look at my ill-gotten gains in my box and I was willing to display my children's war bonds, and they went away.

Now, sir, when the list of 72 stations had shrunk to 50 as a direct result of this campaign, I was approached by one of the few people in radio who recognized that there was a great deal of smoke here, but no fire, meaning that there were no charges against me. By this time I had been assured by some high-ranking executives in the radio and television industry that I was on a blacklist of the FCC, an opinion which is maintained to this very day.

This one executive, Mr. Robert Pauley of the American Broadcasting Co., tendered me a network contract because he resented what was going on. He said that he was justified in giving me the contract on the basis of competence as a broadcaster but the other considerations were also in his mind.

When that news was announced in the daily press three Food and Drug Administration agents whose names I have never been able to get walked in on the

ABC network and announced that the U.S. Government considered me to be an unfit broadcaster.

Senator LONG. Just a minute.

Mr. Rankin, you heard this statement. I would like you to supply me the names of those three agents.

Mr. RANKIN. I heard the statements and I will make an investigation, Mr. Chairman.

Senator LONG. It is not in litigation now, I presume, and there should be some record in the food and drug department and the chairman of this committee asks that you furnish this information.

Mr. RANKIN. If there is any record. I have never seen it. I will have a search made and refer it back to the committee.

Senator LONG. Can you give us more information as to the time and place, Doctor?

Dr. FREDERICKS. I can pinpoint it for you — it was just after I signed the contract. I can get the data from that and we will know.

However, I can also give you the name of the men they went with. They were two and a half hours there.

Mr. RANKIN. Mr. Chairman, it would save a tremendous research through many files if we may wait until the witness pinpoints the date as approximately as he can, or as definitely as he can before starting our search.

Senator LONG. I am sure the doctor will give you that definite time——

Mr. RANKIN. Thank you.

Senator LONG. As soon as he has the information.

Dr. FREDERICKS. When the FDA agents attempted to see the president of the network he sent word back — that network radio broadcasting was not under the legal province of Food and Drug Administration and he refused to see them. So they took themselves to another officer's office of the network, a lesser officer, Mr. William Raphael, and they spent two and a half hours with him and Mr. Charles DeBore, an ABC attorney — he told me directly — attempting to persuade them to cancel the program. Mr. Raphael asked the agents how they could so strongly disapprove a program which had not been on the air as yet and for which there was no scripts in existence. The answer to that question he did not get. He asked for a written complaint. This they never sent. (Mr. Raphael remembers this visit as having been made approximately in the latter part of July or the early part of August 1963.)

They returned from the network to Washington, apparently because there was a call subsequently, either that day or the next day, from Mr. Goldhammer of the FDA to someone at the ABC network reurging them that the network consider canceling the broadcasts.

Senator LONG. Who was that?

Dr. FREDERICKS. Mr. Goldhammer or Mr. Milstead.

Senator LONG. Who is he?

Dr. FREDERICKS. Mr. Goldhammer was formerly——

Senator LONG. Who was he at that time?

Dr. FREDERICKS. He is resigned now. He was Chairman of the Enforcement Division——

Mr. FENSTERWALD. Yes, he is still working for the Food and Drug.

Dr. FREDERICKS. He or Mr. Milstead was the man who made the call.

Now, in addition to this, however, the Food and Drug Administration began to write letters to the medical societies and the dental societies, sent out releases to the newspapers — in other words, renewing the campaign which had started in 1950 in which I was portrayed as having a criminal record and that as being incompetent and the point of the incompetence is a rather important point.

I had been refused permission to take nutrition courses because I was incompetent to teach and I did teach. This the FDA said was a mistake in judgment on the part of the university because I was obviously incompetent.

Senator LONG. What is this criminal record that they referred to?

Dr. FREDERICKS. That charge of practicing medicine and dispensing vitamins.

Mr. FENSTERWALD. Were you convicted?

Dr. FREDERICKS. I pleaded guilty because my attorney said that the publicity would ruin the radio broadcaster. That is not, however, my real motivation for having pleaded guilty. I think I had better give you the rest of the details.

These women took these slips of paper on which I recommended a doctor and got rid of them. They (the slips) disappeared from the case. They then went to a drugstore and ordered some vitamins. The druggist asked them who had suggested that they take the vitamin supplement. They gave my name. He knew me. He also knew a physician in the building. It was a professional building and he knew he could charge more with a prescription label than an over-the-counter label. He put a prescription label on the bottle and put on the prescription on the label the name of one of the doctors in the building.

The doctor, when he found out about this called me and he said, "Look, it is only vitamins, I will take the responsibility for my name being on the label."

I said, "You will also take the responsibility for losing your medical license. Because there is enough hostility for that here."

Senator LONG. Do I understand the situation, and Mr. Fensterwald here if he tells me my pulse is one thing, and that I should take one vitamin instead of two that he is practicing medicine?

Dr. FREDERICKS. If he recommends a loaf of enriched bread for you he is giving you three vitamins.

Mr. FENSTERWALD. That is quackery?

Dr. FREDERICKS. That is cultism.

So at any rate, this is the hue and cry of the criminal record.

I pleaded guilty, not only because the publicity can ruin the radio broadcaster, but if I attempted to allow the physician to intervene I might have jeopardized his license and I did not think I was justified in allowing that to happen.

I would like to point out that my record as a citizen is completely clean on both sides of this incident. I have had speeding tickets.

To come back — since I entered the case at Varna, Ill., on the ground that I knew nothing about the company there and my book was being slandered and the book was not being used for customers unless that company only had 12 customers because they only had 12 books. They were using it for salesmen to educate them. The FDA seized a target where they had more possibility. I was technical director of a vitamin laboratory in New York City. So they seized some $80,000 worth of merchandise at that laboratory and announced that the merchandise was misbranded by virtue of or by malice, of the editorial content of my broadcasts on the grounds of a nexus in that I was a consultant to the company, because the company did not advertise in my broadcasts.

This came to litigation and the litigation has ended. (An appeal has been entered by the defendant company in 1965.)

The important point of the action for the purposes of this committee is, that again, a spate of press releases went out with four lines on the company and three pages of Dr. Fredericks and faithfully reprinted in the newspapers throughout the United States describing me as an individual offering a diet for clubfeet, describing me as offering a diet for cancer. In the scientific community there is no faster way of hanging a man who is supposed to have competence as an interpreter of science and putting him in the position of giving cornflakes or something like this to cure clubfeet, as they know at the Public Relations Department at the Food and Drug Administration.

I found it impossible to break through the wall of silence which insulates this agency from reprisal in which they take advantage of the attitude expressed to me by the science reporter of a major New York newspaper. I asked him, why did you permit publication under your name of the Food and Drug Administration release attributing to me a diet for cancer when all you had to do was pick up the telephone and order a copy of my book which was printed right here in New York City and find out for yourself about what I have said is directly the opposite. He said, which is a very very important point, when it comes in under a Washington dateline with a Government agency's imprint, we do not check the accuracy.

Now, with this unlimited license and credibility, it is fine when handled by an agency with a sense of the rights of the citizen. It is not fine in the hands of the Food and Drug Administration.

At the end of these long series of events I found myself under attack simultaneously and I were so described in the press, FDA, FTC, FCC, Internal Revenue, and CIA was omitted and the Secret Service, by I know not by what error, and I tell you, Mr. Chairman, I rose in the morning and said to my wife on many occasions, "By whom am I being attacked today?"

Senator LONG. It strikes the chairman, as we say back in Missouri, you were a bear for punishment.

Dr. FREDERICKS. Indeed.

As of today, if a salesman wants to sell my program to radio stations he has a job that is unique. He must not only encounter the ordinary hazards, the difficulties and resistances of selling the radio program; he doesn't have the least resistance which would be normal for the sale of the program of a broadcaster who has been on the air 25 years, but he must also climb an invisible mythical wall on which is painted, "blacklisted by FCC and FDA." And there are many times when I had to remind myself that with all the semantics about technical violations by certain corporations with which I have nothing to do, and in the presentation of my program to stations, there are many times when I had to remind myself that in the past 25 years all I did was to sit at a microphone. I didn't do anything else. But I will tell the chairman frankly, that if I were at the Food and Drug Administration I would resent some of the broadcasts, too, because unfortunately, the information was accurate and it was damning.

A typical illustration, and I think in fairness I should give it, is what occurred at the time there was a symposium on cancer at the Biltmore Hotel in New York City.

Dr. Roy Hertz of the National Cancer Institute had remarked that female hormone is a cancer-producing substance and a woman who takes it is playing with fire. Commissioner Larrick was present and the press were aware that the female hormone is a constituent of the birth control pills and the Food and Drug Administration had just given a license for the sale of the birth control pills. So a reporter asked Commissioner Larrick, what do you have to say about Dr. Hertz' allegations about the carcinogenic properties of Estrogen hormone in view of the fact that your agency has just licensed the sale of birth control pills containing the hormone? The Commissioner replied that "he was not up on the technical details."

I remarked on the air and in my newspaper column I could understand that he would not be up on it possibly because he had been too busy stamping out vitamins; and that agency for the past 15 years has been engaged in precisely that.

That brings me to the point which I wish to leave for the consideration, if I may with the committee.

Senator LONG. The committee will be glad to hear you.

Dr. FREDERICKS. In the community of science when you find an area of science in which there is no argument, you are looking at a dead science. I happen to be quoting from Dr. Irvin Page of the Cleveland Clinic. He is a well-known heart specialist, but this remark is a truism for all sciences. When controversy ends there is no more progress.

As Griswold of Yale said, the strife in the arena is the source of productivity in science.

The effect of the attitudes of the Food and Drug Administration, with particular regard to the field in which I operate has been to end controversy. How? By setting up a series of dogma which is error No. 1, and by insisting that those who deviate from this credo in nutrition are cultists or crackpots or faddists or dispensers of nutritional nonsense and in that list they include Albrecht of the University of Missouri who is world famous for his knowledge of soils, Martin of California who is a physician and Curtis Woods and many other people who have good training and good competency.

Now, as a direct result of this it is impossible to get off the ground in the majority of universities today in any real and new pioneering investigation in the field of nutrition, because if you did succeed in getting the money, which would be most difficult because most of the money comes into universities today from two sources, Health, Education, and Welfare, which automatically is going to proscribe funds which would go into research which might demonstrate that FDA could possibly be wrong, and the rest of the funds come from manufacturers of a group of foods which I will describe as pretty poor nutrition. They are not likely to subsidize anything which might lead to invidious comparison and as a result of this it is amazing to look over the university scene and find out how little original work is being done in the field of nutrition with respect to vitamins.

The Food and Drug Administration has noted that the 190 million Americans are well fed. This despite the fact that the definitive survey of American diet which was done by the Department of Agriculture in 1955 indicates, as you might expect, that we have well fed Americans, we have moderately well fed Americans, and we have some very badly fed Americans, and the law of averages would work out that way.

On the basis of a non-existant check of 190 millions of Americans, they are now in a position to take action against a vitamin manufacturer who is advertising that Americans might be malnourished and who may need a vitamin supplement.

By the same token, the action of the Administration in employing its acceptance by newspapers and other media has allowed them to grow so arrogant and so, to misuse this privilege, that we have at the present time the most glaring dichotomy that I have ever seen in a single Government agency in releases by the FDA to radio stations and to newspapers.

On the air there was an FDA spot which is heard from coast to coast saying the best protection for the consumer is to be alert and well informed, read labels. This is the FDA's own statement with which we must heartily coincide.

Simultaneously there is a booklet from the FDA stating that there are 35 classes of food products for which standards have been written whereby the manufacturers are excused from giving any information whatsoever on the labels, with the result that, and this becomes serious, if you, sir, should happen to be allergic to dextrose — some people are — or corn starch — you would have to write to Washington and get the standards to find out whether you are swallowing it; if you are buying it in any one of these 35 different classes of food products.

I submit this only as an example of the kind of contradiction which an agency permits itself when it has grown completely reckless in its use of the media of mass communications.

In the State department of education in Connecticut, and I cite this not with reference to Connecticut, but as an example of how this attitude permeates from the Federal level to State, we have in the State department of education there a list of books not recommended for reading by the public, and is it pornography? No. Nutrition. What is the sin of these books? They disagree with the Food and Drug Administration.

I will give you an example of one of the books listed by the State department of education in Connecticut as not recommended reading — "Silent Spring," by Rachel Carson.

Another, "Nutrition in a Nutshell," by Prof. Roger Williams, who was the former president of the American Chemical Society, was decorated for his discovery of calcium pantothenate. Why? Because he believes there are some people in this country who are not ideally fed, and this disagrees with the dogma of the Food and Drug Administration.

So I submit to the committee the following:

The use of prejudging publicity has been criticized by individuals and agencies more competent than I. I believe the Hoover Committee commented on it. I think the Ribicoff Committee had something to say about it, too. In England, an officer of the Government agency who releases prejudging publicity prior to litigation can find himself in jail. I think this would be salutary here. Because a government agency can ruin an innocent person who subsequently is exonerated in a trial but nobody reads the exoneration. The exoneration is one paragraph. The slandering stories are three pages.

My second suggestion is that the U.S. Food and Drug Administration should be prevented from making pariahs, deriding a substantial group of American citizens who don't want to eat vegetables with insecticides on them, who are concerned about the safety about some of the more dubious food additives and who thereby try to shop a little more intelligently than the average consumer. These are the people labeled as food faddists. They have a right to their beliefs. They have a right to buy the foods they want. They should not be put in that category and made half criminals.

The third point: No listing of workers in the field of nutrition under the heading of "Dispensers of Nutritional Nonsense" should be permitted.

The fourth point: There should be no book burning, whether it is done by this business of making the book part of the labeling or it is done in the basis of not recommended lists of reading. We have not reached the point the Nazis reached. There are many books though on nutrition on the market, Mr. Chairman, which I would like to see off the market. And I will defend to the death their right to be on the market.

Still another point: When the U.S. Food and Drug Administration writes letters concerning a private individual to the public at large, the executive of the agency, the employee who is responsible for that letter should be subject to the laws of libel as much as any private citizen would be, because you have absolutely no way as a private citizen to defend yourself against this. If this agency decides that a nutritionist is a dispenser of nutritional nonsense he can find himself without employment. He can find himself without the possibility of pursuing his livelihood. He may be an M.D.; he may be a D.D.S.; he may be a Ph. D.— it matters not to this agency.

In short, I should suggest that this agency not be permitted to function as a court, which in many of its activities it seems to have moved toward, and that the powers given to it by the Congress to control our food and pharmaceutical supply, which are the powers that were aimed at a constructive purpose, be confined to that purpose. Nobody has yet given to this agency the right to put on the American dining table what it thinks we should eat; and yet that is the trend of what they are doing.

I want to thank you very much for the opportunity to appear here.

Senator LONG. Thank you, Doctor, very much for your very helpful statement.

INDEX

Acne,
  vitamins for, 254
Additives, food, *see* Food additives
Aging,
  health problems associated with, 127–29
  vitamins and, 130–36, 138, 140–43, 179–81
Air pollution,
  Vitamin E and, 7
Alcoholism,
  hypoglycemia and, 115–17
  sex drive and, 25
  vitamin treatment for, 115
Alexander, Dr. Franz, 45
Allergies,
  in babies, 225, 228, 229, 231, 243
  diet and, 17
  niacin and, 260, 262
American Baking Association,
  vitamin content of white flour and, 181

American Chemical Society,
  BHT and, 148
American Medical Association (AMA),
  nutrition and, 11, 20
  vitamins and, 18, 109, 131–32, 257
  yogurt and, 217, 243–44
Amino acids,
  need for, 15
Anatomy,
  individual differences in, 16, 19
Antibiotics,
  in chicken, 1
Aphrodisiacs,
  superstitions about, 238–39
Apple fritter,
  recipe for, 84
Apple juice, organic, 212
Apple juice, hot spiced,
  recipe for, 81
Apples,
  pesticides on, 157–58, 165–66
Arachidonic acid, 214

Arteries, diseases of,
  niacin in prevention of, 259–62
Arteries, hardening of, 256
Arthritis,
  calcium and, 243
Aslan, Dr. Anna, 140–42
Asparagus vinaigrette,
  recipe for, 80
Aspartic acid, 196

Babies,
  nutrition of, 224–34
  superstitions about nutrition of, 240–
    41, 243
  weight loss during first 24 hours by,
    103–4
Baby foods,
  salt in, 226, 258–59
  self-prepared, 226–27
Baked custard,
  recipe for, 74
Baker's yeast, 214–15
  distinguished from brewer's yeast,
    185–86
Beef,
  diethylstilbestrol in, 165, 207–8
BHA, *see* Butylhydroxyanisole
BHT, *see* Butylhydroxytoluene
Bioflavonoids, 196, 200
Birth-control pills,
  cancer and, 7, 31–32, 297–98
  diet and, 27, 31, 176
Birth deformities,
  nutrition and, 100–2
  thalidomide and, 103, 239, 293
Biskind, Dr. Morton, 32
Blackstrap molasses, 217
Blood,
  action of vitamins in, 175
  fats in, 18, 135
  sugar in, 42–44, 56–57, 62
Bone meal, 265–66
Bread,
  for babies, 229–31, 233
  Cornell formula, 210, 281–82
  white, 39, 181, 193
  whole-wheat, 181, 193, 208–9
Breakfast cereals, *see* Cereals, breakfast
Breast feeding, 224–25, 243
Breasts,
  cysts in, 23, 24, 26, 28–31

Brewer's yeast, 215, 244
  for babies, 233–34
  for diabetes, 60, 61
  selenium in, 138
  trivalent chromium in, 201
  Vitamin B Complex in, 35–36, 138–
    39, 183, 185–87
Brown-rice crackers, 67
Buttermilk,
  calcium in, 219
Butylhydroxyanisole (BHA),
  in foods, 145, 150, 213, 214, 247–48
Butylhydroxytoluene (BHT),
  in foods, 145–50, 213, 247–48

Café au lait,
  recipe for, 81
Caffeine,
  consumption of, 50, 62
  low blood sugar and, 43
Calcium,
  arthritis and, 243
  in buttermilk, kumiss, kefir, and
    yogurt, 219
  loss of, 178–79
  requirement for, 13–14, 66, 142–43
  spinach and, 242
  suggested supplement of, 202–3
Calcium propionate, 247
Cancer,
  aluminum utensils myth about, 241–
    42
  birth-control pills and, 7, 31, 297–98
  cystic mastitis and, 30–31
  diethylstilbestrol and, 165
  food additives and, 151, 155, 166
  smoking and, 6
Carbohydrates,
  diet low in, 93–98
  fruits and vegetables, content of,
    92–93
  in weight-reduction diets, 67–68
Carob, 215–16
Carrot sticks,
  recipe for, 73
Carrots,
  organic, 211
Carrots, verithin,
  recipe for, 72
Carrots anise,
  recipe for, 82

Carson, Rachel, 149, 165, 299
"Caveman diet," 69–85
Celery stick, stuffed,
  recipes for, 75, 273–74
Cells,
  regenerative abilities of, 129
  senile pigmentation of, 130–31
Cereals,
  for babies, 227
  mixed, 237
Cereals, breakfast,
  food value of, 10, 147, 150, 166
  in health-food stores, 209
Certified raw milk,
  cheese made from, 209–10
Cheese-hearted hamburgers,
  recipe for, 79–80
Cheraskin, Dr. E., 14
Chewing gum, 149–50
Chicken,
  antibiotics in, 1
Chicken, broiled in orange juice,
  recipe for, 74
Chicken liver and mushrooms, sauté,
  recipe for, 75
Chicken soup, 236
Chinese,
  mixing of cereals by, 237
Chinese pork with vegetables,
  recipe for, 83–84
Chinese restaurant syndrome, 17
Chinese spinach,
  recipe for, 80
Cholesterol,
  eggs and, 8–9
Choline, 195, 200, 267
Clam-tomato soup,
  recipe for, 77
Clams,
  Vitamin B Complex and, 242
"Clinker" cells, 130–31
Cobalamin, *see* Vitamin B$_{12}$
Coffee whip, frozen,
  recipe for, 78
Common cold,
  Vitamin A for, 22, 255–56
  Vitamin C for, 191, 192, 254–56
Connecticut,
  apple industry of, 165–66
Cornell formula bread, 210
  for babies, 233
  recipe for, 281–82

Cornmeal, 212
Corticosteroid adrenal hormones,
  production of, 104
Cott, Allan, 125
Cottage cheese omelet,
  recipe for, 77
Coupe au black cherry,
  recipe for, 70
Cranberry sherbet,
  recipe for, 85
Cream of spinach soup,
  recipe for, 82
Custard, baked,
  recipe for, 74
Cummings, Bob, 22
Cystic mastitis, 23, 26
  breast cancer and, 30–31
  diet and, 24, 28, 29, 31

DDT,
  in breast milk, 224
  Carson and, 149
  in liver, 187–88
Dewey, John, 256
Diabetes, 54–63
  hypoglycemia and, 15, 62
  niacin precaution for, 261
  oral drugs for, 55–56
  sex drive and, 30, 59–60
  trivalent chromium for, 201
  Vitamin-A deficiency and, 190
Diet,
  aging and, 129
  allergy and, 17
  babies' individual needs in, 224, 226,
    232
  "Caveman's," 69–85
  constructive reducing, 86–98
  fertility and, 22
  for hypoglycemia, 271–77
  individual needs in, 6, 9, 12–18, 20,
    22, 64, 169, 270
  low carbohydrate, 93–98, 248
  menstrual cycle and, 27–29, 278–80
  NASA attempt at standardized, 14
  sex hormones and, 24–25
  for weight reduction, 86–98
  women's needs in, 33–39
Dietary deficiency, 169–71
Diethylstilbestrol,
  cancer and, 165, 207–8

Doughless pizza,
  recipe for, 73, 273
Dried stomach and colon tissues
  (supplement), 268
Dubos, René, 217, 244

Eggplant,
  myth concerning juice of, 235
Eggplant, shoestring,
  recipe for, 74
Eggs,
  for babies, 227–29
  cholesterol in, 8–9
  organic, 210
Eggs in nests,
  recipe for, 72
Eggs poached in tomato juice,
  recipe for, 79
Encephalitis,
  nutritional treatment for, 254
Estrogen,
  cancer and, 7, 31–32, 297–98
  diet and, 29
  folic acid and, 196, 280
  in men, 24–25, 30, 60
  menstrual cycle and, 26–27, 280
  Vitamin B Complex and, 27, 29, 35,
    280
Eyesight,
  vitamins and, 21, 22

Fats,
  in blood, 18, 135
  differences in body reactions to, 19
  digestion of, 135
Fats, saturated,
  in diet, 133
Fats, unsaturated,
  in cell structure, 130–33
  in diet, 133–34, 136, 253
Fertility,
  diet and, 22
Fish,
  mercury in, 1
Folic acid, 195–96, 269
  estrogen and, 280
Food additives, 1–2, 145–67, 247–48
  in ice cream, 10
  lists of, 152–55
  in peanut butter, 207

in root beer, 2, 151
Food and Drug Administration (U.S.),
  diethylstilbestrol decision of, 207
  food additives and, 146, 150–55, 166,
    208, 283
  pesticides allowed by, 156–66
  public and, 10–12, 283
  vitamins and, 18, 136, 139, 173, 188–
    89, 195–97, 204, 284
  yogurt and, 217, 244
Food colors,
  toxicity of, 151, 152
Food industry,
  additives and, 146–55, 166–67
  grants to universities by, 11
  pesticides used by, 156–67
  revenue of, 11
Formaldehyde,
  in maple syrup, 1–2, 218
Freud, Dr. Sigmund, 12
Fruits,
  carbohydrate content of, 93
  organic, 210–11, 248
  pesticides on, 156–66
Funk, Dr. Casimir, 189, 284

Gall-bladder syndrome,
  body-type prevalent in, 8
Garlic,
  superstitions about, 243
Gelatin, 219
Glutamine, 197
Glutathione,
  Vitamin C and, 138
Glycine, 197
Grains,
  Vitamin B Complex in, 34, 36
Gyland, Dr. Stephen, 43

Hair, loss of,
  sex hormones and, 25
Ham and mushrooms,
  recipe for, 71
Ham horn,
  recipe for, 70, 273
Ham slice with orange,
  recipe for, 77
Hamburgers, cheese-hearted,
  recipe for, 79–80
Hardening of the arteries, 256

Harris, Dr. Seale, 43
Health,
    definitions of, 2–3, 223
Health-food stores, 207–23
Heart disease,
    niacin in prevention of, 259–62
    Vitamin E and, 136–37
Heart failure, 256–58
    vegetable oils and, 133
Heart pot roast,
    recipe for, 80
Heparin,
    niacin-activating, 260–61
Hertz, Dr. Roy, 31, 297–98
Hesperidin, 196
Hitler, Adolf, 236
Hoffer, Dr. A., 109–10, 112
Honey, 37, 216–18, 246
Hoobler, Dr. B. Raymond, 233–34
Hooton, Prof. Ernest, 167
Hormones,
    in meat, 1
    see also Estrogen
Hydroxycobalamin,
    for schizophrenia, 121–22
Hyperbaric treatment,
    for senile dementia, 126
Hypoglycemia (low blood sugar), 42–48,
    50, 53, 62
    alcoholism and, 115–17
    diet for, 271–77
    glycine for, 197
    neurosis and, 124
    overweight and, 68
    pancreas and, 15, 42–43
    schizophrenia and, 109, 114, 117–19
    symptoms of, 47–48
Hysterectomies, 32–33

Ice cream,
    for babies, 230–31
    sugar and additives in, 10
Impotence,
    diabetes and, 59–60
    nutrition and, 30, 101
Infants, *see* Babies
Infertility,
    nutrition and, 3, 17, 101, 102
    obesity and, 33
Inositol, 195, 200

Instinct,
    diet and, 4–5
Insulin, 54–61
    niacin interaction with, 261
    overdosage of, 56
    overproduction of, 43
    possible side effects of, 55, 57, 59
    production in pancreas of, 15, 43, 55
Iodine,
    suggested supplement of, 203
Iron,
    in blackstrap molasses, 217
    menstrual cycle and, 26, 174
    suggested supplement of, 203

Jams and jellies, 217–18
Jewish penicillin, 236
Jolliffe, Norman, 254
Junket,
    recipe for, 82

Kefir, 219
Kidneys with wine,
    recipe for, 78
Kuglemass, Dr. I. Newton, 228–29
Kumiss, 219

Laetrille, *see* Vitamin B$_{17}$
Lamb dolmas,
    recipe for, 80
Langstroth, Dr., 169
Lecithin, 197, 269
    for digestion of fats, 135, 197, 214
Life expectancy, 5–6, 128
Liver,
    concentrates of, 36, 59, 185–88
    DDT in, 187–88
    diabetes and, 55, 58–60
    in diet, 34
    sex hormones and, 25, 27, 29–30, 32,
    35
Liver strips, sautéed,
    recipe for, 69–70
London broil,
    recipe for, 82
Loss of hair,
    sex hormones and, 25
Low blood sugar, *see* Hypoglycemia

Lung cancer,
  smoking and, 6
Lysine, 196–97
  allergy in babies to, 18
Lysosomes,
  unsaturated fat and, 132

Macaroons,
  recipe for, 75
Magnesium, 263
  suggested supplement of, 203
Manganese,
  suggested supplement of, 203
Manitol,
  as a carbohydrate, 209
MAO inhibitor (tranquilizer),
  possible side effects of, 8
Maple sugar, 218
Maple syrup,
  formaldehyde in, 1–2, 218
Maraschino cherries,
  dye in, 2, 151
Mass action, law of (chemistry),
  vitamin absorption and, 175
Meals,
  timing of, 66
    for babies, 231–32
Meat,
  for babies, 229
  diethylstilbestrol in, 165, 207–8
  hormones in, 1
Megavitamin treatment,
  for schizophrenia, 110–13, 115, 119,
    184
Men,
  estrogen in, 24–25
  reproductive organs of, 17
  role in conception of, nutrition and,
    100, 102
Menopause,
  Vitamin E and, 118
Menstrual cycle,
  diet and, 23–24, 26–29, 176
  diet for, 278–80
  sugar and, 7
Mental illness,
  nutrition and, 40–53, 108–126
  see also Schizophrenia
Mercury,
  in fish, 1

Milk,
  for babies, 224–25, 231–32, 240, 243
  certified raw, 209–10
  kumiss and kefir forms of, 219
  nonfat, 222–23
  superstitions about, 238, 240, 244–45
Mineral water, 223
Minerals,
  supplements of, 201–5
Molasses, blackstrap, 217
Monosodium glutamate (MSG),
  Chinese restaurant syndrome and, 17
Morning sickness,
  vitamin use to prevent, 21, 106
Mushroom salad, raw,
  recipe for, 78
Mushrooms,
  pesticides in, 10
Mussolini, Benito, 236
Myoneuropathies,
  nutrition and, 252–53

National Aeronautics and Space
    Administration (NASA),
  attempt at standardized diet of, 14
Neapolitan zucchini,
  recipe for, 78
Neurosis,
  hypoglycemia and, 124
Newbold, Dr. H. L., 121–23
Niacin, 269–70
  deficiency of, 52–53
  in prevention of heart and artery
    disease, 259–62
Niacinamide, 193, 200
  alcoholism and, 117
  niacin compared with, 259
  schizophrenia and, 109, 111–14, 117,
    118
Nonfat milk, 222–23
Nut butters, 218–19
Nutrition, *see* Diet

Oils,
  cooking and salad, 212–14
Old age,
  health problems associated with,
    127–29
Omelet, cottage cheese,
  recipe for, 77

Orange juice,
   Vitamin C and cofactors in, 182
Organic fruits and vegetables, 210–11, 248
Ornithine,
   schizophrenia and, 114, 197
Orthomolecular psychiatry, 120, 126
Oxidation of cells,
   vitamins and, 131–32, 134, 137–38
Oxygen,
   aging and, 129, 131–32

PABA (para-aminobenzoic acid), 22, 139–43, 197–98, 200, 270
   as an aphrodisiac, 238–39
   estrogen increased by, 280
Paccini, 19
Page, Dr. Melvin E., 133
Palate,
   importance of width of, 106–7
Pancreas,
   insulin production in, 15, 43, 55, 58, 62
Pangamic acid, *see* Vitamin B₁₅
Pantothenate, 193–94, 200
Pantothenic acid, 193, 200, 263, 264
Para-aminobenzoic acid, *see* PABA
Paracelsus, Philippus Aureolus, 132
Parathyroid glands,
   calcium and, 14
Pauling, Dr. Linus, 14, 122, 126, 192, 254–55
Peanut butter,
   additives in, 207
Pears with ginger jelly,
   recipe for, 80
Pellagra,
   porphyrin and, 124–25
Pepsin,
   production in body of, 15
Pernicious anemia,
   Vitamin B₁₂ and, 120–21, 123, 124, 194, 195
Pesticides,
   on fruits and vegetables, 1, 10, 155–67
   leukemia caused by, 150
   lists of permitted, 157–64
Phenylalanine,
   feeblemindedness and, 18

Phosphorus,
   suggested supplement of, 203
Pie,
   sugar content of, 1
Pineapple-lime salad,
   recipe for, 74
Pizza, doughless,
   recipe for, 73, 273
Poison ivy,
   Vitamin C for, 250
Pork with vegetables, Chinese,
   recipe for, 83–84
Porphyria,
   Vitamin E and, 125
Porphyrin,
   pellagra and, 124–25
Pot roast, heart,
   recipe for, 80
Potassium,
   sodium ratio, 259
   in vegetable juices, 220
Potatoes,
   Vitamin C in, 230
Pregnancy,
   nutrition and, 99–107, 239–40
   superstitions about, 239–40
Price, Weston, 100
Procaine,
   PABA in, 140–43
Propionic acid, 247
Propylgallate,
   in oils, 213
Prostaglandins, 252–53
Protein,
   diabetes and, 30
   menstrual cycle and, 26, 27, 29
   need for, 15, 68
   in weight-reduction diets, 68
   in a woman's diet, 33, 34
Protein factors, 196–97
Psychotic children,
   vitamin treatment for, 125–26
Pyridoxin, *see* Vitamin B₆

Radiation,
   aging and, 129–30
Randolph, Dr. Theron, 150
Raw milk, certified,
   cheese made from, 209–10

Riboflavin, 192, 200
Roasted sweet peppers,
    recipe for, 85
Root beer,
    foaming agent in, 2, 151
Royal jelly, 216, 263–64
Rutin, 196, 200

Saccharin,
    safety of, 151
Salzer, Dr. Harry, 43
Saturated fats,
    in diet, 133
Schizophrenia,
    hypoglycemia and, 109, 114, 117–19
    nutrition and, 109–10
    vitamin treatment for, 108–13, 184
    see also Mental illness
Selenium,
    Vitamin E and, 138
Seligmann, Dr. Wolfgang, 59
Selye, Dr. Hans, 57, 252
Senile dementia,
    hyperbaric treatment for, 126
    Vitamin B₁₂ and, 124
Senile pigmentation,
    Vitamin E and, 130–31
Sesame tomatoes,
    recipe for, 72
Sherbet, cranberry,
    recipe for, 85
Sherman, H. C., 143, 173, 190
Shock lung, 151
Shock treatment,
    Vitamin-E treatment compared with, 118
Shrimp delectable,
    recipe for, 71
Shute, Wilfred, 100–1, 257–58
Silent Spring (Carson), 149, 165, 299
Sinuses,
    varying shapes of, 16
Skim milk,
    in weight-reduction diets, 66–67
Smoking,
    lung cancer and, 6
    vitamin requirements and, 7
Snow pudding,
    recipe for, 76

Sodium,
    potassium ratio, 256
Somogyi, 56, 57
Sorbitol,
    as a carbohydrate, 209
Soskin, Samuel, 58
Soy flour, 221–22
Spies, Dr. Tom, 36, 51, 52, 184–85, 249
Spinach,
    calcium and, 242
Spinach, Chinese,
    recipe for, 80
Spinach soup, cream of,
    recipe for, 82
Stammering,
    Vitamin B₁ and, 20–21
Starches,
    body's reactions to, 19
Stare, Prof. Frederick, 181
Stress adaptation syndrome, 57
Stuffed celery stick,
    recipes for, 75, 273–74
Stuffed tomato with crabmeat,
    recipe for, 82
Sugar,
    average intake of, 7, 15, 50, 217
    in blood, 42–44, 56–57, 62
    body's reactions to, 19
    brain's need of, 42, 43, 50, 61
    digestion and metabolism of, 15–16, 57–58
    false need for, 237
    maple, 218
    menstrual cycle and, 7
    quantities in foods of, 10, 48–50
    turbinado, 216
Suicide,
    of college students, 4
Sukiyaki,
    recipe for, 76
Sulfur dioxide,
    in dried fruit, 219
Swartz, Dr. Harry, 98
Sweet peppers, roasted,
    recipe for, 85
Swiss cheese eggs,
    recipe for, 83
Synergism,
    of Vitamins C and E, 138
Tahini, 218
Taller, Dr. Herman, 65

Teen-agers,
  medical problems of, 4
  nutritional needs of, 240
Thalidomide,
  birth defects and, 103, 239, 293
Thiamin, *see* Vitamin B₁
Thyroid glands,
  weight reduction and, 65
Tired-housewife syndrome,
  hypoglycemia and, 45
Tocopherol, *see* Vitamin E
Tomato with crabmeat, stuffed,
  recipe for, 82
Tomatoes,
  as aphrodisiacs, 235
Tomatoes, sesame,
  recipe for, 72
Tongue-cheese horn,
  recipe for, 273
Torula yeast, 138, 186, 215
Tranquilizers,
  side effects of, 8, 110
Trivalent chromium,
  for diabetes, 201
  in sugar, 216
Tryptophane,
  "psychological state" and, 120
Turbinado sugar, 216

Unsaturated fats,
  in cell structure, 130–33
  in diet, 133–34, 136, 253
Uterine fibroid tumors, 23
  estrogen and, 32–33

Vanadium,
  for cholesterol, 201, 204
Vegetable juicers, 219–20
Vegetable oils,
  manufacture of, 132–33, 212–14
Vegetables,
  carbohydrate content of, 92–93
  organic, 210–11, 248
  pesticides on, 1, 156–66
Vegetarianism,
  Vitamin B₁₂ and, 123, 194
Vitamin A, 190, 199, 265
  common cold and, 22, 255–56

requirement for, 15
sinuses and, 17
smoking and, 7
toxicity of, 200–1
Vitamin B₁ (thiamin), 192, 200
  in brewer's yeast, 183
  deficiency of, 51–53
  requirement for, 172
  stammering and, 20–21
Vitamin B₂, 266
Vitamin B₆ (pyridoxin), 193, 200, 264–65
  babies' need for, 16
  morning sickness and, 21
  schizophrenia and, 111–13
  in white and whole-wheat flour, 181
Vitamin B₁₂ (cobalamin), 142, 194, 200, 265
  in brewer's yeast, 215
  electrical activity of heart and, 258
  nervous system and, 120–24, 195
Vitamin B₁₅ (pangamic acid), 204
Vitamin B₁₇ (Laetrille), 204
Vitamin B Complex, 34–36
  borderline deficiency of, 169
  clams and, 242
  cleft palate and harelip prevented by, 102
  crying attacks and, 12–13
  diabetes and, 30, 57–61
  estrogen and, 32, 280
  in grains, 58
  headaches and, 13
  menstrual cycle and, 26, 27, 29, 280
  PABA in, 22, 139, 142–43, 197, 238–39
  removal from food of, 62
  sugar and need for, 216
  unknown factors in, 183, 185
  Vitamin-A toxicity reduced by, 201
  in a woman's diet, 33, 34–36
Vitamin C, 191–92, 200, 266–67
  bioflavonoid, hesperidin, and rutin protection of, 196
  cofactors of, in orange juice, 182
  for common cold, 191, 192, 254–56
  oxidation of cells and, 137–38
  for poison ivy, 250
  requirement for, 14
  schizophrenia and, 111–13
  smoking and, 7

Vitamin D, 191, 199
  calcium and, 202, 203
  requirement for, 14
Vitamin E (tocopherol), 194–95, 200,
    268–69
  aging and, 130–36, 179
  air pollution and, 7
  anticlotting agent in, 16
  as antioxidant in oils, 213
  anxiety and, 114
  as aphrodisiac, 238
  birth deformities prevented by, 100–1
  in grains, 36, 58, 132, 137
  heart attacks and, 257–58
  menopausal symptoms controlled by,
    118
  oxidation of cells and, 131–32, 134,
    137–38
  porphyria and, 125
  removal from food of, 2, 131–33, 136,
    181
  requirement for, 133–34, 136–37
  schizophrenia and, 111–13
  senile pigmentation and, 130–31
  supplements of, 134–35, 137
  unsaturated fats and need for, 131–33
  in a woman's diet, 33, 34
Vitamin K,
  destroyed by freezing, 166
Vitamin deficiencies,
  borderline cases of, 169
  emotional stress causing, 179
  list of conditions that might cause,
    177–78
  mistaken for nervous breakdown, 50–
    51
Vitamin supplements, 180–206
  for babies, 233, 240–41
  Food and Drug Administration and,
    173, 188–89, 195–97, 284
  natural and synthetic, 181–83, 198–
    99, 238
Vitamin toxicity, 200–1, 245–46
Vitamins,
  absorption of, 175
  list of conditions that might increase
    requirement for, 177–78

Water,
  purity of, 10, 223
Wheat germ, 181, 220–21
  for babies, 227–28
  Vitamin B Complex in, 36–37, 172–73
  Vitamin E in, 36, 137
Wheat-germ oil,
  for neuromuscular diseases, 253, 258
White, Dr. Phillip, 131–32
White bread,
  tastelessness of, 39
  vitamin content of, 181, 193
Whole-wheat bread, 208–9
  vitamin content of, 181, 193
Williams, Dr. Roger, 13, 15, 19, 116, 299
Women,
  birth-control pills used by, 7, 27,
    31–32, 176
  breast feeding by, 224–25, 243
  cancers in sex organs of, 31–32
  diet during pregnancy of, 104–7
  menstrual cycle of, 7, 23–24, 26–29,
    176, 278–80
  nutritional needs of, 33–39, 278–80
  pregnancy of, 99–107
  reproductive organs of, 17
  Vitamin E for menopausal symptoms
    in, 118
World Health Organization, BHT and,
  146

Yeast, baker's, *see* Baker's yeast
Yeast, brewer's, *see* Brewer's yeast
Yeast, torula, *see* Torula yeast
Yogurt, 37, 217–19, 243–44

Zinc, 270
  in diet, 189
  suggested supplement of, 203
Zucchini, neapolitan,
  recipe for, 78